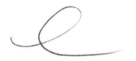

Leopold's
PRINCIPLES AND METHODS
OF
PHYSICAL DIAGNOSIS

HENRY U. HOPKINS, M.D.

Professor of Clinical Medicine,
The School of Medicine,
University of Pennsylvania

THIRD EDITION

W. B. SAUNDERS COMPANY

Philadelphia and London

Reprinted January, 1966

Principles and Methods of Physical Diagnosis

PREFACE TO THE
THIRD EDITION

With the untimely death of Dr. Leopold his plans for revising this book lay dormant for many months, but at the request of his family I agreed to attempt to complete this unfinished task. This revision is my tribute to Dr. Leopold, in memory of the many hours I was privileged to spend with him. He was my friend, my teacher and my mentor for over twenty years. I never ceased to marvel at his breadth of medical knowledge, his keen mind and his diagnostic acumen. Much of this was based upon his almost uncanny powers of observation and his skill in physical examination. He *listened* to the patient's story; he *examined* the patient. Only then would he request such ancillary studies as he considered essential to confirm his diagnosis.

The primary purpose of this book is to provide an introduction to the basic procedures of history taking and the performance of a physical examination. Whenever possible we have attempted to state *what* should be done, describe *how* it should be done, explain *why* it should be done and then indicate the results or findings that would be considered within the normal range in a healthy person. Some of the innumerable variations found in disease are mentioned but only a few of these are discussed. Here again an effort has been made to help the student correlate the abnormal findings with the underlying physiologic or pathologic changes responsible for them.

Those familiar with previous editions of this book will find that many changes have been made. A brief chapter has been added on "Examination of the Skin"; part of this material was formerly included in other areas. Many chapters or sections have been condensed; others have been expanded. A number of new charts and photographs have been inserted; some of the older ones have been deleted.

The desirability of some of these changes had been discussed with Dr. Leopold shortly after the second edition was published. Others were

suggested by members of our staff, so many of whom have given gener-
ously of their time and talent in our cooperative teaching program. Some
are based upon my personal contact with small groups of students during
the many years that I have participated in the actual teaching of this
course, as well as acting as supervisor and coordinator of the instruction.

To my collaborators who aided in the revision of their chapter or
section I extend my gratitude and thanks. The credit is theirs if this book
proves helpful to the student as he struggles to gain an understanding
of the fundamentals of this life-long indispensable art. Any deficiencies—
and there are many—are mine and mine alone.

To N., who has aided and encouraged me during the long lonely
hours required for this revision, who has patiently, quietly and lovingly
helped me whenever she could, this revision is dedicated.

HENRY U. HOPKINS

Philadelphia, Pennsylvania

CONTENTS

final

final

1

The History

Obtaining an accurate, adequate, concise history is essential in the study and treatment of any patient. In clinical practice this usually precedes the physical examination, but in many medical schools the order of instruction is reversed. The student is first taught how to do the examination; later he learns how to take a history. To justify this, it is stated that a good history cannot be obtained unless the examiner is acquainted with the manifestations of a variety of diseases; usually such instruction is not given until the third or fourth year. When much or all of the formal course in physical diagnosis is given during the second year, the student may seem unprepared to obtain the information essential for a good history, and he may be unable to evaluate or integrate the few facts that he does elicit.

However, those who criticized this chapter when it first appeared overlooked an important point. The neophyte has to be taught the fundamental procedures of the examination—inspection, palpation, percussion and auscultation. He is taught to differentiate the normal from the abnormal. We have found that he can be taught the basic principles of obtaining a history, and he is encouraged to practice this early in the course when he begins to examine patients. The record will be crude, but so are the first attempts at percussion; proper supervision plus increased medical knowledge will lead to improvement in both fields. Moreover, information concerning the sequential development of symptoms helps the student correlate the abnormal physical findings with the pathologic process and the physiologic response it produces; thus all are fixed more firmly in his mind.

For the first few periods it is desirable, if not essential, that the student be assigned to a patient who is hospitalized and who has definite symptoms as well as physical signs that are easily elicited. The patient should be able to give a reasonably concise, coherent history and should be willing to submit to examination.

1

By the end of the course the student should know the routine to be followed in obtaining a history. He should have developed a moderate amount of manual dexterity, be able to perform a physical examination and recognize grossly abnormal findings. He should attempt to arrive at a physiologic or pathologic diagnosis even though the etiologic differential diagnosis may be unknown at this stage of his education. No one expects him to be skilled in any of these fields. As a matter of fact, no one, either student or professor, ever takes a perfect history; to do so would require a more complete knowledge of medicine than anyone possesses.

An outline form will be needed at the start of this work; one such guide appears on page 11. This was originally prepared for our third and fourth year students to assist them in their ward and outpatient assignments. It is now distributed to all second year students at the start of our course in Methods of Clinical Diagnosis. It is by no means complete; no outline can be. It is designed merely to suggest a general plan for the interview; it cannot attempt to cover the possible variations that may arise.

THE INTERVIEW

Preliminary Preparation. Before you are assigned your first patient, read the outline form several times. Although you may then think that you are reasonably familiar with it, you should take it with you to the patient's bedside. Glance at it occasionally to refresh your memory and to help you avoid omissions. After you become more proficient you will seldom refer to it and eventually you will be able to work without it.

Physician-Patient Rapport. When you start to talk to a patient you should realize that your attitude toward him and your reaction to his complaints will create more of an impression than your technical skill or medical knowledge. The ability to be interested, unhurried, careful, tactful and considerate, rather than amused, supercilious, distracted, bored or inconsiderate of his sensibilities might well be called the essence of the art of medicine.

Never mistake common sense and tact for dishonesty and deceit, but always remember the possible dire consequences of showing the pity which you may feel for an incurably ill patient, and the tragedy that may result if he, rather than a responsible member of his immediate family, is frankly told the truth when hope alone may be the feeble flicker that sustains life.

The importance of first impressions is often overemphasized, but it must never be overlooked. The patient may be watching you closely. Your general appearance, your dress, your actions, your attitude, your words and even the tone of your voice will all have an effect, favorable or otherwise. You may have seen an experienced physician attempting to size up the patient as he approaches the bedside; he will vary his opening remarks in accordance with this first impression. It is usually advisable to rely upon a simple introduction in a friendly tone such as: "Mr. Jones, I am Dr. Smith." Hesitate, watch the patient, and try to take advantage of any remarks he may make. Forget momentarily that you're the doctor and he is the patient; be sociable, as you would with any other stranger. At a propitious moment you can continue with some remark such as: "Now tell me all about your troubles." Never ask him what his "symptoms" are. Don't ask: "What's wrong with you?" or "What brought you here?"; that is what he wants you to tell him. Just give him an opportunity to talk and to tell his story in his own way.

Patient Personalities. A physician must learn to recognize the personality traits of his patients and to guide his questions and evaluate the answers accordingly. A person who feels that you underestimate the severity of his symptoms or the gravity of his disease can often be "spotted" by the fact that he has pain or other symptoms anywhere you may suggest. It must not be forgotten, however, that these garrulous neurotics who often exaggerate or imagine irrelevant symptoms may also have serious organic disease.

To avoid leading questions, which too often receive an affirmative reply whether correct or not, it is sometimes useful to reword the question in an opposite manner and repeat it later. For example, if you desire to know whether walking or other physical exercise produces pain in the chest, you might say: "Does walking help your pain?" If the patient replies emphatically, "That's when I get it," his answer is probably reliable.

One patient may have a sense of pride or a feeling of superiority because he knows that he is able to diagnose his own illness; he is merely allowing you to confirm this intuitive knowledge. Another will insist that the last thing he did or what he ate at that party is responsible for the symptoms. Don't bother to argue the point; evaluate the evidence and proceed. With tact and "tests" you may be able to change his mind.

The stolid, stoical, taciturn patient may resent questioning and be slow to reply; you must be painstaking and unhurried if an accurate and informative history is to be obtained.

Terminology. Make sure that you and the patient understand each other. Try to appraise his educational background; use words or phrases that he can comprehend, rather than medical terms that may be meaningless to him. "Substernal oppression" sounds erudite and impressive, but a phrase such as "something squeezing like a vise" or "like someone sitting on your chest" is more likely to elicit a prompt and accurate reply. Few women can answer a question about the "menarche" but they can tell you when their periods began. "Dysuria" would be meaningless to most patients; "pain when you urinate" or "when you pass your water" should get a reply. At times it may be necessary to descend to the vernacular of the lowest type to obtain the desired information. It is equally important to be sure that you find out exactly what the patient means when he uses an expression such as "indigestion," "gas" or "nervousness," or when he says that he has "palpitation." Is he aware of his heart because it seems rapid? slow? forceful? Does it seem to "skip a beat" or "flop over" at intervals?

The Chief Complaint (C.C.).   A patient goes to a doctor because he knows or suspects that something is wrong in some part of his body. Even the person who "just dropped in for a check-up" may be trying to hide some worry or fear. The presenting symptom may be almost anything. Pain is frequently the complaint; other common ones are fever, chills, weakness, headache, cough, breathlessness, palpitation, nausea, vomiting, diarrhea, abnormalities of urination, swollen or painful joints, or a "lump," swelling, discharge or bleeding from any site.

Many patients will have more than one symptom, or symptoms apparently unrelated and arising from more than one organ system or disease process. You may have to defer your decision as to which is really the *chief* complaint; as the story unfolds, one of these will eventually predominate and should be used. Palpitation, shortness of breath and pain around the heart may be present, all due to heart disease. Probably the pain was what influenced him to seek medical advice, but the shortness of breath may well be the most troublesome symptom, or the *chief* complaint. To these same symptoms there might be added abdominal discomfort or gastrointestinal disturbance; they too could be due to passive congestion from circulatory failure. On the other hand, the patient with heart disease or circulatory failure can also have a peptic ulcer, gallbladder disease or carcinoma of the colon. If the history suggests two *different* disease processes, there could be two "chief complaints."

The Present Illness (P.I.).   Encourage the patient to tell the story in his own way. Usually this narration will be incomplete and inadequate, but do not interrupt it except to ask questions if he seems to falter. You will get a broad perspective of the problem first; you can fill in the details later.

No attempt should be made to write much at this time. Jot down important items such as dates or time intervals, and a few words about each symptom he mentions. If you write too much or stop him too often he may think that you are more interested in your notes than you are in his problem. When he has finished, start asking the questions that have been occurring to you. Now you can take more copious notes, and begin to compile a rough draft of the history. Cover each symptom he has mentioned, digging out everything you can about it.

You will find that the answers depend not only on the way you ask the questions, but also upon the patient's personality. One will reply "Yes" to almost anything, but don't jump to the conclusion that he is neurotic. Maybe he is, but possibly he doesn't understand the question and is ashamed to admit it. He may think that you expect such an answer, so he is trying to cooperate. Possibly he is too frightened or confused to say "No." Sometimes he may hope to confuse you. Occasionally a patient may not admit having some symptom which you think he should have. If you rephrase your question and repeat it later, you may evoke the true reply.

The specific line of questioning for each particular complaint is something that you will learn gradually as your education progresses, but certain general suggestions seem in order.

DURATION.   When did the first symptom appear? With some chronic diseases the patient may find this difficult to answer; ask him how long it has been since he really felt well. With more acute processes you should be able to determine the exact date or even the hour. Give the day of the week (in addition) only if it seems significant, or if symptoms tend to recur on that particular day. Headache may be present only on Fridays, when the weekly report is due; backache may be much worse on Mondays, after a weekend of sports or gardening.

LOCATION.   Where did the pain first appear? Did it remain there, spread to adjacent areas or seem to move to an entirely different site? Where is it now? Ask the patient to put *one finger* on the painful spot. Can he do this, or does he use the whole hand, or run his fingers vaguely over the entire abdominal wall or thigh?

SEVERITY.   Did the pain increase in severity? How rapidly? How severe is it now? Has it been worse? Pain can range from an annoying or nagging discomfort, as in mild arthritis, to the agonizing or incapacitating pain of renal colic or of myocardial infarction. Remember that pain is a subjective symptom; some people will tolerate severe pain quietly, while others will complain bitterly about some minor discomfort. Watch the person's expression and actions. He may appear to be suffering while he is discussing his pain, but will become cheerful and carefree if you start talking about something that interests him.

TREATMENT.   What was the first thing that he did or the first remedy he tried? Did it help? What else did he do? Did the symptoms disappear completely for a time, only to recur later, or did they merely decrease somewhat in severity? Have any new symptoms developed? When? What changes have occurred in them? When did he first see his physician? Why? Does he know what medication he received, how often he took it, how much he had? Often you will have to call his doctor to obtain or verify this information, especially if you suspect that the patient has been taking potentially toxic drugs.

GENERAL SYMPTOMS.   Has there been fever, chills, sweating, headache or weakness? Has he lost his appetite? Has he lost weight? What effect has the illness had on his daily routine? Has he been forced to limit his activities, give up his work or remain in bed? Does he know why he came to the hospital? Was there no improvement? Was he getting worse despite treatment? Did his physician decide that the patient required facilities for diagnosis or treatment that were not available in his office or in the home?

Never forget to find out what the patient thinks of his illness. The history you have obtained may be prejudiced by what his family, his friends and his doctor have told him. In his opinion, what brought on this trouble? Did anything unusual immediately precede the first symptoms? A big meal of rich foods may be blamed for an attack of biliary colic; being caught in a downpour might seem to have initiated his joint pains. Does he really think that he is getting better, or worse? What does he think you should be able to do, and what does he hope you might be able to accomplish? Usually the answers can be predicted in advance, but occasionally a patient will have confidence in you by this time and will disclose additional information, or his reply may suggest an unsuspected emotional problem that requires further investigation.

The System Review (S.R.).   When you are sure that you have obtained every scrap of information about the present illness, you should inquire about the functioning of other organs or systems. The outline form suggests the most important items, but others will occur to you as the interview proceeds. This review will furnish a sketch of the general health of the patient. It may give additional clues to the present illness, or it may suggest other unrelated diseases or defects that warrant investigation or require medical attention.

Past Medical History (P.M.H.).   Next, you should inquire about previous illnesses, injuries or operations; get the exact date whenever possible. Ask about symptoms, treatment, complications and sequelae. Was the attack of "pneumonia" probably pneumonia, or was it a chest cold that "might have turned into pneumonia"? Were the symptoms of appendicitis fairly typical, and did they develop rapidly? Or did he have "chronic appendicitis" manifested by a variety of vague gastrointestinal symptoms? Did the operation relieve him? In other words, treat each of them as though it were his present illness and obtain enough information to give you a definite impression as to its importance, duration and severity.

Get the names of physicians who have treated him. If the patient has been hospitalized, be sure to find out where and when; you may want additional information from those records. If the patient is a woman, ask whether she was hospitalized under her present name; there may have been one or more changes in the intervening years. Even a man occasionally alters his surname or drops his first name or initial.

The Family History (F.H.). Inquire about the health of the patient's family and ancestors. This may seem useless in some instances, but it is a part of any complete record. Some medical conditions show a high familial incidence; this is particularly true of certain neurologic diseases. The man whose father and grandfather died suddenly from heart attacks or "acute indigestion," as it was often called in those days, is more liable than the average man to have coronary atherosclerosis or thrombosis. Hypertension is frequently a familial trait, with a stroke, Bright's disease or heart failure given as the ultimate cause of death. Allergic diseases in their various manifestations have a definite hereditary factor. Ask about the familial incidence of such conditions as cardiovascular, renal, pulmonary, gastrointestinal, metabolic or mental disease, allergy and blood dyscrasias.

Record the age and health of the parents, or the cause of death (and age) if they are dead. Often it is advisable to obtain similar data about grandparents, aunts and uncles. Note the ages of living brothers and sisters and their health, with the cause of death and ages of any who have died, and similar facts for the marital partner or partners and for children.

If there have been no children after an adequate period of married life, it may be advisable to inquire discreetly about this. One partner or both may have wished to avoid the responsibility and burdens that inevitably arise when there are children. Financial difficulties may be cited as the primary obstacle. In some instances there may be relative or total sterility or sexual incompatibility of a serious degree. This information will be relatively unimportant if the patient has pneumonia, but may be significant in diseases in which emotional factors often play an important part, as in hypertension or duodenal ulcer. If the patient (or his wife) has no children, you can say casually: "Were you trying to have children, or trying not to have any?" Subsequent questions must be based upon the response to this first remark.

Occupational History (O.H.). With the tremendous advances made in all fields of human activity the exact occupation of the patient has become a factor of increasing importance. Volumes have been written describing the physiologic and pathologic changes that can occur as a result of exposure to an ever-increasing number of chemical and physical hazards.

Some definite plan must be followed in obtaining such a history. You can start with the present job and work back, or start with the first job and work up to the present one. If the occupation is unfamiliar to you, you can flatter the patient and add to your knowledge by asking him to explain his work to you. Never accept a broad term such as "laborer," "truck driver" or "clerk"; find out exactly what he does or what he handles. The laborer with neurologic problems may have shoveled some powder which happened to be white lead. Even a "housewife" is not immune; dry cleaning compounds, detergents, furniture polish and waxes, ant paste, roach powder, insect sprays, bleaches, dyes and caustic cleaning compounds are some of the potentially harmful substances to which she may have been exposed.

The attitude of the patient toward his work, his employer and his associates should also be considered. An apparently innocuous job may be responsible for his digestive symptoms or his headache if he hates his work or thinks that the boss is not treating him fairly. Often such information cannot be obtained at the first interview, but comes out later when the patient trusts you and is ready to confide in you.

Social History (**S.H.**). Finally you inquire about a group of items that might be called miscellaneous, or habits. If not previously discussed, ask about such things as the use of tobacco, alcohol, coffee, tea and soft drinks; the amount of sleep and whether the patient considers this adequate; recreation, hobbies and other activities such as church or civic work; family harmony or friction.

Never overlook the financial aspects; medical care or hospitalization costs money. Does he have hospitalization insurance, or will he have to dig into his savings? Also, many insurance plans will cover only a portion of the total costs. How are other members of the family meeting expenses while the wage-earner is ill? Do they have to pay a housekeeper or maid while mother is hospitalized, or are friends or relatives taking care of the children? In large hospitals the Social Service worker can help, but in your private practice you will be the one to whom the patient and his family will turn for aid and advice.

By the close of the interview you should have some definite impression concerning the reaction of the patient to his illness. He may be depressed; why did this have to happen to him? He may secretly rejoice; now he is the center of attention. He may be worrying about the immediate problem, or he may be wondering what the final outcome will be. Will he recover completely or will his health be permanently impaired? Will he have similar attacks in the future? Can he go back to his usual occupation, or must he seek some other type of work? The psychiatric evaluation of the patient is discussed in greater detail in Chapter II.

Having obtained the information necessary for the history, you should proceed with the physical examination. Again it is advisable to jot down the important positive and negative findings, but make no attempt to write a complete record. When you have finished, go to some quiet spot. Review all the items in the history and attempt to correlate them with the results of the examination. If there are obvious discrepancies or omissions, go back and question the patient again, or re-examine the area concerned. Then make a brief outline summarizing the outstanding points. Arrange these in logical order, both as to time and as to their relative importance. With this framework you are ready to start writing the history.

THE WRITTEN RECORD

The following outline is given to each second year medical student and is used then and during the next two years.

For the guidance of others who will read your record but may not know the patient, it is advisable to begin with a statement concerning the source of your information, and your estimate of the reliability of the informant. Does the patient recall details exactly and clearly, or are his statements vague? Does he seem to minimize symptoms or to exaggerate them? Does he contradict himself frequently? Is he apparently confused? Was the history obtained from some other person such as a daughter? Does she live at home, or did she tell you what she had heard or observed when she dropped in occasionally? Is she merely repeating what the neighbors told her? You can indicate this by a brief statement such as: "Informant, patient; reliable" or "Informant, daughter; 50% reliable."

The Identifying Data.   The necessary information should be recorded on the first sheet of your record (p. 11).

Chief Complaint.   Remember that this is merely the headline; the history will supply the details. Keep it brief. Give symptoms, not diagnosis. If the patient's description is suitable, use it; he might say "Spells when I wheeze and can't get my breath." Don't alter this or interpret it as "Attacks of asthma." If he says he has "gallbladder trouble" ignore the time-worn exhortation to "use the patient's own words." Give the symptoms: "Belching and pain in the stomach whenever I eat fried stuff."

The Present Illness.   After recording the chief complaint stop for a moment and recall certain basic requirements which should be met, such as brevity, clarity, coherence and emphasis. Give due space to the important items; subordinate those of less significance. Never omit *facts*.

however contradictory they may seem to be. A history may contain too little information, but a *well written* history never contains too much.

System Review.   Until you acquire familiarity with the outline, make specific statements concerning each item mentioned; thus you will learn to remember them and to ask about them each time you take a history. Later in your training you will not be required to record answers to all of them, but there should always be specific statements concerning the conditions which are *in italics*.

Past Medical History and Family History.   Follow your outline and the suggestions given above when you write these parts of the history. Complete sentences are not required: "No serious injuries; no operations" or "Father 65; healthy" is sufficient.

Occupational History and Social History.   These should be sufficiently detailed so that the reader will have an adequate picture of all the important points.

Summary.   When you have completed the history, add the summary that you have already prepared, either in the original form or revised if that seems necessary. Keep this as brief as possible; the details have already been recorded. For example, you might write: "Head cold began one week before admission (March 5th). Felt miserable yesterday afternoon; went to bed immediately after dinner. Awoke with severe chill at 5 A.M. today (March 12th). Had pain in the left side of chest, shortness of breath and cough. Family doctor saw him at 7 A.M.; admitted here at 8:30 A.M."

The Physical Examination.   In writing this part of the record you should follow the outline on page 11. At first you should make specific statements about all the items mentioned. Later you may be permitted to omit some of these, but your record must contain information concerning each system and those items that are *in italics*.

At the conclusion there should be a brief summary of the significant findings, normal as well as abnormal. For example, a normal blood pressure and pulse rate, normal heart sounds and absence of murmurs would be significant in a patient who seems to have circulatory failure, but would not be included in the summary if the patient's complaint were severe diarrhea of twelve hours' duration.

The Diagnosis.   By this time you should have reached some conclusion as to the nature of the disease process that is present. This is your Tentative Diagnosis; put it down. Keep in mind other explanations, but pick the one that seems most logical and most probable. Remember what you learned in Anatomy, Bacteriology, Physiology and Pathology. Acute rheumatic fever is most commonly seen in young persons; it is rare in the elderly. Chronic cough, weight loss and blood-streaked sputum in a man of sixty suggest bronchogenic carcinoma; in a boy of sixteen you would suspect pulmonary tuberculosis or bronchiectasis.

After you have made your first choice you can put down other conditions that should be considered in the Differential Diagnosis. The record may seem to indicate that the patient almost certainly has a duodenal ulcer, but since he is over sixty you should consider the possibility that he has a gastric carcinoma. If he were twenty-five, that would be unlikely.

Secondary Diagnoses.   List any important abnormalities unrelated to the present illness under this heading. These could be dental caries, poor vision, chronic sinus infection, hay fever, chronic constipation or any number of other conditions that might be amenable to appropriate therapy, but that are not contributing to the present illness.

Studies.   Now you must decide how *you* would handle this problem. What studies or tests should be obtained? In what order should they be done? Try to prove or disprove the most probable diagnosis first. Go over the list again. Can you justify each test? Will it help you treat the patient more effectively or more intelligently? Will it help him, or at least will it do him no harm? Or are you wasting his money for useless "routine" tests that will contribute nothing?

HISTORY

NAME	ADDRESS
DATE OF ADMISSION	HOSPITAL NUMBER
AGE M F S M W D Sep.	RACE NATIVITY
REFERRED BY	ADDRESS

Informant (patient, relative, friend); *Reliability* of informant.

Chief Complaint (C.C.).   This should be a brief statement of the symptom or symptoms for which the patient is seeking medical care, using his own words if appropriate. Pain is frequently the presenting symptom; other common ones are fever, chills, fatigue, weakness, cough, breathlessness, palpitation, nausea, vomiting, diarrhea, abnormalities of urination, swollen or painful joints, or a "lump," swelling, discharge or bleeding from any site.

Avoid vague expressions such as "stomach trouble" or "kidney disease." Find out what the patient really means; "pain after eating" or "pain on urination" are more specific. Avoid diagnostic terms such as "bronchitis," "gallstones" or "asthma." The patient who says he has asthma may have dyspnea, cough, wheezing and other "asthmatic" symptoms due to some entirely different cause.

Present Illness (P.I.).   This is an amplification of the chief complaint. It should begin with the first symptom that seems pertinent. Dyspnea of one month's duration may be due to rheumatic heart disease; start with a description of the attack of rheumatic fever in childhood. Record the first symptom that might indicate heart failure, and the progression of symptoms *to the time of admission.* Use *dates,* not days of the week. Include the symptoms that *are* present, and also make specific statements concerning the *absence* of symptoms that commonly accompany the disease the patient seems to have. For example, if renal disease is suspected, you might need to state: "No colic, pain or cramps; no smoky or bloody urine."

Find out the patient's opinion as to the cause of his symptoms, and the apparent relationship of exacerbation or improvement to therapy or other factors. Include a statement explaining why the patient came to the hospital, such as failure to improve, exacerbation of the disease or the appearance of new symptoms.

If the disease is one that is characterized by recurring episodes, such as migraine, biliary colic or angina pectoris, it is not necessary to give all details of every attack. Give the date of onset, the frequency of recurrences and any change in their general characteristics, and describe the most severe or the most recent episode in detail.

Readmissions.   If the patient has been hospitalized here previously, or has received treatment in any Outpatient Section, get his chart from the Medical Record Library; review this before writing your history. If the previous admission was for an illness *unrelated* to the present one, include it under Past Medical History (below). Thus, a patient who now has lobar pneumonia had an appendectomy five years ago; that belongs in the P.M.H. If the previous illness seems to be related to the present illness, make a *brief* summary of the pertinent information. Following this comes the Chief Complaint, or the reason for the present admission, and an Interval Note which outlines the course of the illness since the patient was last seen here. This takes the place of the usual History of the Present Illness.

System Review (S.R.).   This covers minor symptoms referable to the systems and organs not involved in the present illness; do not repeat information given above. It also serves as a guide to the general health, past and present, of the patient.

GENERAL SYMPTOMS.   Weakness; chills or fever; changes in weight and probable reasons therefor; *present* weight; *previous* weight.

NERVOUS SYSTEM.   Headache; vertigo; nervousness; convulsions; weakness or paralysis; sensory changes; other neurologic manifestations.

SKIN.   Hives; rash; sores; eczema; "athlete's foot"; other lesions.

EYES.   Acuity of *vision;* photophobia; excessive lacrimation. If glasses are worn, date of last refraction.

EARS. Acuity of *hearing;* discharge; tinnitus; otitis media, mastoiditis.

NOSE. Nasal or postnasal *discharge;* frequency and severity of *head colds;* attacks of sinusitis and treatment given; nasal operations; epistaxis; excessive sneezing; allergic rhinitis (seasonal or perennial); change in sense of smell.

MOUTH. Toothache; abscessed teeth; dentures; sore tongue or mouth; difficulty in chewing or swallowing. *Sore throat; tonsillitis;* quinsy. Decreased or excessive salivation. Change in sense of taste.

LUNGS. *Cough; expectoration* (character; twenty-four hour volume); *hemoptysis; dyspnea;* pain; wheezing; frequency and severity of *chest colds;* attacks of pneumonia or pleurisy; bronchitis or "congestion of the lungs." Date of most recent chest roentgenogram; report, if known.

HEART. *Exercise tolerance* (how much dyspnea with what exertion); palpitation; precordial pressure or *pain* (exact location and character); *orthopnea* (number of pillows used). Edema; cyanosis; leg cramps; vertigo; syncope. History of *"heart trouble," "murmur"* or *"blood pressure"* (high or low).

GASTROINTESTINAL. *Appetite; digestion;* pain; nausea; vomiting; belching; heartburn; hematemesis. Sample *diet* if gastrointestinal complaints are present. Food idiosyncrasies. Frequency, consistency and color of *bowel movements,* and any recent change; laxatives. Hemorrhoids; melena; rectal bleeding. *Jaundice* at any time. Regularity of meals; rapidity of eating.

GENITOURINARY. *Urgency; frequency; dysuria; polyuria; nocturia. Hematuria;* cloudy urine. Difficulty in stopping or starting stream; dribbling; stress incontinence. *"Sores";* urethral discharge; venereal disease. History of kidney or bladder disease, or of abnormal urinalyses.

MENSTRUAL HISTORY. *Age* at menarche; *frequency; duration; amount* of flow. *Pain* (before or during period); severity; treatment. Intermenstrual *discharge* or spotting; midmenstrual pain ("Mittleschmerz"); premenstrual tension.

EXTREMITIES. Pain or swelling of joints; "rheumatism," "neuralgia" or myalgia. Numbness, tingling or other paresthesias. Muscular power. Difficulty in walking or in performing other movements.

Past Medical History (P.M.H.). *Infections:* Measles; mumps; pertussis; varicella. Scarlet fever; diphtheria; rheumatic fever; "growing pains"; chorea; "flu" or "virus"; pneumonia; pleurisy; tuberculosis or a "spot on the lung"; typhoid, venereal diseases (usually by symptoms, rather than by name). "Nervous breakdown" or other mental illness. Record date, duration, severity and complications of any diseases that the patient has had.

Operations: Full details—what, when, where, why. Symptoms preceding operation; acute or chronic; complications; result.

Fractures; serious *injuries.*

Immunization procedures: Smallpox vaccination; diphtheria; pertussis; polio; tetanus; other immunizations. Allergy desensitization procedures; give full details whenever possible. Antitoxin or other serum injections; reactions.

Drug sensitivity, known or suspected; manifestations. (Drug therapy of present illness to be included under P.I.)

Transfusions: Number, date and reasons; transfusion reactions.

Family History (F.H.).   *Age* and *health* of mother, father, brothers, sisters, marital partner or partners, children; if dead, give age at death and cause. If indicated, similar data concerning grandparents, aunts and uncles. *Familial* incidence of allergic manifestations; blood dyscrasias; cancer; cardiovascular, gastrointestinal, renal, pulmonary, metabolic, mental or nervous diseases.

Occupational History (O.H.).   Specific *details* concerning the exact type of work done and length of time in each job. Often advisable to start with the first job, and record complete occupational history. Exposure to dust, fumes or chemicals. Abnormal temperature; hazardous work; poor ventilation; poor working conditions. Attitude toward job, employer and fellow workers. *Armed Forces:* duration and geographical sites of service; injuries, illnesses or service-connected disability.

Social History (S.H.).   Use of tea, coffee, milk, soft drinks; alcohol; tobacco. Sleeping habits; sedatives or hypnotics. Exercise; hobbies; outside interests such as church, civic or youth organizations.

Reaction of patient to his illness; disruption of family life; financial stress. Future plans, especially if the disease is chronic or disabling. Consultation with Social Service Worker often valuable to the extern and to the patient.

Summary of History.   A *brief* summary of the pertinent facts.

PHYSICAL EXAMINATION

Give particular attention to the part of the body that seems to be the site of the patient's disease. Except in General Description of patient, telegraphic style is permissible.

Height (inches). **Weight** (pounds). **Vital Signs:** Temperature (T.); unless oral, specify route. Pulse rate (P.); if rhythm is irregular, record apical *and* radial rates. Respiratory rate (R.). Blood pressure (B.P.) in each arm; indicate whether the patient was seated or recumbent.

General Description.   Write a *paragraph* covering such points as: general appearance (healthy, ill, in pain); apparent age; habitus;

nutrition; musculature; skeleton. Mental state: orientation, memory, attention, intelligence. Station; gait; posture. Tremor; tics; athetoid movements. Speech; language barriers.

Skin.   *Color:* pallor, flush, cyanosis, abnormal pigmentation, jaundice. *Texture:* atrophic or elastic; moist, dry; cool, warm or hot; smooth, rough; soft, hard; edema, dehydration. *Lesions:* macules; papules; vesicles; pustules; blebs; ulcers; scales; crusts; desquamation; scars; keloids; nodules; moles; warts; fibromas; keratoses; birthmarks; petechiae; ecchymoses; purpura. *Hair:* scalp; face; axillae; pubic area; trunk; extremities; hirsutism. Nails.

Head.   SKULL.   Size, shape; abnormalities.

SCALP.   Scars; lesions.

EYES.   Eyelids; conjunctivae; sclerae; irises; *pupils* (equality; outline; reactions to light, accommodation and convergence). Ocular *rotations* (extraocular movements); nystagmus; exophthalmos or enophthalmos; intraocular tension. Estimate amount and character of correction if glasses are available. *Ophthalmoscopic:* lens; media; optic disks; macula. Retinal *vessels:* caliber; light reflex; regularity of lumina; sclerosis; arteriovenous compression or nicking; *hemorrhage; exudate.*

EARS.   *Hearing* (watch or voice test); cerumen; discharge; appearance of canals and *drums.*

NOSE.   Congestion; discharge; obstruction; mucosa; turbinates; nasal septum; polyps; tenderness over frontal or maxillary sinus areas.

MOUTH.   *Lips:* color; moisture; herpes; rhagades. *Mucosa:* color; pigmentation; ulcers; leukoplakia. *Gums:* pyorrhea; bleeding. *Teeth:* number present; roots; devitalized teeth; crowns; bridgework or dentures (plates); dental hygiene. *Tongue:* movement; tremor; moisture; coating. *Tonsils,* if present: size; crypts; exudate; subtonsillar adenitis. Hard and soft palate; uvula. *Pharynx:* lymphoid tissue; postnasal drip; gag reflex; swallowing. Abnormal *odor* on breath: acidotic; fetid; uremic; alcoholic.

Neck.   Movement; position of trachea; *thyroid;* lymph nodes; salivary glands; scars; vascular pulsations; venous distention (estimate venous pressure).

Thorax and Lungs.   Size; shape; symmetry; equality and degree of *expansion.* Estimate vital capacity; *measure* it if pulmonary symptoms are present. Type of respiration (thoracic or abdominal); depth; rate; rhythm. *Fremitus. Percussion* note; diaphragmatic excursion. *Breath sounds;* voice sounds. *Rales,* friction or other adventitious sounds. Describe sputum if any is seen.

Breasts.   Size; contour; symmetry; scars; consistency; masses; tenderness. *Nipples:* contour; retraction; discharge; lesions.

Cardiovascular.   HEART.   Character of cardiac impulse; abnormal pulsation or retraction; shock; thrill. *Location* of point of maximum impulse (PMI) and of apical impulse (AI), by interspace and number of centimeters from midsternal line. Area of cardiac dullness (*measurements*) in each interspace. Character of heart *sounds;* intensity; rhythm; rate. *Murmurs:* location; time in cardiac cycle; character; pitch; intensity (Grade I to VI); direction of transmission; changes with change in posture or after exercise. Friction; other adventitious sounds.

PERIPHERAL VESSELS.   Thickening, tortuosity, elongation, beading or other *abnormalities* of temporal, carotid, brachial, radial, femoral or popliteal arteries. *Character* and synchronicity of *pulse.* Pulses in *dorsalis pedis* and *posterior tibial* arteries; if absent, indicate the most distal point at which the pulse can be felt. If blood pressure is elevated, record character of pulsations in *femoral* or popliteal arteries, or measure the blood pressure in the legs.

Abdomen.   *Contour;* relative size; shape. Visible peristalsis; prominence of veins; striae; abnormal pigmentation; location of *scars.* Panniculus. Involuntary resistance or *rigidity;* voluntary resistance. Hyperesthesia, *tenderness,* rebound tenderness; tenderness in costovertebral areas. Abnormalities on percussion; shifting dullness. Size, shape and all other characteristics of liver, spleen, kidneys, bladder, uterus, cecum, sigmoid or other palpable *organs.* Abdominal *masses:* size; shape; consistency; sensitivity; fixed or movable. *Hernia:* epigastric; umbilical; femoral; inguinal; ventral (incisional). Size of inguinal *rings;* impulse on cough. Character of peristaltic *sounds.*

Genitalia.   *Males.* Hair distribution; development of external genitalia. *Lesions* or scars; urethral discharge; phimosis. Scrotal contents: size, consistency, tenderness of testes, epididymides, spermatic cords; varicocele or hydrocele; masses (transilluminate).

Anus and Rectum.   *Males.* Hemorrhoids; skin tabs; perianal excoriation or skin lesions; fissures; fistula. *Digital* palpation: sphincter tone; masses; Blumer's shelf. *Prostate:* size; consistency; nodularity; tenderness; secretions; fixation; seminal vesicles. Character of *feces* on glove; blood (guaiac test).

Pelvic and Rectal.   *Females: With Intern or Resident Only.* Labia; lesions; scars; Bartholin's and Skene's glands; hymen; urethra. Vaginal *discharge,* amount and character; vaginal walls; cystocele; rectocele; enterocele. *Cervix:* position; appearance; lacerations; erosion; eversion. Size, shape and position of *uterus,* adnexa, ovaries; tenderness; masses. *Rectal,* as for males (above).

Spine.   *Deformities;* kyphosis; lordosis; scoliosis; *mobility;* tenderness.

Extremities.   *Deformities* of bones or joints; bowlegs; knockknees; saber shins; flat feet. *Muscle* development and power; hypertrophy; atrophy; weakness; paralysis; tremors. *Joint* swelling; limitation of motion. Varicose veins; edema; cyanosis; phlebitis; phlebothrombosis; lymphangiitis. Clubbed fingers or toes.

Lymph Nodes. Number, size, shape, consistency and fixation of occipital, posterior and anterior cervical, axillary, epithrochlear, inguinal and femoral nodes.

Nervous System. *Record* as markedly increased, increased, normal, decreased or absent (++++, +++, ++, +, 0): Achilles, patellar, biceps, triceps, abdominal, corneal and gag reflexes; cremasteric in males. If the patient has evidence of neurologic disease do a complete neurologic examination.

Summary. List *briefly* the important positive and negative findings.

Diagnosis. *Primary* Diagnosis; use Standard Nomenclature.

Differential Diagnoses. Less probable causes of the present illness that may have to be ruled out.

Secondary Diagnoses. Abnormalities unrelated to the present illness, such as poor vision, dental caries or flat feet.

Studies. Laboratory, x-ray and special procedures, in the *order* in which they should be performed.

Orders. Activity, diet, medication, nursing care, special instructions.

II

Psychiatric Survey

The psychiatric survey encompasses the evaluation of the total personality of the patient, his customary method of adjustment to the problems of life, and his specific ways of reacting to situations caused by the current illness. To accomplish this survey adequately, one must develop the ability to describe clearly the behavior characteristics of the patient's thinking and emotions in simple and meaningful terms, first to himself and then to others. Each of us perceives intuitively many facts concerning another person; these must be made explicit and verbal. It must be remembered that what is termed "intuitive" has its foundation in the prior knowledge and experience of the interviewer. Much of the knowledge that is helpful in understanding another person has been gained through the various experiences of the interviewer.

Current psychodynamic concepts of personality are only a few decades old and therefore have not been delineated with finality. Nonetheless, information obtained from clinical experience is adequate to enable one to formulate useful and nondoctrinaire concepts of the structure of the emotional life of a human being.

PERSONALITY

Personality can be viewed as consisting of three parts. These divisions are made for purposes of convenience and are difficult to distinguish in emotionally healthy persons. In psychologic illnesses, however, there may be gross distortion, and the divisions are easier to understand. They are as follows:

1. The *ego* is conceived to be the conscious, controlling and integrating part of personality. Understanding of the ego is facilitated if one regards it as the entity which is represented by the phrase "I as I

18

know myself." A person normally thinks of himself as having certain physical and mental attributes, as having a continuity of past experience, a role and status in present life with all its material and interpersonal aspects, and future plans. "I as I know myself" includes all of those aspects of living that a person knows and thinks of as they relate to himself. The ego operates in accordance with the reality-principle. It learns to delay pleasure, and even to withstand pain, for the well-being of the individual. It is also that characteristic part of the personality that is most in contact with others and is best known to them.

2. The *super-ego* is usually called the conscience; this has both conscious and unconscious components. The super-ego develops during early life as one aspect of identification (p. 24) with the prohibitions of parents, teachers and the community. These prohibitions are necessary so that the child will not get himself into a situation in which he might be harmed physically, or so that he will not transgress against the mores of the community. For example, the conscience of a five-year-old child in our culture usually will not permit him to defecate in the street. The environmental demands may be presented in a nonpunitive and not overrestrictive way, or may be harsh, unrealistically demanding and punishing. The super-ego also has positive values, and represents aspirations, goals, tendencies and expectations.

3. The *id* is conceived to be the seat of primitive emotional and psychologic needs and drives. This is the basic, instinctual part of personality, and here reside hunger and thirst, hate and love, aggression and destruction. The id is completely selfish and self-seeking, and operates on what Freud called the pleasure-principle: "The pleasure I want, I want *now*." The consequences of this are never considered. Pain (discomfort) is to be avoided at all costs. The id is the least amenable to conscious control, and through defense and repression it is often not accessible to conscious awareness. Its importance and its strength can be appreciated by observing children two or three years old at play. It will become apparent quickly that they are self-oriented and pleasure-seeking and continually strive to avoid pain.

The ego has the extremely important function of effecting compromises among the demands of the primitive drives from deep within the person, which clamor for immediate discharge regardless of consequences, the demands, often punitive, of the conscience, and the stark realities of everyday life. The ego must permit each of us sufficient gratification to satisfy our emotional needs without incurring either the wrath of the super-ego or the penalties inflicted by the outside world for inappropriate behavior by the id.

The ego is partially but not completely conscious or a part of our awareness. The id is unconscious; it is not available to conscious recall, and not a part of our awareness. The super-ego is largely unconscious.

The transitional area between conscious and unconscious is termed pre-conscious.

DEFENSE MECHANISMS

The ego is aided in these tasks by mechanisms of defense. For the most part, these are normal healthy methods by which disproportionate tension and anxiety can be avoided. These have been clearly and simply described by Anna Freud. Some of the more important of these mechanisms in the healthy person will be discussed; this list is not complete. It is important to remember that several mechanisms are usually operating simultaneously.

Repression. This is the unconscious act of pushing out of awareness any conflict-laden thoughts and feelings. For example, suppose that a young man works for an older person whom he likes and respects. However, were the older man to die, the younger one would take over his position. The thought of wishing harm to the older person is unacceptable to the young man, since it would make him feel guilty and anxious, yet it is an idea that will recur intermittently. But as the thought occurs, before the young man is consciously aware of it, it is pushed from the consciousness; it is repressed. Once repressed, constant energy must be expended to keep it out of consciousness. The act of maintaining repressions can be compared to pushing a rubber ball below the surface of the water. It requires energy to do this. If the hand is removed the ball rises; to keep it submerged constant pressure must be maintained. All persons expend energy continuously in perpetuating repressions.

Sublimation. This is the conversion of unacceptable primitive drives into mature socially and personally acceptable feelings. For example, children normally derive pleasure from looking and observing, and these acts are essential if they are to learn. In adult life, looking must be diverted from the infantile goals of looking at some other person's body to more socially acceptable uses, such as looking at art works or heavenly bodies. The pleasure gained in sublimated looking, however, has much in common with childhood pleasures. When sublimation of the act of looking fails to take place, the kind of disturbance known as voyeurism ("peeping Tom") may occur.

Reaction Formation. This is the turning of an unacceptable feeling into its apparently opposite acceptable feeling. A person who has many unconscious cruel and destructive feelings toward people and animals may handle these feelings by becoming an ardent antivivisectionist, or unusually scrupulous, or overanxious about the welfare of others. In this way the unconscious cruelty is turned into a kind of over-beneficence.

Displacement. Displacement of feelings may be from dangerous to less dangerous objects. A youngster may dislike and fear his father, and know that it would be foolhardy to express his feelings directly. Indeed, he probably would not be consciously aware of these emotions. If he had a male teacher who in any small way resembled his father, the youngster might develop a great hatred for the teacher. So far as the teacher is concerned, this would seem unjustified, but it is completely understandable in terms of the displaced feelings for the father. This mechanism unconsciously forms the basis of many irritations and prejudices that even doctors hold against others.

Projection. This is the casting off to others of one's own short-comings. In a golf match the player who would like to "forget" a few strokes of his own may attribute to his opponent the desire to cheat. Projection is also a mechanism in major psychologic illnesses such as paranoid schizophrenia, in which an unconscious, overwhelmingly threatening feeling such as homosexual desires, for example, is projected to others. Projection is seen in the use of "scapegoats."

Purpose. Admittedly, all these mechanisms and several others can be misused at times of physical or psychologic stress, or even in illness. In conversion hysteria, for example, the anxiety is first repressed; if the repressing forces fail, the psychic energy may be displaced to a symbolically important part of the body. This was well demonstrated in a young woman with an unconscious fear of her impending marriage. Prior to it, she developed a functional paraplegia. This prevented her from "walking to the altar" and was for her a way of symbolizing her attitude toward her marriage.

The individual need for these various mechanisms of defense can be understood, in part, by the realization that in all people there resides a kind of energy that is both physiologic and psychologic. This energy has been termed the *libido* by Freud, and the "élan vital" by Bergson. It is derived from the soma itself, and appears to be the driving force of life. The libido constantly strives to keep tensions in balance so that the physiopsychologic equilibrium can be maintained at the least painful and most pleasurable level. This does not imply that the healthiest life is one in which tensions are absent. Rather, it indicates that such tensions, both pleasurable and painful, are dealt with as they arise, so that a relatively peaceful balance results.

As a person matures, he develops increasingly well-integrated means of maintaining this equilibrium with appropriate feeling, thinking and acting. Illness, somatic or emotional, tends to disrupt this balance. One can understand the real meaning of an illness to any person only by comprehending the degree and extent of the disturbance of this equilibrium and the distribution of energies.

Source of Personality Concepts.   These concepts of the structure of personality were developed from two primary sources: first, from an understanding of the psychologic processes of emotionally ill adults, and second, from the study of both well and disturbed children. Sigmund Freud was the first physician to realize and emphasize the great significance of unconscious factors in influencing conscious, apparently rational behavior, and to point out the importance of the role of the balancing of psychic energy. During his early work he felt this energy to be primarily sexual. He modified his views later in life, so that he came to feel that both sexual and especially aggressive impulses were of prime importance. Anxiety, he believed, was a danger signal indicating that aggressive or erotic impulses were liable to get out of bounds.

His work has been carried forward by an increasing number of workers, including his daughter Anna Freud, and by Ernest Jones, Franz Alexander and many others. Carl Jung originally agreed with Freud, but has come to believe that Freud's concept of the unconscious drives is too narrow and too much limited to the sexual sphere. He believes that the unconscious contains not only the memories and drives of the individual patient, but also the collective experiences of mankind. Alfred Adler, like Jung, believed that Freud overemphasized the libidinal drives, and Adler saw the "drive to mastery" as the dominant theme. Adolph Meyer attempted to synthesize these varying levels of reaction in the concept of his "psychobiological approach" to human problems. Edward Strecker and Kenneth Appel have attempted to integrate psychobiologic and psychoanalytic concepts into current "standard" psychiatric thinking. Harry Stack Sullivan pioneered in the application of psychodynamic concepts in the treatment of psychotic patients. Schizophrenic patients, as well as persons with psychotic elation or depression, had previously been considered beyond therapeutic reach. Sullivan demonstrated that the application of psychoanalytic principles was useful in helping these patients, and emphasized that well persons and psychotically ill patients form an emotional continuum. Sullivan called attention to cultural and environmental factors in the development of illness. He also stressed the importance of these psychodynamic concepts in everyday interpersonal relationships. Sullivan's concepts have been extended by Fromm-Reichman, Thompson and Rosen. Historically, all these workers emphasized the importance of unconscious drives and of the various devices by which they are handled.

EMOTIONAL DEVELOPMENT

To understand the emotional configuration of adult life more clearly, some knowledge of emotional development is helpful. It is obvious that the infant is born with certain and undifferentiated drives that could hardly be called conscious according to adult concepts. Nevertheless the infant instinctively reacts to certain stimuli, including the proffering of suitable food, the receiving of warmth and the administration of tenderness and affection, as well as the reverse. During this early time in life the infant appears to be both emotionally and physically a passive, receiving being. It can readily be understood that if he is not able to have his needs met with reasonable promptness and with reasonable love, in later childhood or adult life he may feel that he can not or will not receive those things and feelings to which he is entitled.

As the infant reaches the third or fourth month of life the conscious ego apparently begins to develop. From then on the child successively, albeit slowly, learns to distinguish self from non-self, active from passive, and eventually male from female. During the second six months of life the baby changes from a passive, receiving being to a more active and outgoing person. This is determined physiologically by the better command of his limbs, and more particularly by the development of the teeth. It is during this time that the mouth is used for exploring and biting, and sometimes for swallowing both actual things other than nourishment, and symbolically, the world around him. It is important that during this phase of development the child be given considerable freedom to explore, but some limits must be placed on the amount of aggression the outside world will tolerate. Aggression at this age is expressed mostly in oral terms. Failure to effect reasonable compromise during this period of life may result in difficulties in handling certain types of aggressive impulses in adult years.

As the child continues to grow, the world and especially the home begin to put demands on him in terms of the control of his bowels and bladder. This is usually the first time when the parents exert definite, unyielding control. If the child fails to please the parent, the parent is liable to threaten in return that the child will lose his love. This is a period in which there is marked struggle for control between the child and the parents. It is not unexpected that many habit patterns of later childhood and adult life, and some psychologic illnesses, appear to have their origins in this period when the struggle for control is so important. Acquiescent, submissive, rebellious or antagonistic attitudes to authority, control, duty and what is "right" have their origins in these years.

After sphincter control has been learned the child slowly enters the period of "family romance." The five- or six-year-old boy becomes even more attached and attentive to his mother, while the six- or seven-year-old girl finds that her father has become a most attractive man. During this period son competes with father, and daughter with mother. But the break with the parent of the same sex is by no means complete, since son still needs father's love as desperately as daughter needs mother's. This mixture of love and anger is termed *ambivalence*. It is obvious that the boy is neither big enough nor mature enough to win mother away from father, nor can the girl usurp mother's role with father. However, by living through this period of "romancing," each child learns something about how to become a giving and receiving man or woman. Eventually the child gives up, at least temporarily, the struggle with parents and slips into the period of latency in which intellectual and musculoskeletal activities with one's own sex become predominant. Each child needs the experience of the struggle of the "family romance" to become prepared for his or her renewed struggle in adolescence.

Adolescence recreates in a rather different way the same struggle of aggression and passivity, and male against female, which in a less mature way was characteristic of the period of "family romance." This whole conflict can be resolved finally only when the son realizes that he does not have to replace his father, and the daughter that she does not have to replace her mother; each finds that he can be, in his own right, as mature a man or woman as the parents. Only then can the individual be said to have "grown up," for then he is able to form a realistic and mature relationship with the parent and with other individuals.

A word should be said about the vital process of *identification*. Human beings can learn in one of two ways. The first, trial and error, is an unsatisfactory and painful method of learning. The second, identification, means placing one's self in another person's position for purposes of learning what that person has already learned; it is a necessary psychologic requisite for physical and emotional growth. Psychologic development may be viewed as a group of layers or superimposed identifications or oppositions (reaction formations). The child identifies with the parents, with teachers, with siblings, and indeed with all emotionally meaningful people. He says: "I will do this thing this way because Father does it this way." In adult life these identifications become less strong, but are always operative to some extent. Thus, a patient who initially has no personal knowledge of the physician to whom he goes will intuitively identify the physician with some previously known person. By so doing he may then attribute to this unknown physician major characteristics of a previously known person. This phenomenon is known as *transference*.

It should be clear from the foregoing that the people encountered in everyday life and in medical practice operate in a complex variety of ways (repression, sublimation, reaction formation, displacement, conversion, projection). When one learns to recognize the importance of nonrational elements in daily life, and realizes that these nonrational elements inevitably become important during the tortuous course of development from infancy to maturity, it becomes less surprising that what the patient *thinks* and what he *feels* may be vastly different. If a patient is asked: "What is troubling you?" he may not know. He may have no conscious access to the source of his real difficulties, which may lie in the area of his feelings, hidden from him by various mechanisms described above.

EMOTIONAL REACTIONS TO ILLNESS

Physical illness, especially when sudden or severe, causes an adult in reality to be in a dependent position. When he is dependent, he necessarily recalls both consciously and unconsciously that earlier time of life when he was in fact dependent upon those around him. It is probable that he will react, not as the mature adult that he is, but as a dependent child. He is liable to think of the physician and other medical personnel as parents. He expects them to treat him as though he were a child, and in accordance with the way in which he was treated when young. He may expect the doctor to act in a certain way, but what the patient expects is not known to the doctor. If the doctor acts like one of the patient's parents who had acted in an unreasonable way, one would expect the patient to be overrebellious, overfrightened or overpassive. Only if the physician can maintain a position of interested and benevolent objectivity can he help the patient to understand the reality of the current illness as divorced from past experiences, and to regard the doctor as part of the current situation.

It must be remembered that the physician is also human. He has had an early life, and this early life has left its imprints upon him. He also has learned to react in unconscious ways to the people about him, not only his family and friends, but also his patients. Medical students and doctors sometimes feel what they recognize as irrational annoyances with certain patients, and ease and comfort with others. When one's own reaction is observed to be out of proportion to the actual clinical situation, one must seek within one's self for the explanation. Just as patients have expectations of wondrous things from their physician, so the physician may feel that it is necessary for him to cure his patients in some magical way. Certain illnesses are not curable at present, and the physician may find himself considering the hopelessly ill patient a "bad" patient, one who will not do him credit since he will not get well. Sometimes a patient will not follow strictly the recommended regimen; this disobedience may displease the doctor, especially a young one. The patient-doctor relationship has within it all aspects of the other relationships in both the patient's and the doctor's lives, and has as its background the emotional lives of both. Thus the apparently simple relationship between doctor and patient is actually an emotionally complicated one. It must be the subject of considerable thought on the part of the physician, and often a discussion with the patient will lend valuable clues to the patient's illness and his manner of reacting to it. Physical illness, with its attendant discomfort and enforced dependency, results in disturbed relationships with one's fellows. These disturbances are mirrored in the doctor-patient relationship and need to be understood within the framework of this relationship.

On this basis it becomes clear that simply to tell a patient something or to ask him something may not be sufficient. The patient must have the opportunity to bring to the surface his feelings about his illness, about how he feels concerning important persons and relationships in the present and in the past, about what he expects of the doctor, and about what the doctor expects of him. In this way, a purely intellectual approach to emotional problems can be lessened, and a process of emotional working-through of problems, a rubbing-off of emotional disturbances and excesses, can be facilitated.

THE PSYCHIATRIC INTERVIEW

In the light of these psychodynamic concepts the importance of the psychiatric interview should be obvious. Although there is a considerable difference between the technique of conducting a medical and a psychiatric interview, many of the essentials are similar. Taking the history becomes more than a simple question and answer period; the patient may not consciously know the most relevant parts of his history, which are partly hidden from him.

During the interview both the physician and the patient should be seated comfortably. Neither should be looking into a bright light. Most psychiatric interviews last forty-five to sixty minutes; if less time is available, one should tell the patient. It is disturbing to him if he begins to speak of emotionally important matters, and then has to stop abruptly.

Much can be learned by listening to the patient, and by trying to understand not only his words but also the feelings behind his words. Several interviews may be necessary before you can understand not only the patient's illness, but also the *person* who is ill. The patient should be encouraged to tell his story in his own words; specific questions should be reserved until later. Sufficient time must be allowed to permit the physician to learn something of the meaning *to the patient* of his medical or surgical illness.

The formal recording of information should be kept at a minimum; take as few notes as possible in the presence of the patient. If you are busy recording copiously what he says, you may not actually listen to him and appreciate the feelings involved. If you record only at certain *apparently* important times, he may try to emphasize this aspect; unfortunately, this may not be his primary concern. Whenever possible, nothing but brief notes of pertinent material should be made during the interview; a full report can be prepared after the patient has left. To illustrate this, tell an emotionally important story such as that of a serious illness of your own to a colleague, and have him compulsively record every detail. Then tell the same story to a colleague who is really listening, and see how much easier this is. Although competent psychiatrists differ as to the notes they take, the principles enunciated above generally hold true.

In recording the physical examination, some note should be made of the patient's emotional status. For example, if the patient has difficulty in speaking, this should be recorded. If the patient is tense and anxious during the recounting of the story, or particular parts of it, this should be a matter of record. By writing a summary concerning the patient's intellectual and emotional condition, the examiner helps to bring to his own awareness the salient features concerning the patient's personality make-up.

There are times when the patient is too ill or too upset to give more than an inadequate understanding to the physician of his illness and its surrounding situations. Under these circumstances interviews with members of the family may help you understand the complexities of the illness. Under most circumstances the patient should be told of these interviews, so that he does not feel that the doctor is going behind his back.

MENTAL STATUS

Determination of the mental status of the patient can be divided into several categories. When the patient is psychiatrically ill, these can be used for a rather thoroughgoing systematic summary of the patient's emotional state.

General Attitude of the Patient. This means the total picture that the patient presents and the impression he makes on the examiner. Note first the state of consciousness—whether the patient is alert, lethargic or semistuporous—and also the way in which he carries himself and how he walks and talks. The facial expression is often indicative of his attitude toward himself and toward others; it may also give considerable insight into underlying disease processes. It may be particularly valuable to note the limited play of facial muscles in the patient who is depressed. The tone of voice and the speed with which the patient talks often mirror his attitude toward the treatment situation.

The degree of motor activity should be evaluated. Is the patient restless or agitated, or does he sit quietly or stolidly in his chair? For example, the person who fingers his watch or jewelry or plays with a book of matches betrays his underlying tension even though his voice and facial expression are well controlled. Notice whether he is dressed carefully and neatly, or in a slovenly fashion; even the way in which a woman wears her makeup may suggest what her attitude toward herself may be.

It is very important to note whether the patient is accessible. Does he understand the examiner and the general situation, or does he refuse to recognize the examiner's presence, and fail to follow his instructions? The patient may be accessible, but suspicious and evasive.

The degree of attentiveness should also be evaluated as a part of the determination of the general attitude. Patients may be inattentive for many causes; an explanation should be sought.

Does the patient talk readily and spontaneously about his problem, or is he overaggressive and self-justifying, or aloof and seemingly disinterested?

This list, of course, is not all-inclusive. It merely suggests that all aspects of appearance and attitude are of value in determining the patient's mental state.

Memory.   In many instances memory need not be tested directly. As the patient relates his story the clarity of his memory is usually evident. When he apparently does not remember important events and dates, one can test memory more specifically by asking the names of parents, children and spouse, and by asking him to recall specific dates and events in his life. Occasionally it may be necessary to have members of the family verify his statements. Memory is often impaired in patients with organic disease of the nervous system.

Orientation.   This means the knowledge of the correct time (day, month, year or hour), place (state, city, building) and identification of his own person (name, spouse's name, approximate age). In most examinations there is no need to ask the patient specifically for this information, since it will be apparent that the patient is well oriented. With states of altered consciousness, or when there seems to be confusion for any reason, it is advisable to attempt to get specific information from the patient.

Stream of Thought.   Under this heading one evaluates the patient's story as he tells it. It is essential that he be allowed to tell his story in his own words, with a minimum of interruption. When he stops talking, he should be encouraged with noncommital phrases such as: "What happened then?" or "Won't you tell me more about that?" Only when no more information can be obtained in this way should leading questions be asked, but questions liable to increase the anxiety of the patient should be avoided, especially in the early interviews.

Attempt to estimate the clarity of the stream of thought, its direction and its speed. Note whether the patient uses words in common usage, and whether these words appear in an orderly fashion, so that what he says is clear to you. It is obvious that the way in which he actually tells a story will be determined largely by his educational background. Care must be taken to use his cultural background, not yours, as a frame of reference.

In determining the direction of the stream of thought, note whether the patient starts his story at a given place and attempts to reach a goal or climax, or whether he becomes distracted either by his own words or by stimuli in the environment, so that he loses the trend of his story and stops short or wide of his main goal. Here again there is a wide normal variation that is both cultural and emotional; however, most patients eventually reach their goal. Failure to do so despite aid from the interviewer is suggestive of organic brain disease or schizophrenia; when combined with excessive speed of production, it is suggestive of the hypomanic or manic stage of manic-depressive psychosis.

The speed with which the stream of thought is produced varies considerably. Watch for marked slowness of thought production, especially when there are long pauses between sentences or thoughts. The depressed patient speaks slowly, and at times his stream of thought may seem to be retarded, but usually the phrase or sentence will be completed. The hypomanic person shows pressure of the stream of thought, speaks quickly, and is distracted by his own words (*flight of ideas*). *Blocking* occurs not uncommonly in the schizophrenic and occasionally in the depressed patient. He attempts to start a phrase, or actually does utter a few words, but appears prohibited from continuing and does not finish the thought.

Disturbances of Perception. When a person is awake, mental activity is concerned with the perception, sorting and interpretation of countless numbers of stimuli from the outside world. In most instances correct evaluation of these stimuli is performed largely unconsciously and is reasonably accurate. In some individuals, especially those who are mentally ill, there may be disturbances or falsification of the perceived phenomena.

An *illusion* is a false perception of some definite external stimulus. For example, if the patient hears a clap of thunder and says: "They're shooting at me," and at the same time performs appropriate acts to take cover from the shooting, he has perceived falsely what has actually occurred and is acting on this. However, it must be noted that the question of social acceptance plays a role in the evaluation of illusions. If an object in the sky is thought to be a "flying saucer" by the patient, and if many of the people around him substantiate this idea, he may be mistaken but not necessarily suffering from an illusion.

A *hallucination* is a false perception without an outside stimulus to account for it. For example, if a patient states that he hears voices in a noiseless room, and is able to recount the stories the voices tell him, he probably is having hallucinations. These are most often auditory or visual, but may be olfactory, gustatory or tactile. Often these disorders are obvious, but sometimes a patient is sufficiently in contact with the world so that he does not wish to betray himself. Be cautious when questioning a patient about hallucinations and illusions. If he seems to be listening to a sound that you cannot hear, ask him: "What do you hear?" rather than: "Are you hearing voices?".

Association of Ideas.   This means the way in which ideas follow one another in speaking or writing. Normally, one person can follow the sequence of thought of another person; what the first one says seems fairly coherent and relevant. All people will be distracted occasionally from what they are saying, but the cause of this will generally be apparent.

In organic or toxic states the association of ideas may be incoherent; in schizophrenic reactions one sees the great defect in the association of ideas. In these patients, phrases are spoken subsequentially but appear to have no connection one with the other. Instead of a smoothly running stream of speech, phrases seem to fall in separate droplets. The associations may depend purely upon the sound of the words, rather than upon their meaning. New words are often constructed, or sounds repeated many times. What is said may be irrelevant or inappropriate. In hypomanic or maniacal reactions one may see the flight of ideas mentioned previously.

Judgment.   This may be defined as the ability to perceive the elements of a situation, and then integrate past experience with current perceptions so as to act in a rational and realistic manner. In essence, good judgment can be equated with the popular concept of "common sense." A person's judgment is, in some measure, determined by his previous education and training and by his cultural background. One must consider the patient's previous life experiences, social and racial ties, and actual current status before attempting to evaluate the integrity of his judgment.

Often a definite opinion should not be given after a single interview. Judgment is evaluated from the historical data available, from the patient's statements and reactions during the interview, and often by corroboration from other sources. A person with good judgment should be able to conduct his affairs with moderate caution and discretion and should get along fairly well with other human beings. There are, of course, many people whose judgment appears marginal. From the viewpoint of medical evaluation it is well to have some written record of your estimate of the patient's judgment.

Gross disorders of judgment occur in delusional states and when ideas of influence are present. A *delusion* is a false belief based on wrong premises, usually held by one person alone, and not correctible by argument or reasoning. Thus if a man is certain that his wife has been unfaithful to him repeatedly, and clings stubbornly to this belief even after he has been shown that all of her time and effort are accounted for in other ways, he can be said to have a delusion regarding his wife's fidelity. Bleuler points out that delusions are incorrect ideas created by "an accidental insufficiency of logic, but out of inner need." There are many types of delusions; those of grandeur, persecution, hypochondriasis or impoverishment are examples. It is essential that one evaluate the real situation carefully before deciding whether or not the patient has a delusion.

Ideas of *influence* are a specialized form of delusion. The patient believes that other people are able to influence his thoughts or acts by external and often by magical means, as through air waves or through radiators, for example. These delusions may be difficult to elicit, especially if the observer overlooks the possibility that they exist. Often a momentary disturbance of facial expression while the patient is recounting his story can be the clue that will lead to these ideas of influence.

Mood.   Evaluation of the patient's mood is perhaps the most important part of the study of the mental status, yet it is the most difficult to discuss objectively. One is concerned both with the predominant mood exhibited during the interview, and, of equal importance, with the appropriateness of the relation between the expressed thought content and the mood itself. It is convenient to classify mood into four basic types: anxiety, depression, apathy and elation. All other feeling tones are permutations or combinations of these.

ANXIETY.   Clinically, anxiety is of great importance. It may be defined briefly as a state of uneasiness, apprehension, worry or misgivings about what *may* happen. Anxiety is to be differentiated from fear. The latter is a reaction to a real or threatened danger, whereas anxiety is more typically a reaction to an unreal or imagined danger. Anxiety consists of a somatic physiologic side manifested by such signs as motor restlessness, excessive perspiration, rapid respiration or tachycardia, and a psychologic side with perception of specific unpleasurable feelings and sensations, and of apprehension. Most patients display variable amounts of anxiety, restlessness or agitation during the initial examination; indeed, some anxiety is probably appropriate on these occasions. In addition, the symptoms that bring a person to a physician are often of the kind that one would expect to create anxiety. Excessive anxiety may be indicative of either organic or psychologic dysfunction. When considerable anxiety is present, its purported cause should be investigated by appropriate laboratory tests and also by detailed psychologic study.

APATHY.   This can be defined as a state of disinterest on the part of the patient in himself and in his surroundings. It is decidedly not the usual reaction to a medical interview and examination; when it is present, an explanation for it should be sought. Many physical illnesses, especially malignancy, certain endocrine dysfunctions and many chronic diseases associated with cachexia, are accompanied by an apathy which often appears beneficial to the patient. In the absence of grave somatic disease, apathy may be seen in severe depressions and in the simple forms of schizophrenia.

DEPRESSION.   In psychiatry, this term may either denote an element of mood or be a diagnostic label for a specific psychiatric syndrome. The term is used here to denote a mood element.

All individuals normally experience a certain amount of depression and a certain amount of elation; a more or less rhythmical oscillation between these two is not uncommon in a normal person. Even in the well person, feelings of mild depression or elation cannot always be correlated with the conscious mental life and are related to unconscious processes.

Abnormal degrees of depression may be observed in serious physical illness or in the psychoneuroses, but they are most pronounced in the depressed phase of manic-depressive psychosis and in mental illnesses occurring in middle life (*involutional depression*), where they are accompanied by a sense of inadequacy and by self-blame. The depressed patient appears downcast, usually sits with his gaze fixed on the floor rather than on the examiner's face, speaks slowly and in a monotonous tone of voice, and may on occasion cry. He may speak of the hopelessness of his life situation, of the fact that he is guilty of neglecting his family or of misusing material goods. Although motor activity may be decreased, agitation may be seen. The depressed person, especially in the involutional period of life, may show great concern with bodily functions in general, and those of the gastrointestinal tract in particular. Any patient who shows marked depression should always be considered a potential suicidal risk, and it must be realized that the person who talks of "hurting" himself often does carry out his threat.

ELATION.   This is the opposite of depression; it is a mood characterized by a false sense of well-being. An elated person speaks quickly and often liltingly, but usually displays poor judgment. Often there is marked motor activity, great sexual drive or activity, and the need for less than the usual amount of sleep. It may be difficult to detect minor degrees of elation when seeing the patient for the first time; if you suspect it, talk to a member of his family. Elation may be seen in the organic psychoses, especially in paresis, and in the manic phase of manic-depressive psychosis; it may also occur in schizophrenia.

OTHER MOODS.   It is well to watch for some of the more complex feeling tones, such as hostility, suspiciousness, shyness and withdrawal. Resentment and hostility, either overt or masked, are commonly seen in psychoneuroses. One should attempt to decide whether the mood is appropriate to the thought content. When a patient speaks of severe headache, does his facial expression and the tone of his voice suggest anxiety and realistic concern, or are there indications that he is reciting these symptoms only to elicit sympathy? Wide discrepancies between the mood and the expressed thought content occur in the schizoid and schizophrenic group of illnesses, and are therefore of great importance.

Special Preoccupations.   It is to be expected that the patient will be concerned mainly with the symptoms for which he consults the physician. In certain cases, however, one gets the impression that there is over-concern about some one symptom or a single organ or group of organs; he seems to have fixed his attention on these rather than on his problem as a whole. In extreme cases such preoccupations may indicate hypochondrial delusions, and are significant in evaluating the illness. Also, he may have preoccupations which do not relate to bodily functions, such as delusions, hallucinations or other special problems. Whenever preoccupation is encountered, every effort should be made to find out more about its meaning.

Phobias, Obsessions and Compulsions.   These are psychologic mechanisms that attempt to avoid, disguise or solve problems of anxiety.

A *phobia* is a fear, not related to a threat in the outside world, but rather to a set of circumstances that are specific for the patient. The formulation of a phobia is generally the result of his need to compartmentalize anxiety. For example, he may be afraid to go outdoors alone. He realizes that nothing will happen to him if he does, but the fear is so great that he remains indoors. The fear in this case is not related to the threat of what really will happen if he goes outside, but rather to inner restriction and tension which find an outlet in the phobia.

An *obsession* is an irresistible thought, the absurdity of which the patient recognizes; nevertheless, he must pursue this thought to avoid the development of anxiety. Although the obsession creates anxiety, this is usually less severe than it would be without the obsession. For example, a woman fears that she will kill her child. She knows that this thought is ridiculous but she cannot control it; therefore it is quite painful. However, she is still able to say that she loves her child and that the thought of hurting him is really foreign to her way of thinking and acting. Thus the obsessional thought may be considerably less painful to her than the recognition that unconsciously she really does have tremendous hostility toward either her child or some other person who has been emotionally important in her life.

A *compulsion* is an irresistible act, the absurdity of which the patient recognizes; nevertheless, he must perform this act to avoid anxiety. Often a patient will go to great lengths to hide the absurd act from his fellows. Compulsions vary in severity, and range from mild to incapacitating.

When a patient appears to be unduly tense the interviewer needs to learn more of his patterns of feeling; it may be advisable to ask the patient whether he has any specific fears. Common fears are those of height, crowded places, open spaces and water. The presence of a single phobia need not be of diagnostic significance unless it incapacitates the patient or makes him obviously uncomfortable. Patients with obsessions or compulsions can usually be expected to describe their symptoms because of the amount of discomfort involved.

Phobias, obsessions and compulsions are manifestations of the group of disorders known as *psychoneuroses*. These are emotional disorders characterized by anxiety, phobias, compulsions, obsessions or somatic disorders which may partially or almost completely disable the patient. The symptoms, however, are more or less compartmentalized; the patient is able to maintain contact with reality and often has some insight into the nature of his illness. Here the ego has partially failed in its synthetic integrative function, and must take neurotic measures to insure some measure of freedom from anxiety.

Insight.   This is the ability of the patient to admit that he is ill and that he needs help. It is a means by which one evaluates his understanding of the fact that he is ill, of the nature of his illness, and of what the possible consequences of his illness may be to him and his family. Some patients appear to have a clear intellectual grasp of the situation, but are unable to accept their illness emotionally. Only with experience can one learn to evaluate accurately the true degree of the patient's emotional understanding of the problem he has.

Throughout your medical life you will collect information which is helpful in the understanding of other human beings. This chapter has attempted to summarize a few of the basic data concerning the ways in which these clinical impressions can be classified in an orderly fashion. Symptoms of mental illness are beyond the scope of this chapter, but in every routine examination you should attempt to gain an understanding of the person as a whole, to recognize major emotional abnormalities and to make a carefully organized record of your observations. If this is done the patient can then be evaluated as a total human being— physically, emotionally and socially.

III

Preliminary Observations;
Vital Signs

To perform a satisfactory examination one must learn to use his senses of sight, touch, hearing and smell and to coordinate the findings obtained through these senses. The four basic procedures, usually performed in the order indicated, are:

Inspection. This requires more than a casual glance or a vacuous stare. You must learn to look for and to recognize a vast number of variations from the average or normal, and thus initiate the differentiation of physiologic from pathologic processes.

Palpation. This is the use of your tactile senses to determine the physical characteristics of tissues or organs; with experience you will learn to detect abnormalities.

Percussion. By striking a blow, you produce vibrations in the tissues; the analysis and interpretation of the characteristics of the sound so produced gives valuable information concerning the structure of the underlying tissue.

Auscultation. Listening to the sounds produced as various organs function will provide helpful clues, especially in the examination of the heart and arteries, the lungs and the gastrointestinal tract.

Not all of these procedures are applicable to every area. For example, one would inspect and palpate the extremities, but percussion or auscultation would not ordinarily be necessary or even helpful. Under exceptional circumstances this is not true; auscultation would be indicated if an arteriovenous fistula were suspected, for example, or if there were abnormal grating when a limb was moved.

Before starting the examination one must remember that the patient is not only a human being, but an *individual* human being. He is probably ill, either physically, emotionally or mentally, or he would not have come to the hospital. He will show certain variations from the "normal" or average, but these may be unimportant; other changes, even though

35

minor, may be of great significance. Skill plus experience will enable you to detect and evaluate these changes; you will not acquire these talents in a few short class sessions.

PREPARATION FOR THE EXAMINATION

The examining room should be comfortably warm; so should your hands, your stethoscope and any other instruments you use. Daylight is the preferred type of illumination; minor degrees of jaundice, for example, cannot be detected if incandescent lights are used. The daylight-type fluorescent tube is a satisfactory substitute if natural illumination is not available. The bed or examining table should not be near or against a wall; free access to any position simplifies the examination and increases its accuracy.

PREPARATION OF THE PATIENT

For a *complete* physical examination the patient must disrobe; an examining gown should be provided. There are numerous types of these, but the most practical are those that permit adequate examination of every area in turn without unnecessary or undue exposure at any one time (Figs. 1, 2, 3). A patient may be somewhat nervous or apprehensive when he knows that he is going to be examined. Some patients, especially women, resent disrobing even when they visit a physician. A competent nurse or office assistant can frequently secure cooperation; it is advisable to have her remain in the room if a woman is being examined.

Always bear in mind the comfort of the patient. If dyspneic, he may be unable to lie flat for any length of time; if very ill, he may be too weak to sit up very long. Do as much of the examination as possible with him in the most comfortable position. Never make a patient sit up *in bed* for any length of time without support; try this and see how uncomfortable it is. Let him sit on the edge of the bed, or on a chair or stool. If this is not possible, have someone support him in bed.

Although the complete examination must include all parts of the body, it is not always necessary or desirable to adhere to a fixed outline or routine. For example, if a diabetic patient has just developed an ulcer on his foot, it may be preferable to examine the feet first, and then proceed to other areas. This will show him that you are really interested in the presenting problem; you can then say that you want to be sure that "everything else is all right."

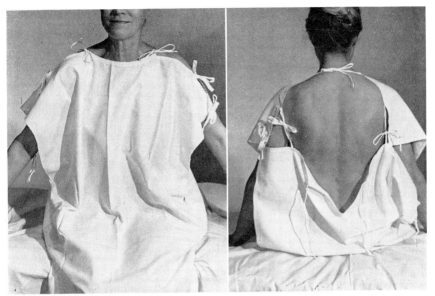

Fig. 1   Fig. 2

Fig. 1. One style of easily adjusted examining gown.

Fig. 2. By varying the position of the straps that are tied over the shoulders or around the neck it is possible to obtain an adequate view of the back without undue exposure. For examination of the chest anteriorly one side can be exposed, then the other.

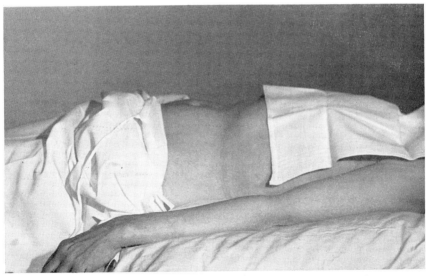

Fig. 3. The abdomen can be bared, using a towel to cover the breasts.

INSPECTION

> *Don't touch the patient—state first what*
> *you see; cultivate your powers of observation.*
>
> Osler[1]

Inspection is the first step. While you were taking the history you should have formed certain general impressions about the patient as an individual merely by watching him and listening to him. If he is ambulatory and walks in to see you, additional facts can be learned. If he is hospitalized or bedfast, look at him but look around him as well. Make a mental note of the oxygen tent, mask or catheter; the drainage bottle at the bedside; the mouth gag within easy reach; the aspirator nearby; the oscillating bed or foot cradle; the cane or crutches at the head of the bed and all other clues. Look at the bedside table; medication or special equipment may be there. Even such things as flowers or "Get Well" cards may be significant.

Now look at the patient again. Does he appear fairly healthy, or does he look sick? Does he prefer to sit or lie in some specific position, presumably because it is more comfortable? Is he propped up, or can he lie flat in bed? Estimate his age and compare that with the stated age; chronic illness, or even acute disease, may make a person look much older than he really is.

Habitus

Classify the general body build or *habitus*. The asthenic person (the *ectomorph*) has "a lean and hungry look." He is usually thin, wiry and active. The bones are relatively small; the limbs are long in proportion to the trunk. The chest is thin, with an acute costal angle; the clavicles and ribs are prominent. The abdomen is flat; the buttocks are small.

The sthenic individual (the *mesomorph*) has larger bones; the face and even the entire body seem more square-cut. The neck, shoulders, abdomen, buttocks and extremities all show muscular masses.

The hypersthenic or pyknic person (the *endomorph*) has a large, soft, bulging, rounded body. The trunk is relatively long; the extremities are short and thick. The musculature may be good, but inspection alone cannot differentiate muscles from masses of fat.

The general nutritional status must be taken into consideration. A patient of any habitus may be weakened and wasted to skin and bone, but the general architecture of the framework remains unchanged. Record the nutritional status, as well as the habitus.

[1] Sir William Osler, Canadian, American and British physician, 1849–1919.

Modifications.   The body type or configuration is modified by the secondary sex characteristics. The masculine body tends to be angular and rugged. The thorax is well muscled. The arms are relatively straight. The shoulders are wider than the hips. There is usually a space between the thighs, and the calves curve inward. The lower abdomen is relatively flat, and a triangle of hair extends from the suprapubic area to the umbilicus.

The feminine characteristics are roundness and softness, with relatively more subcutaneous fat. The muscles are ill-defined. Hyperextensibility is seen at the elbows, and a more obtuse carrying angle is present. The hips are wider than the shoulders. The thighs tend to overlap in the midline and the calves curve outward. The lower abdomen is more protuberant; the upper limit of pubic hair forms a transverse line.

In certain endocrine disorders alterations of the secondary sex characteristics may be striking; the general habitus of the individual may mimic that of the opposite sex. Even in the absence of overt endocrine imbalance wide variations occur, such as the rugged he-man *vs.* the effeminate type, or the mannish woman *vs.* the ultrafeminine type.

Deficiency of male sex hormones may result from partial or complete destruction of the testes or from atrophy secondary to pituitary insufficiency. Complete loss of testicular function gives rise to *eunuchism;* partial loss produces *eunuchoidism.* When either of these occurs before puberty and is the result of a pituitary tumor, cyst or other abnormality, it gives rise to Fröhlich's[2] syndrome. The legs become abnormally long, the general body configuration may resemble that of a female, and moderate or pronounced obesity of the trunk is usually present. There is hypoplasia of the genitalia and the breasts may seem well developed (*gynecomastia*). Unfortunately this diagnosis is often applied incorrectly to any boy who shows delayed puberty due to any cause, especially if he is fat. Usually it is the caloric intake and not the pituitary gland that is responsible for this picture.

In the female, ovarian insufficiency results in short stature, infantile sex organs and lack of development of the secondary sex characteristics.

When the preliminary inspection of the patient is completed, it is customary to determine his height and weight if he is ambulatory and the vital signs—temperature, pulse rate, respiratory rate and blood pressure.

Height

Height is usually expressed in inches, but centimeters can be used. Multiply inches by 2.5 to obtain the height in centimeters; multiply centimeters by 0.4 to convert to inches.

[2] Alfred Fröhlich, Viennese physician, 1871–1953.

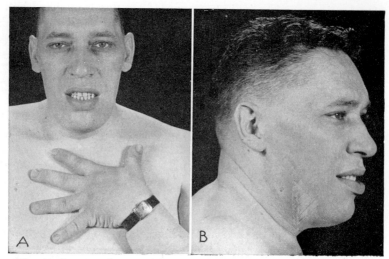

Fig. 4. Acromegaly. Note the large and elongated head, large nose, ears and lips, and the large broad hand. Prognathism and slightly increased interdental spaces are also present. (From Williams, R. H.: Textbook of Endocrinology. 3rd ed. Philadelphia, W. B. Saunders Co., 1962.)

The average range for adult males is from 60 to 74 inches; for females from 58 to 72 inches. The shaft and epiphyses in long bones usually become fused by the time a person is 20 years old; further increase in height is rare after that age.

Several factors influence the height that an individual will eventually attain. Racial variations occur; northern Europeans tend to be taller than persons from southern Europe. Climate may play a part; persons of the races inhabiting a region of moderate temperature tend to be taller than those in a very hot or very cold environment. Nutrition during childhood is important. Also, there has apparently been a gradual increase in height as the centuries pass. Richard Coeur de Lion,[3] reputedly the tallest man in England, was probably little more than 5 feet 8 inches in height; his suit of armor would be of little use to most of the present-day basketball players. Statistics also show that the average height of members of the Armed Forces of the United States during World War II was definitely greater than in World War I.

Abnormalities. Excessive height or _gigantism_ is thought to be due to the production of excessive amounts of growth hormone by the anterior lobe of the pituitary gland. If this occurs before the epiphyses and shafts of the long bones become fused, the individual becomes

[3] Richard Coeur de Lion (Richard the Lion-Hearted), 1157–99. As King Richard I of England (1189–99) he went on the Third Crusade to the Holy Land with Philip II of France, but subsequently fought against him and died of battle wounds incurred in France.

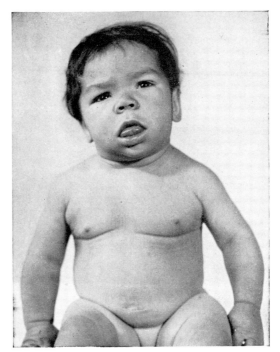

Fig. 5. Cretinism. The outstanding features are an appearance of mental dullness and a tongue so large that it protrudes from the mouth. The bridge of the nose is low, producing the naso-orbital configuration of a younger infant. (From Howorth, M. B.: A Textbook of Orthopedics. Philadelphia, W. B. Saunders Co., 1952.)

abnormally tall; sexual development may be retarded or absent. If overactivity of the pituitary occurs after epiphyseal union is completed, the extremities enlarge and acromegaly develops. The hat becomes too small; a jutting crag-like jaw develops; the nose may rival that of Cyrano de Bergerac;[4] the hands and feet can become monstrous (Fig. 4).

Lack of height (*dwarfism*) can be caused by a variety of diseases. Ateliotic dwarfs are normally proportioned but never attain normal stature; this condition is due to a deficiency of the anterior pituitary growth hormone. These are the midgets of the circus side-show.

In *achondroplasia* the epiphyseal cartilages of the long bones are at fault. The head and trunk develop normally; the arms and legs are short. The dachshund has the same defect.

If the thyroid hormone is congenitally deficient or absent, *cretinism* results. It becomes apparent within the first year that the child is not developing physically or mentally. Unless treatment is instituted the child will become a sluggish, sleepy, good-natured, mentally deficient dwarf (Figs. 5, 6).

Heart disease, either congenital or acquired, may stunt normal growth; mental retardation may accompany this (Fig. 7). Surgical cor-

---

[4] Savinien Cyrano de Bergerac; French author, 1619–55. His swaggering personality and protuberant proboscis were romanticized in 1897 by the French poet and dramatist Edmond Rostand (1868–1918).

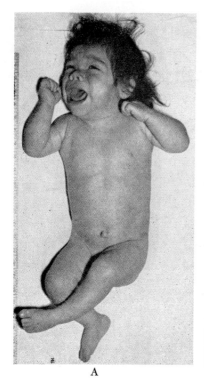
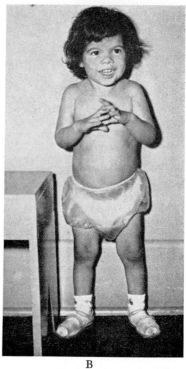

A   B

Fig. 6. *A*, Cretin, untreated; age 3 years, 10 months. *B*, The same child after 14 months of optimum treatment with thyroid. (From Williams, B. H., and Cramm, C. J.: Hypothyroidism in Early Childhood. M. Clin. North America, *39:*1135, 1955.)

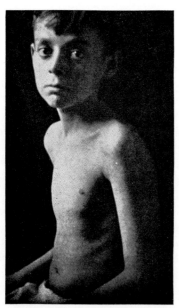

Fig. 7. Stunted growth and bulging of the precordium resulting from mitral stenosis and insufficiency in a boy of 15.

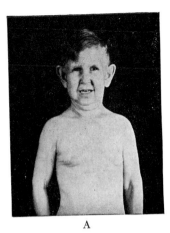 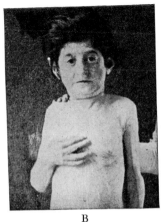

A B

Fig. 8. Progeria in a boy of 5 (*A*) and in a girl aged 8 (*B*). (From Thoma, K. H., and Robinson, H. B. G.: Oral and Dental Diagnosis. 5th ed. Philadelphia, W. B. Saunders Co., 1960.)

rection of congenital defects in infancy or early childhood may be followed by remarkable improvement in the physical and mental development. Chronic renal disease that results in abnormalities of calcium and phosphorus metabolism can cause dwarfism; this is called renal dwarfism, renal osteodystrophy or renal rickets.

Progeria is rare but unexplained. Growth is stunted, the skin is wrinkled and the facies of old age develops in childhood. Such a child usually dies before the age of puberty (Fig. 8).

Weight

The weight is usually recorded in pounds; kilograms (Kg.) are sometimes used in this country and commonly in many other countries. To convert kilograms to pounds, multiply by 2.2.

A person's weight depends largely upon the amount of bone, muscle and fatty tissue that he has; the weight of the viscera is relatively constant and unimportant. The thin, wiry, active person with small bones and muscles will weigh much less than a person of the same height who has a large, heavy skeleton and massive muscles. In either type it is usually the amount of fat that determines the individual fluctuations in weight; the bone and muscle mass remain constant in health.

Many of the tables purporting to give "average" or "ideal" weight for a given height fail to take this into consideration. Others attempt to do so, and are more accurate, but even these are based upon the *average* weight of a large number of individuals. Minor deviations from the normal or ideal weight may not be significant; a rapid change of weight, either gain or loss, may be very important. Such changes should have been recorded in the history.

Temperature

Galileo[5] is said to have invented the thermometer, and Santorio[6] described a clinical thermometer in 1625. For the next two centuries this phase of diagnosis seems to have been entirely overlooked and forgotten. Wunderlich[7] became interested in "body heat in disease" and published the results of his extensive studies in 1868; this marked the beginning of systematic temperature records in health and disease.

There are three methods used clinically to determine the body temperature—oral, rectal and axillary. The oral method is convenient and is used most frequently. Be sure that the top of the mercury column is well below the "normal" mark. Place the bulb under the side of the tongue, not merely between the lips, and leave it there for the specified time or longer; three minutes is often required for an accurate reading. This method is inaccurate if for any reason the patient must breathe through his mouth, or if he cannot or will not keep his mouth closed. Recent ingestion of hot or cold food or liquids will also alter the oral temperature. This method is unsafe with uncooperative patients and also with very young children, who may bite and break the bulb.

The rectal method is more accurate; a special thermometer with a short stout bulb is used. The reading is 0.5° to 1° F. higher than that obtained by the oral method. The axillary determination is least accurate. Place the thermometer bulb high in the axilla and hold the arm against the chest wall for several minutes. The axillary temperature is about 1° F. lower than the oral temperature.

⅄ **Normal Temperature.**   The average is 98.6° F. or 37° C. In a healthy person, the temperature may vary by a degree or more during any 24-hour period. It is usually higher in the late afternoon than in the early morning, especially on a hot summer day. Temperature readings that are persistently slightly elevated usually indicate the presence of some hidden disease, but may be physiologic. Also, some healthy persons have a temperature which is consistently below normal. Exercise, emotional excitement or an excessively warm environment may raise the temperature to 99.6° F. Prolonged exposure to cold or even sleeping with too few bedcovers in a cold room can result in a subnormal temperature. However, accurate oral temperature readings that are per-

[5] Galileo Galilei, Italian scientist, mathematician and astronomer, 1564–1642.
[6] Santorio Santorio (also called Sanctorius), whose work was done at Padua, 1561–1636.
[7] Carl Reinhold August Wunderlich, professor of medicine at Leipzig, 1815–77.

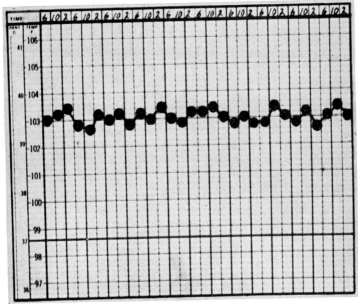

Fig. 9. Continuous fever.

sistently below 97.0° F. or above 99.8° F. should certainly be considered abnormal.

✕ **Chills.** A chill is the physiologic response to some form of tissue injury. It may be minimal—slight "chilliness" or a "creepy sensation down the back"—or it may be extremely severe. Muscular contractions produce heat; peripheral vasoconstriction and inhibition of sweating minimize heat loss; the temperature rises. The rise is roughly proportional to the severity and the duration of the chill, which rarely persists for more than 30 miserable minutes. After a hot, dry phase of variable length, sweating begins and may become profuse; the temperature then falls.

Types of Fever. The temperature record can provide valuable information. In continuous fever (Fig. 9) the temperature may fluctuate somewhat but it never reaches normal during any 24-hour period. In remittent or septic fever (Fig. 10) there are marked fluctuations each day, with no normal readings, whereas in intermittent fever (Fig. 11) the temperature does fall to normal or subnormal values between febrile periods. In relapsing fever there are recurrent episodes of fever for one or several days, alternating with periods of normal or subnormal temperature, as in Pel-Ebstein[8] fever seen in Hodgkin's[9] disease. ⅄

[8] Pieter Klaases Pel, Dutch physician, 1852–1919; Wilhelm Ebstein, German physician, 1836–1912.
[9] Thomas Hodgkin, English physician and Curator of the Museum at Guy's Hospital, London, 1798–1866. His dissertation, prepared in 1832, was ignored for over 30 years.

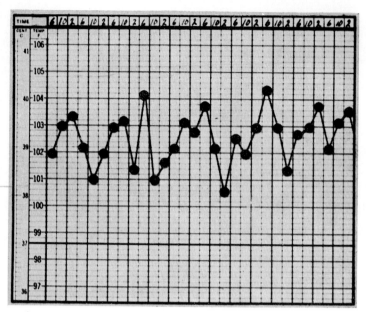

Fig. 10.   Remittent or septic fever.

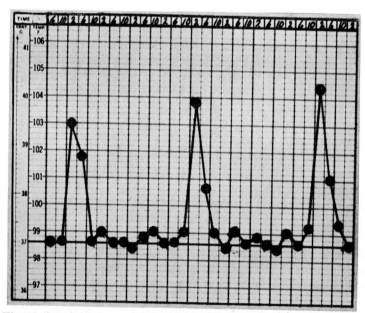

Fig. 11.   Intermittent fever. The patient had benign tertian malaria, with chill and fever at 48-hour intervals.

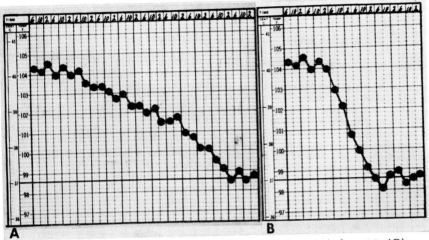

Fig. 12. Elevated temperature returns to normal by lysis (*A*); by crisis (*B*).

When an elevated temperature returns to normal it does so either by *lysis*, with a gradual subsidence over a period of several days, or by *crisis*, a precipitous fall usually accompanied by profuse sweating (Fig. 12).

Pulse

The rate, rhythm and character of the pulse should be determined; this can be done while the temperature is being taken. Any artery can be used if necessary, but customarily the radial artery at the wrist is chosen. Have the patient's arm at rest in a comfortable position; use the tips of your fingers to compress the artery against the bone. Count the pulse for one full minute. If any irregularity is noted, it may be helpful to count the rate during each of four consecutive 15-second periods.

Rate. In adults at rest the normal rate ranges from 60 to 80 beats per minute. In young athletic persons a rate as low as 50 is not unusual. In infants and young children it is higher; 90 to 120 beats per minute is often found and a rate of 130 to 140 may not be abnormal.

TACHYCARDIA. This denotes an abnormally rapid rate. Psychic factors that may not be apparent can increase the rate; even the emotional stress of the medical interview and examination can do this. If the rate is above normal initially, recheck it later or at the end of the examination. Persistent tachycardia is found in certain types or stages of heart disease, or with severe anemia, hyperthyroidism, shock or massive bleeding, either external or internal. In most febrile illnesses the pulse rate rises 5 to 10 beats per minute for each degree (F.) of fever.

BRADYCARDIA.   An abnormally slow rate may occur in persons with heart block, obstructive jaundice or increased intracranial pressure. It is also common during the convalescent stage of many febrile illnesses and when a person faints (*syncope*). Occasionally it is physiologic, as in a well-trained athlete while he is at rest. With certain infections, especially typhoid and influenza, the pulse rate increases much less than one would anticipate from the amount of fever present; this is called *relative bradycardia*.

Rhythm.   In healthy adults the rhythm of the heart and of the pulse is regular (normal sinus rhythm); any irregularity constitutes an *arrhythmia*. Certain cardiac disturbances can be suspected or diagnosed by palpation of the pulse; these will be discussed under the cardiovascular system.

Character.   The character of the pulse is dependent upon the magnitude of the pulse pressure and the rate at which this changes. The pulse may be feeble and barely perceptible; it may be of average intensity; it may be full, forceful and bounding. Here again experience is an important factor in evaluating the significance of the palpable pulsations.

Abnormalities of the Pulse.   Certain abnormalities may be obvious. *Pulsus parvus* (*et tardus*) denotes a pulse wave of small amplitude that seems to rise and fall slowly. It is due to obstruction of the outflow tract, usually narrowing (*stenosis*) of the aortic valve or ring. A *dicrotic pulse* has a small secondary wave immediately following the regular pulse wave. It can often be felt during the course of a febrile illness, especially if the diastolic pressure is low. *Pulsus alternans* has regular alternations; a strong wave is followed by a weak one but this may not be obvious until the blood pressure is taken. As the pressure in the cuff is lowered the stronger beats will be heard; with further lowering of the pressure the weaker beats appear and the rate suddenly doubles. Paradoxical pulse (*pulsus paradoxus*) is one in which the force of the pulse wave decreases or the pulse actually seems to disappear during quiet inspiration; it reappears promptly with expiration. This can be confirmed by inflating the blood pressure cuff to a point 5 to 10 mm. lower than the maximum systolic pressure and noting the disappearance of sounds coincident with inspiration. It is very suggestive of pericardial effusion or constrictive pericarditis, but it may also be found with hyperventilation associated with such conditions as severe pulmonary emphysema, asthma, pneumothorax or massive pleural effusion. Similar variations can be produced in a normal person by rapid forceful respiration, or by compression of the subclavian artery trapped between the clavicle and the first rib.

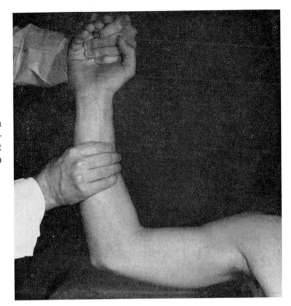

Fig. 13. Eliciting a water-hammer pulse. Elevate the arm with your left hand; compress the forearm with your right hand.

Water-hammer[10] pulse (Corrigan's[11] pulse; collapsing pulse) is a short, sharp, forceful impulse—"a jerky pulse with full expansion, followed by a sudden collapse." It is more easily elicited by holding the patient's hand, raising the arm well above the level of the heart, and slowly compressing the muscular tissue of the forearm with your other hand (Fig. 13). A *diffuse* throbbing will be felt, as all of the arteries and arterioles are suddenly distended, then collapse. This can also be elicited in the legs. Although this type of pulse was originally attributed to reflux of blood into the ventricle through an incompetent aortic valve, this does not seem to be the entire explanation. A similar pulse can often be felt in patients with normal heart valves who have other diseases such as hyperthyroidism, severe anemia, patent ductus arteriosus or other arteriovenous communications, or even during the course of a febrile illness. It is probable that a decrease or loss of arteriolar tone, which is a common factor in all of these conditions, permits the pulse wave to progress almost without resistance to the smaller arteries and arterioles and thus produce the sharp impulse that is so easily felt.

[10] The water-hammer is an apparatus devised in 1805 to illustrate certain physical principles. It consists of a piece of thick-walled glass tube about half-filled with water. The water is heated until it boils; steam displaces the air and the tube is then sealed. When inverted quickly the water falls through the vacuum and produces a short, sharp thud.

[11] Sir Dominic John Corrigan, Dublin physician, 1802–80. As often happens, he was not the first to describe this phenomenon, but as a result of his superb paper, his name seems inseparably associated with this sign. He also described a form of chronic fibroid tuberculosis, which was known as Corrigan's lung.

Arterial Wall. The characteristics of the arterial wall should also be determined. To do so, occlude the artery by firm pressure and palpate the vessel distal to that point. A normal radial artery is soft and pliable. With arteriosclerosis, compression requires more force and the vessel tends to roll under the finger tips; often it is irregular and beaded. Elongation also occurs and the tortuous arteries writhe rhythmically under the skin; this can sometimes be seen more easily in the brachial artery if the forearm is partially flexed ("brachial dance") or in the temporal arteries.

Having determined these characteristics in one radial artery, repeat the process in the other arm. Lesions proximal to the radial artery can cause retardation, weakness or obliteration of the pulse in one wrist or the other. Anomalies are not rare; the radial artery may be abnormally situated, very small or totally absent. In such instances the ulnar artery should be sought and examined.

Respiration

It is advisable to observe respiration and to count the rate while apparently interested in something else such as the pulse. In a nervous person there may be changes if he realizes that he is being watched. The character or type, the rate and the rhythm are all important.

Normal respiration is a composite of two different actions: expansion of the thoracic cage and descent of the diaphragm. In women, the thoracic element predominates; in men, descent of the diaphragm is the major component. Alteration of the normal thoracic:abdominal ratio in either sex may be significant.

Rate. The normal rate for an adult at rest is from 14 to 20 per minute. With fever this increases about 4 cycles per minute for each degree (F.) of temperature elevation.

Abnormal Rate. *Tachypnea* denotes excessively rapid respiration. This may be physiologic after exercise or with emotional stress; otherwise it suggests the presence of fever or of disease of the heart or lungs. *Bradypnea* is an unusually slow rate. Occasionally it is physiologic; more commonly it is associated with uremia, diabetic acidosis, increased intracranial pressure or an overdose of an opiate or other drug that depresses the respiratory center. *Apnea* is total cessation of breathing; if prolonged, the prognosis is grave. *Hyperpnea* indicates increased depth and usually an increased rate, resulting in hyperventilation.

Dyspnea. This actually means difficult or labored breathing; more commonly it is used to indicate the patient's awareness of the act of breathing, or of his need to breathe. He says that he is "short of breath" or "shortwinded." Dyspnea is a relative term; sufficiently vigorous exercise will produce it in a healthy person, but this quickly disappears with rest. When dyspnea follows moderate exertion it is significant; when it occurs with the person at rest it is serious. Dyspnea may be inspiratory, expiratory or both. Inspiratory dyspnea occurs with partial obstruction of the air passages, usually the larger ones such as the larynx, trachea or large bronchi. It also occurs with circulatory failure. Expiratory dyspnea is more commonly due to obstruction of egress of air by narrowing of the lumina of the smaller bronchi and bronchioles; infection, edema, spasm or tenacious secretions can produce this. Loss of normal lung elasticity is also a frequent cause. The inspiratory phase may be relatively normal or even very short, but expiration is prolonged.

Paroxysmal dyspnea occurs with asthmatic attacks, or with paroxysmal pulmonary edema due to sudden left-sided heart failure; the latter often develops during sleep and wakens the patient (paroxysmal nocturnal dyspnea).

Orthopnea means that the patient is dyspneic, or more dyspneic, when recumbent. In a normal adult the vital capacity decreases by 5 to 10 per cent when he lies down; with congestive heart failure the loss may be as high as 30 per cent. With serious heart or lung disease, even a slight decrease may mean the difference between comfort and dyspnea.

Trepopnea indicates that the patient may breathe comfortably while in one position but becomes dyspneic in some other position. He may be able to lie on his back, for example, but not on his right side.

Abnormal Rhythm. Shallow or jerky breathing is observed when pain causes voluntary diminution of the normal depth or rhythm of respiration. Deep sighing breaths interspersed with normal or shallow respiration are usually functional and suggest emotional stress. The patient complains bitterly of her inability to get her breath, and narrates a steady stream of other complaints with only an occasional pause for a deep breath. "See? That's what I mean; I can't get my breath."

Kussmaul[12] described "great loud breathing" in severe diabetic acidosis; deep, sighing respirations are present, usually inconstant in rate. He attributed this to air hunger ("Lufthunger"); that term is more commonly used now to indicate the hyperventilation seen with severe anemia from hemorrhage or other causes.

In *periodic* breathing, apnea of variable duration alternates with breathing; the commonest form is Cheyne-Stokes[13] respiration (Fig. 14). After a period of apnea that lasts from 5 to 40 seconds, respirations begin and gradually increase in depth until the patient appears to be breathing maximally; the rate remains fairly constant. After the peak

[12] Adolf Kussmaul, German physician, 1822–1902.
[13] John Cheyne, Dublin physician, 1777–1836; William Stokes, Regius Professor of Medicine at Dublin, 1804–78. Cheyne's paper appeared in 1818; Stokes amplified the description in 1846.

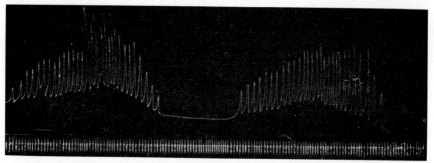

Fig. 14. Cheyne-Stokes respiration in an adult. The upper line shows thoracic movement; the lower line marks the time in seconds. The respiration is rapid, increases in depth, then decreases and finally stops. In this tracing, the apneic period lasts for about 25 seconds.

has been reached there is a gradual decrease in depth until the apneic stage is again reached. This may be physiologic in an infant or in an elderly person with severe arteriosclerosis; in most instances it is of serious import.

A less common abnormality of respiration is *meningitic* or Biot's[14] breathing. There is complete arrhythmia, both in time and in depth; breathing is jerky and irregular. It is an indication of a severe insult to the respiratory mechanism, often calling for mechanical assistance by means of a respirator of some sort.

Other Abnormalities. *Stridulous* breathing has harsh, high-pitched whistling or crowing sounds accompanying inspiration. These are produced by partial obstruction of the larynx; the "whoop" of whooping cough is an example. *Stertorous* breathing is due to vibrations of the soft palate as in snoring, or of secretions in the upper air passages; the latter produce the so-called "death rattle."

Blood Pressure

To determine the blood pressure, either an aneroid or a mercury manometer may be used. The former is more compact but less rugged; it should be tested at least once a year for accuracy. In a mercury manometer, the tube may break or some of the mercury may be lost, leading to false readings.

Procedure. The patient may be seated or lying, but the arm and the forearm must both be bared. The arm should be relaxed, with the forearm slightly flexed and resting on a flat surface if the patient is recumbent. If the patient is seated the forearm can be supported but it

[14] Described in 1878 by Camille Biot, French physician, as a modification of Cheyne-Stokes respiration.

may be more convenient to let it hang at the side. This may change the blood pressure slightly; ordinarily this is of no significance.

Deflate the blood pressure cuff completely; then wrap it snugly around the arm with the lower edge 2 to 3 cm. above the antecubital fossa. Locate the brachial artery by inspection or palpation. In a very obese person the best landmark is the biceps tendon, which can be felt if the patient tenses the muscle; the artery lies just mesial to this. Place the bell of your stethoscope over the artery; it should not touch the bag or the tubes. Close the valve and inflate the bag until all sounds in the artery disappear. Then open the valve and release the pressure slowly. Determine the point at which sounds first appear; this is the *systolic* pressure. Continue the slow deflation to obtain the *diastolic* pressure.

The American Heart Association has recommended that the point at which sounds disappear *completely* be recorded as the diastolic pressure. Others advocate taking the point at which the sounds suddenly become dull and muffled; this averages 5 to 10 mm. higher. It is more easily determined in a noisy area, and is less dependent upon the auditory acuity of the examiner. Moreover, in some conditions sounds can still be heard with the cuff completely deflated or removed. A compromise is to record all three values.

By custom, the blood pressure (B.P.) is expressed in millimeters of mercury and is recorded as a fraction, with the systolic pressure over the diastolic pressure—140/80, for example, or 140/80/75 if both "diastolic" pressures are recorded.

At the initial examination the blood pressure in each arm should be determined and recorded. Normally these values may differ by a few millimeters; with vascular or perivascular disease that interferes with blood flow to one arm the inequality in pressure may be considerable. Since the blood pressure varies somewhat with change of posture, the record should indicate whether the person was standing, sitting or lying down.

X **Auscultatory Gap.** In certain hypertensive patients a phenomenon known as the auscultatory gap sometimes occurs. For example, sounds may first be heard in the brachial artery when the pressure in the cuff has fallen to 200 mm. These will persist until the pressure drops to 180 mm.; then all sounds disappear, only to reappear at 160 mm. and persist until the diastolic point is reached. The gap in this case would be the pressure between 180 mm. and 160 mm. (Fig. 15).

To avoid this error, you can use either of two procedures with such patients. Inflate the cuff until the radial pulse has been completely obliterated; then slowly decrease the pressure until the pulse reappears. This serves as a rough guide to the systolic pressure. A better method is to inflate the bag rapidly until the pressure is 250 mm. or more; then release the pressure fairly rapidly and listen for the approximate points at which sounds first appear and then totally disappear. Wait several

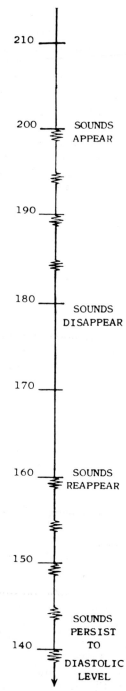

Fig. 15. Auscultatory gap. No sounds heard between 180 mm. and 160 mm.

seconds, and then reinflate the cuff until the pressure is 10 to 20 mm. above the point at which the sounds first appeared. Deflate the bag slowly (2 or 3 mm. at a time) until sounds are heard; this is the systolic pressure reading. Then allow the pressure to drop more rapidly until it approaches the point at which sounds disappeared and agai.. resume slow deflation to obtain the diastolic reading. After a little prac tice, you will find this second method simple and accurate.

Variations in Systolic Pressure. Changes that occur with pulsus alternans and with pulsus paradoxus have been mentioned (p. 48). Certain arrhythmias that will be discussed in Chapter XIV also produce definite changes. With premature ventricular contractions the ventricle becomes adequately filled or overfilled during the compensatory pause; the next normal beat will result in a systolic pressure higher than that of the other normal beats. With atrial fibrillation and a rapid ventricular rate the filling is variable from beat to beat and consequently the systolic pressure fluctuates; this is almost diagnostic. To demonstrate this, apply the cuff in the usual manner and lower the pressure slowly. At some point—140 mm. for example—an occasional beat will be heard. Lower the pressure 5 mm.; more sounds will appear. Each time the pressure is dropped more beats become audible; eventually all of them seem to come through. With fibrillation, it is customary to consider the point at which sounds are first heard as the systolic pressure.

The Legs. Blood pressure in the legs need not be determined routinely, but the pulses in each leg should be palpated sometime during the examination. If there is weakness, absence or abnormality of these, or any suggestion of disease of the aorta or of one of the large arteries in the leg, the blood pressure in the lower extremities must be measured. This can be done by applying the cuff around the lower third of the thigh and placing the bell of the stethoscope over the popliteal artery. Using the standard cuff, which is 12 cm. wide, the systolic pressure in the thigh may be 20 to 30 cm. higher than in the arm; the diastolic pressure shows less elevation. With a wide cuff (18 cm.) there is less discrepancy, and direct (intra-arterial) measurements show little difference in a normal person. If the pressure in the thigh is lower than in the arm, some degree of arterial occlusion probably exists.

Normal Blood Pressure. For adults under 40, most life insurance companies consider as normal a systolic pressure between 110 and 150 mm., with the diastolic pressure ranging from 60 to 90 mm. With advancing age these values tend to rise somewhat. In a study of 15,000 unselected persons ranging in age from 16 to 65 years it was found that after the age of 45, elevated readings were encountered more frequently than some of the so-called normal readings. In a person in the older age group, a systolic pressure of 180 or even 190 mm. and a diastolic pressure of 100 mm. or more must not automatically be considered abnormal.

The pressure obtained at the start of the examination may be unexpectedly high; the patient is often nervous and tense, especially if he has any symptoms that he attributes to "heart trouble." Emotional strain, physical exertion, fatigue and other factors have a definite influence on blood pressure. The history, the findings on physical examination, fluoroscopy, electrocardiography and other special procedures must all be evaluated before one can conclude that the person has significant hypertension just because one or even several determinations gave figures higher than the accepted normal for his age.

× **High Blood Pressure (Arterial Hypertension).**   This implies readings that are consistently above the normal range even when the person is at rest. It is not diagnostic of any one disease. It can be present with renal disease of various types, during pregnancy, with increased intracranial pressure, with disturbances of endocrine glands, with arterial or vascular changes and with other systemic diseases. When no specific cause can be found, the term *essential hypertension* is often used.

In a very obese arm there may seem to be an elevated systolic pressure; usually the diastolic reading is less affected. In such porcine subjects it may be desirable to check the reading by placing the cuff around the forearm and auscultating or palpating the radial artery; the systolic pressure may be found to be definitely lower than the reading obtained in the arm. In elderly persons with tortuous sclerotic pipestem arteries, the elastic tissue no longer cushions its share of the systolic thrust. In such persons the systolic pressure may be well over 200 mm., while the diastolic pressure remains in the normal range. An apparent elevation of the systolic pressure will also be found if the cuff is wrapped too loosely around the arm; the full width is not available to compress the artery as the cuff balloons out.

To the patient, "high blood pressure" has an ominous sound. It is unwise to tell him the actual figures until the diagnostic survey is completed; even then it may be preferable to say that the pressure is "up somewhat" or "a little higher than I had expected."

Low Blood Pressure (Vascular Hypotension).   To the laity, "low blood pressure" is a known cause of fatigue, lassitude, weakness and a host of other vague symptoms. These may occur, but many an adult is perfectly comfortable and happy with a systolic pressure of 90 or 100 mm., and a diastolic pressure of 50 to 60 mm., if he doesn't know this. Clinically significant hypotension is found with a wide variety of conditions such as hemorrhage, adrenocortical failure (Addison's[15] disease), severe myocardial damage, chronic wasting diseases or extensive malignant lesions, or with abnormalities of the autonomic nervous system, either spontaneous, surgically induced or due to drugs.

[15] Thomas Addison, English physician, 1793–1860. He described pernicious anemia (Addisonian anemia) and adrenocortical failure in the same paper in 1849; in 1855 he published a monograph on the latter, which was largely ignored.

⅄ **Pulse Pressure.**   This is the difference between the systolic pressure and the diastolic pressure; normally this value is about one-half the diastolic figure. Increased pulse pressure may be due to elevation of the systolic pressure, lowering of the diastolic pressure or a combination of these. It is seen physiologically as a result of exercise or excitement. Pathologically it is found with such conditions as sclerosis of the large arteries, hyperthyroidism, fever, aortic regurgitation or a patent ductus arteriosus. Decreased pulse pressure is almost invariably due to a relatively low systolic pressure. It occurs with acute vascular hypotension (collapse), or with cardiac abnormalities such as mitral or aortic stenosis, pericardial effusion or constrictive pericarditis.

Venous Blood Pressure

Accurate measurement of the venous blood pressure requires special equipment. A needle is inserted into a vein; a manometer registers the pressure. With the needle at the same horizontal level as the atrium, the venous pressure is normally between 4 and 8 cm. *of water* (40 to 80 mm.); values above 10 cm. are abnormal.

Estimation of the venous blood pressure is less accurate but is relatively simple. Normally, with the person sitting upright and breathing quietly, the column of blood in the jugular vein should not be visible above the clavicle. If it can be seen, measure the vertical distance from the mouth of the superior vena cava (third right costochondral articulation) to the meniscus of the blood column in the vein. If the pressure is very high the visible portion of the vein may be completely filled from the clavicle to the angle of the jaw; this method then becomes useless. With a bedfast patient, Wood[16] has pointed out that the venous pressure can be checked by "slowly raising and then lowering the head of the bed and noting the location of the meniscus." The angle at which the vein is completely filled can be estimated, or the vertical distance can be measured. A third method is to observe the veins on the back of the patient's hand as it hangs at his side. Then elevate the hand slowly; the veins should empty when the hand reaches the level of the gladiomanubrial articulation.

Increased venous pressure with distended neck veins is usually due to heart failure, pericardial effusion or constrictive pericarditis, if obstruction of the superior vena cava or of the jugular veins has been ruled out. With circulatory failure the pressure in the jugular veins can be considered a reliable index of venous pressure throughout the body. When venous pressure appears to be elevated, actual measurement is always desirable.

[16] Francis C. Wood, Philadelphia physician, 1901–.

IV

The Skin

Examination of the skin of the entire body is an essential part of any complete physical examination. Unless the patient's complaint is primarily a dermatologic one it is customary to do this as each part is examined, rather than as an isolated procedure. However, the findings are usually recorded under a single heading in the write-up.

Inspection is the most important procedure; palpation is employed to confirm and amplify the findings. Whenever possible, use natural illumination, and guard against reflected colors from walls or drapes.

INSPECTION OF THE SKIN

The first thing that one notices is the color of the skin. This depends largely upon three factors: pigment normally present in the skin itself; abnormal pigments in the skin; color due to blood in the vessels of the skin.

NORMAL SKIN PIGMENTS

There are marked variations in pigmentation that may be normal, or minor ones that may be significantly abnormal. In Caucasians, the degree of pigmentation ranges from the extreme blond so common among the Nordic peoples to the swarthy complexion of those whose origin is in the Mediterranean littoral. The same variations are seen in other groups such as Negroes or Orientals.

Increased Pigmentation. Increased pigmentation over the entire body is very uncommon. It is seen occasionally in hemochromatosis or in chronic adrenocortical insufficiency (Addison's disease). When present over *most* of the skin it is usually the result of prolonged exposure to

58

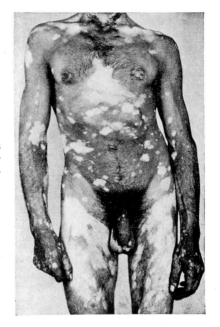

Fig. 16. Widespread vitiligo in a Negro. (From Andrews, G. C., and Domonkos, A. N.: Diseases of the Skin. 5th ed. Philadelphia, W. B. Saunders Co., 1963.)

ultraviolet light, either natural or from a sun lamp, or to roentgen irradiation.

Localized areas of increased pigmentation may result from a variety of causes. Chronic irritation such as heat, scratching or pressure is frequently the cause; impaired venous circulation due to varicose veins or phlebitis is another. In Addison's disease there may be considerable darkening of the skin at sites of irritation. Pregnancy is often accompanied by patchy hyperpigmentation of the skin of the cheeks, forehead and arms (*chloasma gravidarum*); this usually fades after delivery. Similar changes occur with ovarian disorders or during the menopause.

Decreased Pigmentation. This may be generalized or localized. The *albino* lacks melanophores; the skin itself is universally white, but a light pink tinge is seen due to the presence of blood in the vessels of the skin. If only certain areas are involved, the term *leukoderma* is used; this is a congenital abnormality. Sometimes such areas develop later in life, from loss of melanophores; *vitiligo* appears (Fig. 16). This is most conspicuous in deeply pigmented persons but it can also occur in blonds. Such white or pink areas are usually surrounded by a narrow zone of deeper pigmentation.

ABNORMAL SKIN PIGMENTATION

Yellow Skin. Yellowness of the skin (*jaundice; icterus*) is due to the presence in the blood of an abnormally high concentration of bilirubin; this then escapes into the tissues. It produces a color that may range from orange-yellow to yellow or even greenish yellow. Slight degrees may be difficult to detect in dark-skinned persons; look for abnormal color in the conjunctivae and in the oral mucosa. Use daylight or the "daylight type" of artificial illumination; the yellow light from the common incandescent bulb or most fluorescent tubes masks minor degrees of jaundice.

In pernicious anemia the skin may show a lemon-yellow hue which can usually be differentiated from jaundice by the presence of generalized pallor due to the anemia. An excessive intake of carotene (carrots; tomatoes) can result in an orange-yellow color much like that seen in jaundice. Certain drugs may also cause some yellowish discoloration of the skin if taken for long periods of time.

Other Abnormal Pigments. On rare occasions an elderly person with *argyria* may be seen. The skin has a grayish-blue color due to deposition of particles of silver; this may follow prolonged ingestion of silver salts for the treatment of peptic ulcer. Localized argyria has followed excessive use of silver-containing nose drops or eye drops. Bismuth, formerly used to treat syphilis, may produce a similar discoloration. Gold salts used in rheumatoid arthritis may cause a slate-gray or brown pigmentation (*chrysiasis*). The discoloration due to these metallic pigments is most apparent in regions exposed to the sun or other sources of ultraviolet light.

Buried bits of dirt, sand, cinders or other foreign material can be present in scars of abrasions or deeper injuries; they are not always the mark of a former track star. Localized deposits of carbon may persist in scars of injuries incurred by coal miners; these are usually seen on exposed areas such as the face, neck, hands and forearms.

THE VASCULAR COMPONENT

Erythema. When undue redness (*erythema*) is present, try to determine whether it represents a temporary change or something more permanent, and whether it is localized or generalized. Exertion, emotional stress, exposure to heat or cold or the use of certain drugs will produce transient reddening; this is due to dilatation of the superficial vessels and fades when the causative factor is eliminated. Fever is also accompanied by generalized flushing of the skin.

A localized area of redness may be due to radiant energy of any type such as a heat, sunlight or roentgen irradiation; the location or distribution of such areas will usually suggest the causative factor.

An excessive concentration of erythrocytes will also produce redness of the skin. This may be a relative increase as in dehydration, or an actual increase (*polycythemia*). Reduced hemoglobin may also be present in such conditions, adding a certain amount of blueness (*cyanosis*).

Pallor.   Decreased redness is seen in anemia, but it can also be present in those who spend little time out-of-doors and in otherwise healthy elderly persons. In shock there is peripheral circulatory collapse; the patient is usually very pale.

Localized pallor, especially of the face, accompanies emotional states such as fear or anger; these cause temporary vascular spasm. Partial or complete occlusion of an artery can also cause pallor; this is usually seen in an extremity.

 Ⅹ **Cyanosis.**   This is due to reduced hemoglobin in the vessels of the skin or mucous membranes. It does not appear clinically unless there are at least 5 Gm. of reduced hemoglobin per 100 ml. of blood; therefore it is not seen in the severely anemic person. An excessive concentration of erythrocytes (polycythemia or hemoconcentration) can also produce cyanosis; the lungs are unable to oxygenate all of the hemoglobin present. In susceptible individuals cyanosis may follow the ingestion of certain drugs such as acetanilid or some of the sulfonamides.

Cyanosis may be temporary when due to drugs or when chilling causes venous stasis, for example. Persistent cyanosis is more ominous; circulatory failure is the most common cause. Pulmonary disease that results in inadequate aeration of the blood must also be considered; these two conditions may co-exist. A venous-arterial shunt may permit unoxygenated blood to reach the systemic circulation; this shunt may be in the lungs or in the heart (congenital heart disease).

If cyanosis is present the degree of unsaturation can merely be estimated at the bedside; chemical analysis is necessary to determine this accurately.

VASCULAR LESIONS

Certain vascular lesions may be present in the skin. A *spider angioma* (spider nevus; vascular spider) has a central punctate red dot with very small vessels radiating outward for a centimeter or more. Pressure over the central spot results in blanching of the vessels (Fig. 17). These are most commonly seen over the thorax; less frequently they can be found on the head or neck. They seem to be associated with alterations in estrogen metabolism. With cirrhosis or other types of liver disease they may be permanent, but when they develop during preg-

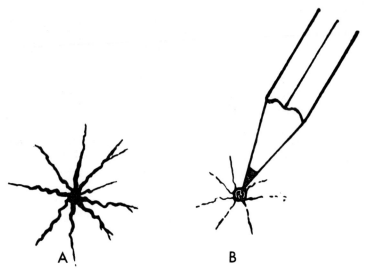

Fig. 17. *A,* Vascular spider. *B,* When pressure is applied at the center, the blood supply is decreased and the radiating vessels become smaller or disappear.

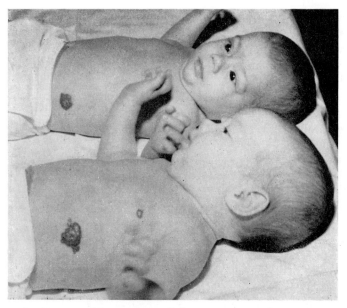

Fig. 18. Hemangiomas in identical twins, age 15 weeks. (Courtesy of E. P. Pendergrass, M.D.)

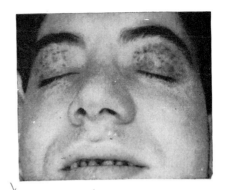

Fig. 19. Pinpoint petechiae on the eyelids in thrombocytopenic purpura. (From Thoma, K. H., and Robinson, H. B. G.: Oral and Dental Diagnosis. 5th ed. Philadelphia, W. B. Saunders Co., 1960.)

nancy they usually fade after delivery. *Capillary hemangiomas* are sometimes present on the side of the face or neck; occasionally they occur elsewhere. Because of their color they are often known as *port wine birthmarks.* Another vascular anomaly is the slightly elevated *hemangioma simplex,* the "strawberry" or "raspberry" birthmark (Fig. 18).

Hemorrhage.   Bleeding into the skin itself may be due to rupture of capillaries, venules or arterioles; the weakest point seems to be the capillary-venule junction. Very small hemorrhages are called *petechiae;* these are only a millimeter or two in diameter. For centuries they were recognized as one of the classical features of what we now call scurvy; the British Navy, accepting the recommendations of Lind,[1] reported that this disease could be prevented if the sailors were given fresh fruits and vegetables, especially citrus fruits. The lack of vitamin C (ascorbic acid) can cause petechiae to appear; so can other vascular disorders, certain blood dyscrasias and some systemic diseases such as subacute bacterial endocarditis (Fig. 19).

More extensive bleeding into the skin (*purpura; ecchymoses*) can result from a variety of diseases but most commonly it is due to trauma. As the blood is reabsorbed the hemoglobin undergoes changes that give rise to the various colors seen; bright red soon becomes blue or purple, then back through the rainbow to a yellow or orange hue, with fading in intensity until the area returns to normal. Blood under the skin will be less conspicuous but there can be similar color changes. Often the actual site of bleeding in such cases is not at the point of discoloration; gravity and fascial planes determine the point at which the pigment becomes visible.

[1] James Lind, a native of Scotland who served as surgeon in the British Royal Navy, 1716–94. He was not the first to record this observation (1754), but this was the first extensive clinical study of scurvy.

PALPATION OF THE SKIN

Having noted the color of the skin and the presence of abnormalities, palpate the skin next—but be sure that your hands are warm.

Temperature and Moisture.   Determine first the relative temperature and moisture. A hot dry skin is found with sustained or rising fever. A hot wet skin usually indicates a falling temperature. A moderately moist skin that is slightly warmer than normal may indicate hyperthyroidism. Localized areas of warmth suggest an inflammatory process such as cellulitis or acute arthritis, for example. A cold dry skin is usually the result of chilling; it may also be present in hypothyroidism. In shock, the skin is cold and wet or "clammy." Cold moist hands and feet are usually due to emotional stress. A cold dry extremity may mean partial or complete occlusion of the arterial blood supply to that area.

Texture and Elasticity.   The next point to be determined is the texture of the skin and its elasticity. It may be smooth or rough, thickened as with edema or in hypothyroidism, or thinned by malnutrition or senility. Loss of elasticity is physiologic in the aged; temporary loss may be present with emaciation or with dehydration.

X **Edema.**   This denotes abnormal accumulation of fluid in the tissues, especially in the intercellular spaces. Most commonly it is demonstrable in the skin and subcutaneous tissues and can be recognized on inspection and palpation. The edematous area loses its normal contours and the landmarks disappear. The skin becomes smooth; normal creases and folds are wiped out. With more extensive edema the skin becomes stretched and glistening; occasionally it actually develops tiny cracks from which fluid oozes.

To confirm the presence of edema and to estimate the amount, make moderately firm pressure preferably over a bony area such as the tibia. Maintain the pressure to allow time for the fluid to be displaced; then lift the fingers. If a depression remains, *pitting edema* is present. This can be classified as slight, moderate or marked, or graded from 1+ to 4+.

Edema develops when fluid escapes through the capillaries more rapidly than it can be resorbed. This can be due to alterations in capillary permeability such as those that occur in anoxic states or in allergic diseases. It can result from altered osmotic pressure relations, as in the hypoproteinemia that occurs with chronic liver disease, with renal disease, in starvation or from other causes. It is most commonly found with circulatory changes, localized or generalized; increased pressure or obstruction of the veins and lymphatics interferes with proper reabsorption of the fluid.

X **Myxedema.**   On inspection, myxedema ("mucus edema") due to a deficiency of thyroid hormone may be confused with edema. Palpation should dispel any doubt; the skin itself is coarse, dry and inelastic. Both the skin and the subcutaneous tissues are swollen and thickened by viscid mucoid material that is not readily displaced; there is little or no pitting on pressure.

BASIC DERMATOLOGIC LESIONS

No attempt will be made to describe and differentiate various skin diseases, but you should have some familiarity with the nomenclature used to describe and classify the basic dermatologic processes.

Macule. This is an area of discoloration without palpable swelling that is not more than a few millimeters in diameter.

Papule. This is a similar area with swelling of the tissues.

Vesicle. This is an elevated lesion that contains a collection of serous fluid, like a small blister.

Pustule. This is a vesicle that contains pus instead of serum.

Bulla. This is a large vesicle or pustule.

Wheal. This is an elevated area of any size produced by edema of the corium. A wheal is often the result of an allergic reaction in the skin; it is usually transitory. *Dermographia* is an induced form of whealing that is seen with vasomotor instability. If the skin is stroked lightly a red line appears; in a few minutes this is replaced by a white wheal.

Nodule. This is a small solid mass in the skin that may project downward, upward or both. Palpation is usually necessary to determine its size, extent and consistency.

Tumor. This is a nodule of larger size, usually 2 cm. or more in diameter.

Secondary Changes. All of these primary lesions may be modified by secondary changes, which include:

Scales. These are flakes of dead skin, small or large; they may brush off easily or be firmly adherent.

Crusts. These are composed of epithelial debris or dead tissue plus dried serum, blood or pus.

Excoriation. This is the result of vigorous scraping or scratching of either the intact skin or a lesion of any type.

Fissure. This starts as a crack in the superficial layer of the skin and may extend to the underlying tissues.

Ulceration. This denotes actual loss of skin tissue; it may be superficial or deep.

Scarring. Replacement of lost tissue by fibrous or connective tissue produces a scar.

Pigmentation. Often this is a late result of irritation; it indicates that the lesion has been present for a long time.

V

The Head

When the preliminary survey of the patient has been completed a careful, detailed examination is begun, starting with the head. The size, shape and symmetry of the bones should be noted. A crooked nose, a lopsided jaw or unusual bumps or depressions can be the result of injuries, or they may be due to other causes such as congenital defects, metabolic disorders, neurologic disease or neoplasm.

THE SKULL

Inspection. SIZE AND SHAPE. The *microcephalic* skull is abnormally small. The forehead is usually narrow and sloping, the vertex is pointed and the occiput is flattened. This smallness is accentuated by contrast with the face, which is normally developed. A congenital defect in the development of the brain is present; severe mental retardation is the rule with microcephalus.

The *macrocephalic* skull is abnormally large; several diseases may produce this. In infants and young children the most common cause is hydrocephalus (Fig. 20). This is due to an obstruction at some point along the cerebrospinal fluid channels, with accumulation of fluid under greatly increased pressure. If the fluid is largely in the subarachnoid space, external hydrocephalus results. More commonly there is increased pressure in the ventricles, producing internal hydrocephalus. A congenital anatomic abnormality is usually responsible for internal hydrocephalus.

The *hydrocephalic* skull is globular. The sutures and fontanels are widely open and bulge. The face is unaffected but appears small by comparison. The brain fails to develop normally, or pressure atrophy occurs; mental retardation or idiocy is present.

Acromegaly. This is due to oversecretion of growth hormone by

66

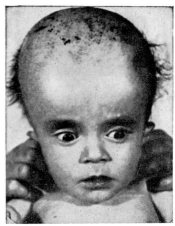

Fig. 20. Hydrocephalus in a boy aged 1 year. (From Thoma, K. H., and Robinson, H. B. G.: Oral and Dental Diagnosis. 5th ed. Philadelphia, W. B. Saunders Co., 1960.)

the anterior portion of the pituitary gland. The entire head enlarges; so do the hands and feet. The ears, nose and lips increase in size; the jaw becomes massive and juts forward (*prognathism*) (Fig. 4, p. 40).

Osteitis Deformans (Paget's[1] Disease). This first appears in middle life. The calvarium becomes thickened and enlarged, particularly in the frontal and occipital regions. The face is usually unaffected. The temporal arteries are often conspicuously dilated to supply additional blood to the diseased bone, where arteriovenous communications may be numerous.

Rickets. This is due to vitamin D deficiency, which interferes with calcium absorption and with mineralization of the bones. The forehead appears high, the frontal and parietal bones or bosses become more prominent and the occiput may be flattened. This square or boxlike contour makes the head appear larger than it really is.

Congenital syphilis may produce enlargement of the frontal bosses; occasionally other cranial bones are enlarged. *Craniostosis* is the congenital or premature ossification of one or more of the cranial sutures. The commonest deformity produced is *oxycephaly* ("steeple head"; "tower skull").

Palpation. This will confirm the abnormalities found on inspection, and may yield additional important information. Unsuspected nodules or depressions may be felt; these may be benign, or they may be due to a fracture or to some disease such as multiple myeloma (plasma cell myeloma), or primary or metastatic malignancy. Additional features to be recorded for infants will be discussed in Chapter XXIII.

Percussion. This is occasionally helpful in hydrocephalus; the water-filled skull yields a peculiar "cracked pot" note. It has been re-

[1] Sir James Paget, English surgeon, 1814–99. In addition to the bone lesions, he described changes in the nipple (also called Paget's disease) that are precancerous or malignant, and similar cutaneous lesions of the penis.

ported that in adults with hyperparathyroidism, percussion yields a peculiar booming, low-pitched "watermelon" sound. Superficial or deepseated inflammation or a mass lesion can occasionally be demonstrated by percussion of the skull; the overlying area is abnormally sensitive.

Auscultation. This is used to detect murmurs or bruits in or within the skull. Such sounds can be produced by vascular malformations such as an atherosclerotic plaque, an arteriovenous fistula or an intracranial aneurysm. They may also occur with a vascular meningioma or if a brain tumor presses on a large artery. In Paget's disease, the affected areas may be extremely vascular and simulate an arteriovenous shunt, or changes in the bones at the base of the skull may compress the vessels at the cranial foramina. Such bruits are always synchronous with the pulse.

Sometimes the bruit is audible to the patient only; if loud enough it can be heard by the examiner. Digital compression of the carotid artery on the same side may alter or abolish the bruit; pressure on the contralateral artery may intensify it as more blood pours through the diseased vessel.

THE HAIR

The color, character and distribution of the hair should be noted. It may be fine or coarse, dry or oily, straight, naturally wavy or artificially curled. In men the observations are usually reliable and may be significant; women often resort to dyes, bleaches, rinses, "permanents" and other beautifying aids which tend to make the hair coarser, drier and more brittle, and subject to change of color without warning.

In hyperthyroidism the hair tends to be fine and soft; in severe hypothyroidism (*myxedema*) it is commonly coarse, dry and brittle, and usually it is sparse over the temples and above the ears.

Alopecia. This denotes partial or total loss of hair. The term X *hereditary alopecia* is applied to premature baldness, seen predominantly in men, and also to the form that appears later in life; over 40 per cent of individuals are affected to some degree. This form begins with thinning of the hair generally, and a receding hair line that remains symmetrical. In the later stages the greatest loss of hair occurs over the vertex and occiput; a fringe laterally and posteriorly usually persists. Although genetic factors seem to play a part, those who are so afflicted may be solaced by the reminder that baldness is said to be unknown in eunuchs.

Toxic or *symptomatic alopecia* denotes a rapid and more or less

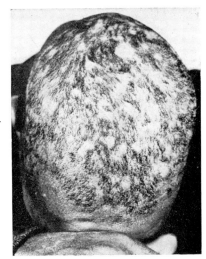

Fig. 21. Alopecia in a man with secondary syphilis. (Courtesy of the Philadelphia General Hospital.)

complete loss of hair that may occur following a prolonged exhausting illness, or postoperatively, postpartum or after a severe emotional strain. Usually there is regrowth of hair after recovery from the illness or stress.

X *Alopecia areata* is characterized by a patchy loss of hair from the scalp or the beard; this often develops rapidly. The margins of these areas are usually well defined; the hair elsewhere remains unchanged. In most instances this condition is temporary.

In secondary syphillis the hair may have a moth-eaten appearance, especially noticeable when the hair is short (Fig. 21). Other diseases of the scalp may also produce temporary or permanent loss of hair. Roentgen irradiation for a brain tumor will have the same effect.

XLice (*pediculi capitis*) are not found frequently, but much to his later embarrassment, the physician may fail to search carefully, especially when examining an uncooperative child. The ova ("nits") are more easily seen than the parasites themselves; they are pear-shaped white bodies firmly attached to the hair shaft with the larger end toward the scalp.

THE SCALP

The scalp should be inspected for lesions such as abrasions seborrhea ("dandruff"), eczema, epidermoid carcinoma, ringworm, sebaceous cysts ("wens"), senile keratoses and warts. Scars may be present; determine the cause of these if that information has not already been recorded. If infection is present the regional lymph nodes may be enlarged.

THE FACE

Facies.   You have already had some opportunity to observe the face; now concentrate on it. The general appearance or expression (*facies*) should give some indication of the patient's personality and may provide clues to his illness. How often have you been asked: "What's the matter with you? Are you sick?" or "What are you worrying about?" Your facial expression provided the clues. The various changes seen in emotional states such as agitation, anger, anxiety, apathy, despair, fear, joy, pain, resignation or worry are difficult to describe but one should learn to recognize them. With more experience one also quickly notes the typical facies of certain diseases such as pneumonia or advanced malignancy. Emotional lability should also be estimated. The stoical patient may be minimizing his symptoms; the agitated or nervous person may be exaggerating.

Symmetry.   Look for asymmetry; normally the two sides of the face are not exactly symmetrical, but gross differences should be recorded. Changes due to neurologic diseases are not uncommon; they will be discussed under The Neurologic Examination (Chapter XXII).

Edema.   This is frequently overlooked if of minor degree; the patient may be the one to call attention to it. When more pronounced it should be obvious. It frequently appears first as a puffiness of the eyelids or just below the orbits, where loose subcutaneous tissues permit fluid to accumulate. It may be most conspicuous when the patient awakens and may disappear during the day. The swelling may be symmetrical but often it is greater on one side if the patient has been lying on that side for some time.

Angioneurotic Edema.   This is also known as giant urticaria or Quincke's[2] disease. It is an allergic form of edema manifested by swelling of the loose areolar tissues, particularly of the eyelids, lips and earlobes; the oral mucosa and the tongue may also be involved (Fig. 22). Laryngeal edema also occurs; it can be extremely serious or fatal if not controlled. Urticarial lesions may also be present over other parts of the body.

Myxedema.   In myxedema the facial appearance alone may be enough to arouse suspicion (Fig. 23). The entire face appears swollen; the eyelids are puffy and the lips are large. There is no pitting on pressure; this helps to differentiate it from edema. The skin is coarse and inelastic, and usually very dry. The person appears somnolent and as a result of the lowered metabolism he may move and speak slowly. This can lead to an erroneous impression of stupidity.

[2] Heinrich Irenaeus Quincke, German neurologist, 1842–1922. He also described the capillary pulse and did much to popularize lumbar (spinal) puncture—with physicians, that is.

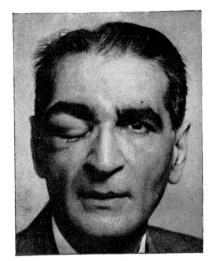

Fig. 22. Angioneurotic edema, cause undetermined. The patient never had urticarial manifestations. (From Cooke, R. A.: Allergy in Theory and Practice. Philadelphia, W. B. Saunders Co., 1947.)

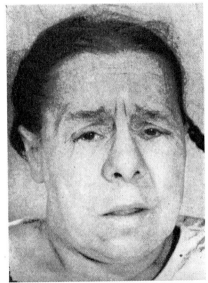

Fig. 23. Typical facial appearance of a myxedematous patient. (From Williams, R. H.: Textbook of Endocrinology. 3rd ed. Philadelphia, W. B. Saunders Co., 1962.)

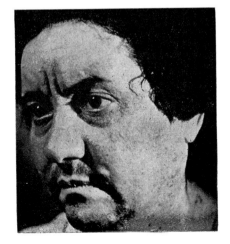

Fig. 24. Cushing's syndrome, with virilism from functioning adrenocortical tumor (carcinoma). (Courtesy of F. Curtis Dohan, M.D.)

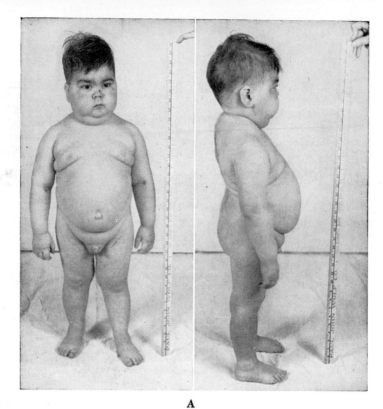

A

B
(Figure 25. See legend on opposite page.)

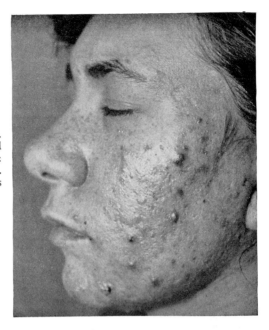

Fig. 26. Acne vulgaris. Note oily seborrhea, scars and pustules. (From Andrews, G. C.: Diseases of the Skin. 3rd ed. Philadelphia, W. B. Saunders Co., 1946.)

Cushing's[3] Syndrome. A typical facies is often present in this condition, in addition to other characteristics. There is rounding of the face ("moon face") as well as excessive hairiness (*hirsutism*), most noticeable in women (Fig. 24). The skin is thin and the superficial vessels are prominent; as a result the person may appear ruddy or plethoric. Formerly this syndrome was thought to occur in association with a basophilic tumor of the pituitary, an adrenocortical tumor, hyperplasia of the adrenal cortex (Fig. 25) or an ovarian arrhenoblastoma. Recently a similar picture in a somewhat milder form has become fairly common; it follows prolonged administration of large doses of adrenocortical steroids, particularly cortisone and hydrocortisone.

The Skin. Examination of the skin has already been discussed (Chapter IV); a few facial lesions will be mentioned. The most common is *acne vulgaris;* it is usually most pronounced and most disconcerting during puberty and adolescence (Fig. 26). In *disseminated lupus erythematosus* the typical eruption may first appear over the malar regions and the bridge of the nose as a "butterfly rash" (Fig. 27). However, the

[3] Harvey Cushing, Boston surgeon, 1869–1939.

Fig. 25. *A,* Child aged 4, with adrenal hyperplasia causing Cushing's syndrome: rounding of the face, hirsutism and marked obesity. *B,* Same child 6 months after bilateral partial adrenalectomy. (Courtesy of Drs. E. K. Rose, E. Rose and J. E. Rhoads.)

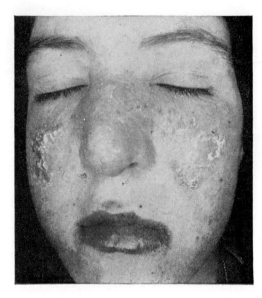

Fig. 27. Lupus erythematosus. (From Thoma, K. H.,
and Robinson, H. B. G.: Oral
and Dental Diagnosis. 5th ed.
Philadelphia, W. B. Saunders
Co., 1960.)

lesions of tuberculosis of the skin (*lupus vulgaris*) may have a similar
distribution, as do the skin lesions of sarcoidosis and erysipelas. With
mitral stenosis a malar flush is often seen; the person appears pink-
cheeked and deceptively healthy.

THE EYES

Systemic disease is frequently manifested by changes in structure or
function of the eyes. Because of the smallness of the components and the
high degree of specialization of the eye, examination must necessarily
be detailed. A routine method of study saves time and helps to prevent
overlooking important variations or abnormalities.

Prominence of the Eyes.   Probably one of the first things noticed
is the relative prominence of the eyes, especially if they appear to be
sunken into the skull (*enophthalmos*) or seem to protrude (*exophthalmos; proptosis*).

X ENOPHTHALMOS.   This is usually due to trauma; it may also result from dehydration or severe wasting disease. The orbital tissues lose
moisture or the fat decreases or disappears, and the eyes sink into the
sockets. Occasionally enophthalmos is congenital.

X EXOPHTHALMOS.   Ordinarily the upper lid conceals a very small
segment of the cornea and iris; the lower lid rests just below the junction
of the cornea and the sclera (the *limbus*). In some people the palpebral
fissures are wider than average; this makes the eyes appear unduly

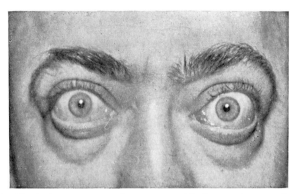

Fig. 28. Typical appearance of a patient with thyrotoxicosis and exophthalmos. (From Adler, F. H.: Textbook of Ophthalmology. 7th ed. Philadelphia, W. B. Saunders Co., 1962.)

prominent. In the nearsighted (*myopic*) person there is actual elongation of the globe; therefore the eye tends to protrude from the orbit. In true exophthalmos there is forward displacement of a normal-sized eyeball; the exact amount must be determined by using an exophthalmometer.

Unilateral exophthalmos is usually due to an inflammatory or neoplastic process involving the orbit on that side; in rare instances it is found with hyperthyroidism. Bilateral exophthalmos can be produced by thrombosis of the cavernous sinus, or by leukemic infiltration or other malignant lesions of the orbit, but the commonest cause is hyperthyroidism (*exophthalmic goiter*) (Fig. 28). Ocular signs of this disease will be discussed later in the chapter.

Palpebral Fissures. Normally the palpebral fissures should be equal; a very slight difference is usually of no significance if the lids move normally. Have the patient close his eyes; the lid margins should meet. If any portion of the globe remains exposed it is liable to become irritated or injured. Then have the patient open his eyes as widely as possible. Both upper lids should be drawn up equally, leaving a small segment of sclera visible above the limbus.

Marked drooping of one upper lid, or inability to open the eye widely (*ptosis*), indicates injury to the third cranial nerve or to the cervical sympathetic nerve supply. Inability to close the lids is seen with weakness or paralysis of the seventh cranial nerve.

HORNER'S SYNDROME. In 1869 Horner[4] described a syndrome which included unilateral narrowing of the palpebral fissure, a contracted pupil, enophthalmos and a decrease or total absence of activity of the sweat glands of the face on the affected side ("little fissure, little pupil, little eye, little sweat"). It is now known that the enophthalmos is more apparent than real; the narrow palpebral orifice gives the illusion of a

[4] Johann Friedrich Horner, Swiss ophthalmologist, 1831–86.

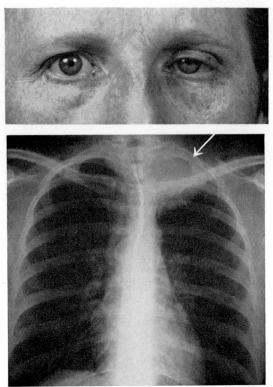

Fig. 29. Superior sulcus tumor (Pancoast tumor) producing Horner's syndrome. The tumor can be seen at the apex of the left lung; the posterior portion of the second left rib has been destroyed. (Courtesy of E. P. Pendergrass, M.D.).

sunken eyeball. This syndrome is produced by paralysis of the cervical sympathetic nerve supply, usually in the cervical chain but occasionally in the spinal cord or the medulla. An aortic aneurysm or an apical intrathoracic tumor is mostly commonly the cause of the peripheral type of paralysis (Fig. 29).

Irritation or stimulation of the cervical sympathetic supply will produce dilatation of the pupil, a widened fissure and increased sweating; this may precede the appearance of paralysis as Horner's syndrome is developing, and may lead the examiner to attribute the inequality to a lesion on the opposite side. In such cases the presence or absence of sweating is a valuable guide to the site of the disease.

Movements. Rotation of the eyeballs (extraocular movements) should now be determined. The most conspicuous abnormality is squint or strabismus, in which one eye deviates from its normal axis; this may be convergent (internal; esotropia; cross-eyes) or divergent (external; exotropia; walleyes). Gross deviations are easily detected (Fig. 30); minor degrees may require more elaborate procedures.

Strabismus may be concomitant or paralytic. In concomitant strabismus the relative position of the two eyes remains constant; the deviating eye can turn straight and fix. This condition usually becomes apparent before the age of three and should be treated promptly. To avoid double vision (*diplopia*), the child quickly learns to suppress the image in the squinting eye, with resulting lack of vision in that eye (*amblyopia*).

Paralytic strabismus is due to paralysis of one or more of the extraocular muscles. It usually appears suddenly; diplopia is always present initially, and may give rise to vertigo or nausea. To determine which muscle or muscles are at fault, have the patient look in various directions or watch your finger tip as it slowly circles the orbital area. More elaborate tests are available for localizing the site of the lesion; they are especially useful when there is weakness (*paresis*) but not total paralysis of the muscle.

Nystagmus. This is an involuntary rapid jerking movement of the eyeballs in a lateral, vertical or rotary direction or a combination of these movements. It may be apparent when the person is looking directly forward, but usually it is most easily seen in one position or another as the eyeballs are rotated in various directions. Nystagmus may occur in a normal person as a manifestation of ocular fatigue or poor vision. Pathologically it is seen with various diseases of the nervous system such as multiple sclerosis (disseminated sclerosis), encephalitis or a strategically situated intracranial mass lesion.

Eyebrows and Eyelashes. Look carefully at the eyebrows. Thinning or loss of hairs, especially in the outer portions, may occur with various diseases such as myxedema, syphilis or leukemia; more commonly it is due to tweezers. Then look at the eyelashes (*cilia*). They

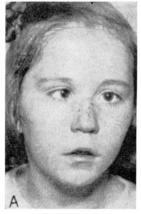 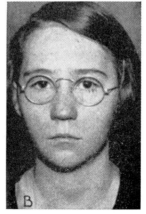

Fig. 30. *A*, Concomitant convergent strabismus. *B*, Result of refraction correction. (From Adler, F. H.: Textbook of Ophthalmolgy. 7th ed. Philadelphia, W. B. Saunders Co., 1962.)

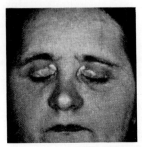

Fig. 31. Xanthelasma. (From Pullen, R. L.: Medical Diagnosis. 2nd ed. Philadelphia, W. B Saunders Co., 1950.)

should be fairly uniformly distributed and should all curve away from the eyeballs. A total absence of cilia may be congenital; more often it is the result of inflammatory disease. Lashes that turn inward irritate the cornea and must be removed.

Eyelids. These should be inspected with certain points in mind, looking especially for deformity or disease. Lacerations or other injuries with scar formation may distort a lid and interfere with its normal movements. Yellowish plaques (*xanthelasma*) may be present, especially near the nasal margins and in the adjacent nasal skin (Fig. 31). They are sometimes associated with disturbances of cholesterol metabolism but frequently occur without other abnormalities, especially in postmenopausal women.

Slight redness, crusting or scaling of the lid margins is associated with mild chronic infection. A localized acute inflammatory lesion is usually a sty (*hordeolum*) due to infection of one or more of the glands of Zeis[5] or Moll[6] at the lid margin. When there is chronic irritation of a meibomian[7] gland, or obstruction of its duct, a *chalazion* develops; usually this produces a relatively asymptomatic nodule that is easily seen and felt.

Inversion of the lid margin (*entropion*) is usually due to scarring of the conjunctiva from previous inflammatory disease. This may force the lashes against the cornea and conjunctiva, causing irritation. Eversion of the lid margin (*ectropion*) may be due to scars in the skin of the eyelid or to seventh nerve paralysis. In the elderly, loss of muscle tone may permit the lower lid to become everted; the tears roll out onto the cheek.

The Lacrimal System. The lacrimal glands lie in the upper outer portion of the orbit. Normally they are not visible or palpable, but they may enlarge as a result of acute or chronic infection (*dacryoadenitis*) or in certain systemic diseases. Tears are constantly formed in small amounts and spread downward over the cornea and conjuntiva. They pass through the puncta of the canaliculi, located near the nasal end of

[5] Edward Zeis, Dresden ophthalmologist, 1807–68.
[6] Jacob Antonius Moll, Dutch oculist, 1823–1914.
[7] Heinrich Meibom, German anatomist, 1638–1700.

the lids, into the lacrimal sac and the nasolacrimal duct, and thence into the nose. Inflammation of these structures (dacryocystitis) will produce a visible and palpable bulge on the side of the nose or beneath the eyelid.

The lacrimal glands are innervated by sympathetic and parasympathetic fibers carried in the lacrimal branch of the first division of the fifth cranial nerve. Excessive lacrimation may occur from direct stimulation of the fifth nerve, or as a reflex from painful stimuli elsewhere; frequently it is due to psychic factors. Abnormal dryness (*xerophthalmia*) may be due to nerve injury; it is also seen with vitamin A deficiency. Excessive formation of tears, or obstruction of the canaliculi or ducts, results in an overflow of tears onto the cheeks (*epiphora*).

The Conjunctiva. The bulbar conjunctiva covers the sclera from the limbus outward and is continuous with the palpebral portion that lines the eyelids.

All except the uppermost portion of the bulbar conjunctiva can be examined by gently holding the lids apart while the patient gazes in various directions. The conjunctiva is transparent; the normal white color of the eye is produced by the underlying sclera. A number of small subconjunctival vessels can be seen entering near the periphery; these points of penetration may be surrounded by very small dots of uveal pigment.

The palpebral conjunctiva of the lower lids can be inspected by pulling down on the skin of the eyelid with a finger while the patient looks upward (Fig. 32). To examine the conjunctiva of the upper lid, the eyelid must be everted. To do this, have the patient look down but not close his eyes. Grasp the cilia of the upper lid between the thumb and index finger and gently pull downward slightly, then forward. With an applicator stick, tongue blade or even a finger, press downward above

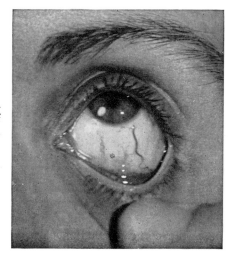

Fig. 32. Eversion of lower eyelid. (From Adler, F. H.: Textbook of Ophthalmology. 7th ed. Philadelphia, W. B. Saunders Co., 1962.)

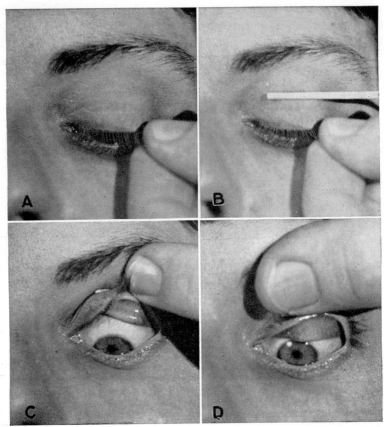

Fig. 33.   Eversion of the upper eyelid. *A*, The patient looks down. The lashes are grasped between the thumb and forefinger. The eyelid is pulled downward and away from the globe. *B*, Applicator stick makes pressure above tarsal plate. *C*, The lid is pulled quickly upward and everted. *D*, The thumb maintains eversion by pressing the eyelashes against the supraorbital tissues. (From Adler, F. H.: Textbook of Ophthalmology. 7th ed. Philadelphia, W. B. Saunders Co., 1962.)

the tarsal plate—a centimeter above the lid margin; this pressure is the force which produces eversion. To maintain eversion, press the eyelashes against the eyebrow with a finger (Fig. 33).

The palpebral conjunctiva normally appears pink. Over the tarsal plate yellow streaks may be seen running at right angles to the lid margin; these are the meibomian glands. With anemia the conjunctiva may be pale, but edema can give a false impression of pallor. With polycythemia the entire surface may be abnormally red; this must be differentiated from vascular congestion. In the latter, the blood vessels appear superficial, are relatively tortuous, will move with pressure, and the redness is most intense around the periphery; it is much less prominent around the cornea. Irritation of any type, infection or allergy are the common causes of congestion; in the latter, fine nodules may be visible. If the congestion is most marked around the limbus, or if it is seen there only (*ciliary flush*), it is indicative of disease involving the cornea or iris.

A benign growth consisting of a triangular fold of conjunctiva containing many superficial blood vessels may extend from the inner canthus out to the cornea or partially over it; this is a *pterygium* (Fig. 34).

SUBCONJUNCTIVAL HEMORRHAGE.   This may occur following an injury, after coughing or sneezing, or without obvious cause. An irregular bright red area several millimeters in diameter suddenly develops. The patient may be alarmed and worried when he sees this but it is of little clinical significance. The blood retains its bright red color for several days, but eventually it is entirely resorbed.

PETECHIAE.   These are often seen in the palpebral conjunctiva when subacute bacterial endocarditis is present. Usually only a few are present at any one time, but new ones may appear as the old ones fade. They may also occur in other systemic infections or in certain hematologic disorders.

The Sclerae.   The normal sclera has a porcelain-white color. In jaundice the yellow color may be apparent here before it is noticeable in the skin. In Negroes, flecks of brownish pigment are often seen, especially in the areas normally exposed; similar spots are occasionally seen in other races. Subconjunctival fat will produce a patchy yellowish discoloration. Quinacrine (Atabrine), an antimalarial drug, may cause a yellowish color; this is most noticeable around the limbus and in the areas normally exposed to light. In carotenemia, which results from an excessive intake of provitamin A, the sclera may be slightly discolored but the yellowness of the skin is the most striking feature. In osteogenesis imperfecta, a rare familial disease, the sclerae are blue.

The Cornea.   A healthy cornea is a smooth, glistening, transparent structure, practically invisible except for reflections from its surface. Oblique illumination is needed to detect the presence of irregularities or opacities; special staining procedures are used to delineate abrasions or other injuries.

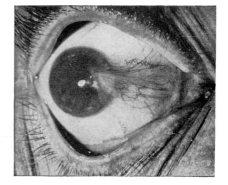

Fig. 34.   Pterygium. (From Adler, F. H.: Textbook of Ophthalmology. 7th ed. Philadelphia, W. B. Saunders Co., 1962.)

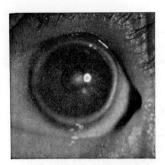

Fig. 35.   Annulus senilis. (From Adler, F. H.: Textbook of Ophthalmology. 7th ed. Philadelphia, W. B. Saunders Co., 1962.)

An *arcus senilis* is frequently seen in persons past middle life. This is a grayish white opaque zone near the limbus but separated from it by a very narrow zone of clear cornea. With advancing age the arc may extend to form a complete ring or *annulus senilis* (Fig. 35). In this age group it is of no significance; if seen in a young adult it may be suggestive of disturbances of lipid metabolism.

In hepatolenticular degeneration (Wilson's[8] disease) a somewhat similar ring of golden-brown granular pigmentation may be seen on the posterior surface of the cornea at the limbus (Kayser-Fleischer[9] ring).

The intact cornea is remarkably resistant to infection; the slightest injury makes it extremely vulnerable. Inflammation of the cornea (*keratitis*) may be due to the presence of a foreign body embedded in the cornea or under one eyelid, or to infection following such an injury. It also occurs with various diseases, especially congenital syphilis, herpes simplex ("cold sores") or herpes zoster ("shingles"). Since the cornea normally contains no blood vessels it does not become red, but the involved area will appear hazy or duller than normal and there will be a ciliary flush. A residual gray scar may persist when the acute process has subsided (Fig. 36).

As part of the neurologic examination, corneal sensitivity is tested by touching the cornea lightly with a wisp of cotton or a hair; the interpretation of the response is discussed on page 427.

The Iris.   The color of the iris of each eye should be determined. Occasionally one is blue and the other brown, or one iris may be part blue and part brown (heterochromia iridis). The markings should be easily visible on each iris. Sometimes an artificial eye (*prosthesis*) does not match the color of the normal eye.

The Pupils.   Normal pupils are round, approximately equal in size if equally illuminated, and become smaller (constrict) if additional light strikes them. Marked inequality of the pupils or an irregular pupil should always be considered abnormal; trauma, localized infection or

[8] Samuel A. K. Wilson, English neurologist, 1878–1936.

[9] Bernhard Kayser, German ophthalmologist, 1869–1954; Richard Fleischer, Munich physician, 1848–1909.

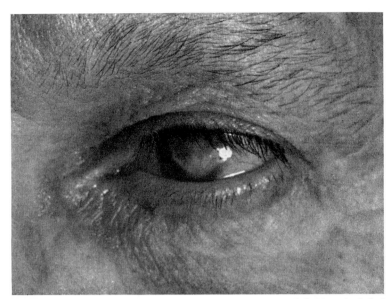

Fig. 36. Dense corneal scar secondary to herpes zoster of the first (ophthalmic) division of the fifth cranial nerve.

central nervous system syphilis are the most common causes, but occasionally a scar or a congenital defect may be present.

SIZE. The size of the pupils may be important. In infancy the pupils are usually small. In childhood and early adult life they are much larger, then decrease in size with advancing age. In persons with dark irides the pupils tend to be smaller than in those with light blue eyes.

Dilatation of the pupils (*mydriasis*) may be seen in fright or other emotional states; it may also be present in patients who are taking belladonna or other antispasmodic or sympathomimetic agents. Untreated glaucoma may also produce mydriasis.

Abnormal constriction of the pupils (*miosis*) is usually due to morphine or one of the other narcotic drugs; these are often called "pinpoint" pupils.* It may also be due to local or systemic use of other drugs such as pilocarpine, or to neurologic disorders.

PUPILLARY REFLEXES. The pupillary reflexes should now be determined. The *direct* light reflex is the constriction that occurs when one eye suddenly receives additional light. Have the patient fix his gaze on some distant object. Cover one eye with the palm of your hand; shine a flashlight into the other eye. The pupil should constrict promptly. Now test the other eye in the same manner. If a flashlight is not available, cover both eyes for several seconds, then uncover one quickly; repeat this for the other eye.

* Originally described by Robert Graves (p. 125n) in 1848 as the "pin-hole pupil."

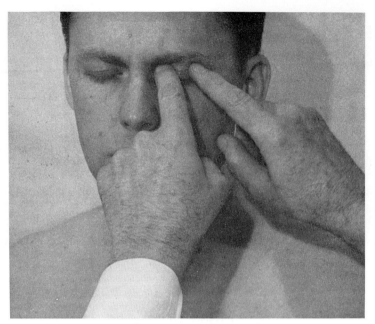

Fig. 37. Tactile estimation of intraocular tension.

The *indirect* or *consensual* reflex is elicited by shining a light into one eye only while observing the opposite pupil; it should constrict moderately.

The reaction to *accommodation* or *convergence* (near point reaction) is less obvious. Hold a finger or other small object a few inches in front of the patient's face. Have him look at the wall directly beyond your finger, then focus quickly on the finger. The pupil should constrict when he focuses on the near point.

✕ ARGYLL ROBERTSON PUPIL.   In 1869 Argyll Robertson[10] described the pupillary changes that still bear his name; he correctly attributed these to syphilis of the central nervous system (tabes dorsalis or tabo-paresis). The important characteristics are: small (miotic) pupils, usually irregular in outline and unequal in size, with normal or even increased contraction at the near point (accommodation) but a marked diminution or total absence of reaction to light, either direct or consensual. With total blindness, of course, the diagnosis cannot be made.

A tonic pupil (Adie's[11] pupil) may be mistaken for the Argyll Robertson type because the reactions appear to be lost. Careful observation will show that the pupil is not miotic and that the light reaction is present but is sluggish, with a very long latent period; the near point reaction is also slow to appear. This abnormality is frequently unilateral

[10] Douglas Moray Cooper Lamb Argyll Robertson, Scottish physician, 1837–1909.
[11] William John Adie, British neurologist, 1886–1935.

and occurs in young people. The cause is unknown but it is not due to neurosyphilis.

The Lens.   Oblique illumination is used to visualize deposits on the surface or opacities within the substance of the lens; preferably, the pupils should be dilated. In elderly persons the lens may look gray by oblique illumination even though there are no opacities.

Intraocular Tension.   A tonometer must be used to determine intraocular tension accurately and to detect minor variations; gross changes can be detected with the fingers. Have the patient look downward without closing his eyes. Place both index fingers on the upper eyelid above the tarsal plate. Press gently on the sclera above the cornea, first with one finger and then with the other (Fig. 37). With experience one can learn to recognize unusual firmness or softness of the globe. In glaucoma the intraocular tension is often increased, sometimes to such a degree that the eyeball feels hard. In diabetic acidosis or coma the globe may become very soft.

OPHTHALMOSCOPIC EXAMINATION

Every medical student should learn to use an ophthalmoscope; recognition of abnormal findings and their significance will come only with experience.

Procedure.   A darkened room will facilitate the examination; a suitable mydriatic may be instilled to dilate the pupils if there is no suspicion of glaucoma. It will help if the patient is cooperative and able to keep his gaze fixed. Select some object across the room or on the ceiling and ask the patient to look steadily at that point.

To examine the right eye, hold the ophthalmoscope as close as possible to your right eye with your right hand; keep the index finger on the milled disk that carries lenses of various focal lengths. Rest your left hand lightly on the patient's head, and with your left thumb lift his right upper eyelid slightly to keep him from blinking or closing the eye. With the "O" lens in place, turn on the light in the ophthalmoscope, direct the beam into his right pupil and move your head closer to his (Fig. 38). When you are within a foot or less the pupil will appear bright red. If the media are not clear this red reflex will vary from dull orange to black.

Now bring your head closer to the patient's, with the +20 lens in position (Fig. 39). This will permit careful inspection of the cornea. As the wheel is turned and lenses of lower power are used the deeper structures come into focus; eventually the fundus is clearly seen. Try not to accommodate; imagine that you are looking at some point far away. If

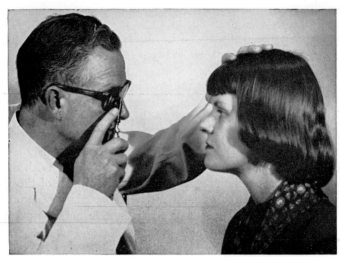

Fig. 38. Ophthalmoscopic examination of the media. (From Adler, F. H. Textbook of Ophthalmology. 7th ed. Philadelphia, W. B. Saunders Co., 1962.)

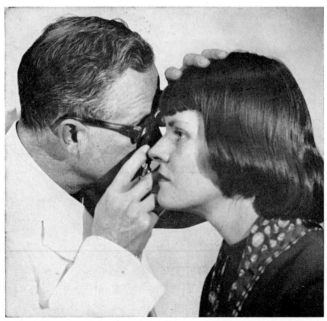

Fig. 39. Ophthalmoscopic examination of the right fundus. (From Adler, F. H.: Textbook of Ophthalmology. 7th ed. Philadelphia, W. B. Saunders Co., 1962.)

at first you cannot relax your accommodation, a concave lense (—2 or —3) may be turned into position. The retinal vessels should now be visible; alter the strength of the lens until they are sharply focused.

Optic Disk.   Look first for the optic disk; this is toward the nasal side. Follow the course of one of the vessels to find it, if necessary. The normal disk is circular or a vertical oval, and appears paler than the retina; the center may be almost white and may show a depression known as the physiologic cup (Fig. 40). The margins should be sharp. With

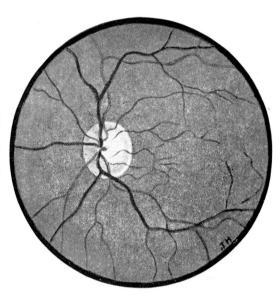

Fig. 40.   The normal fundus with physiologic cupping of the disk. (From Adler, F. H.: Gifford's Textbook of Ophthalmology. 4th ed. Philadelphia, W. B. Saunders Co., 1947.)

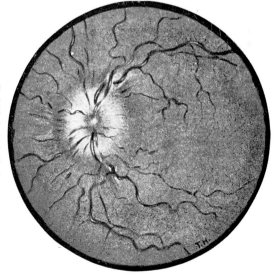

Fig. 41.   Early stage of choked disk, showing blurring of the nasal half, dilated veins and a few small hemorrhages just off the disk. (From Adler, F. H.: Textbook of Ophthalmology. 7th ed. Philadelphia, W. B. Saunders Co., 1962.)

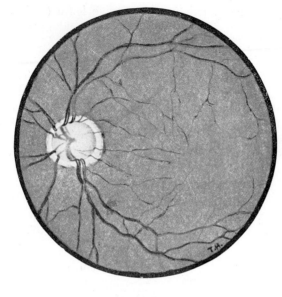

Fig. 42. Cupping of the disk in chronic glaucoma. (From Adler, F. H.: Gifford's Textbook of Ophthalmology. 4th ed. Philadelphia, W. B. Saunders Co., 1947.)

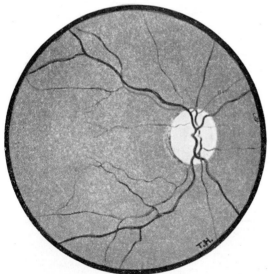

Fig. 43. Simple optic atrophy. (From Adler, F. H.: Textbook of Ophthalmology. 7th ed. Philadelphia, W. B. Saunders Co., 1962.)

choked disk (*papilledema*) there is swelling of the disk with blurring of details. This appears first on the nasal side (Fig. 41), but later the entire area is involved. In chronic glaucoma the cupping becomes much more conspicuous (Fig. 42). With destruction of the optic nerve (optic atrophy) the disks become white (Fig. 43).

VESSELS.   The retinal vessels should now be studied. Usually the retinal artery divides into four branches that spread outward irregularly from the disk; veins weave around the arteries. Arteries are somewhat smaller in diameter (about 4:5) and show a definite narrow, shiny reflex stripe. Follow the course of each artery from the disk to the periphery. To do this it will be necessary to have the patient look upward, downward, to the right and to the left. Normally the vessels spread out in undulating curves; there is no sudden change in direction. As branching occurs the vessels become smaller, but sudden change in caliber should not be present. Look carefully at the points where arteries cross veins; the vein should be visible right up to the artery and should reappear immediately beyond the crossing (Fig. 44).

MACULA.   The macula is now inspected. This lies about two disk diameters (a distance twice the diameter of the disk) from the optic disk itself, on the temporal side. It is usually darker in color than the surrounding retina, with a small dark red spot in the center (*fovea centralis*). No blood vessels are visible in this area, but all of the nearby small branches seem to be converging toward this point. If it is difficult

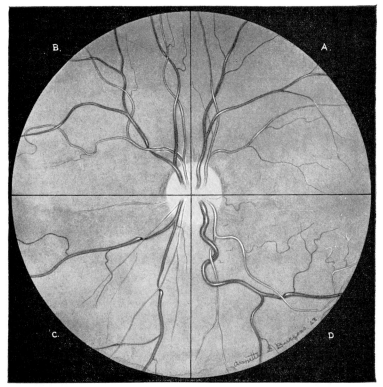

Fig. 44.   Retinal arteriosclerosis. *A,* Normal fundus; *B,* senile arteriosclerosis without hypertension; *C,* retinal arteriosclerosis with hypertension; *D,* retinal arteriosclerosis, showing copper-wire arteries. (After Friedenwald, courtesy of the Wilmer Institute.)

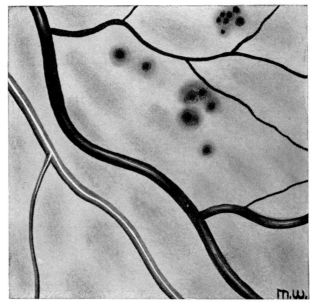

Fig. 45. Round hemorrhages in the deep layers of the retina. (From Adler, F. H.: Textbook of Ophthalmology. 7th ed. Philadelphia, W. B. Saunders Co., 1962.)

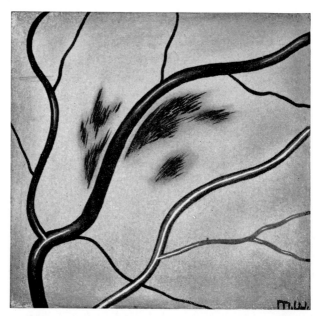

Fig. 46. Flame-shaped hemorrhages in the nerve fiber layer of the retina. (From Adler, F. H.: Textbook of Ophthalmology. 7th ed. Philadelphia, W. B. Saunders Co., 1962.)

to locate the macula, have the patient look directly at the ophthalmoscope light; the macula will then be in the center of your field of vision.

FUNDUS.   The rest of the fundus is now examined. The color
varies with the amount of pigment present; this is roughly proportional
to the patient's complexion. In a blond it will be a light orange-red; a
brunet will have a much darker fundus; in a Negro the fundus may be
slate-gray.

HEMORRHAGES.   These appear as homogeneous dark red areas;
they tend to occur centrally rather than in the periphery. In the superficial layers of the retina they are usually flame-shaped; in the deeper
layers they tend to be round or oval (Figs. 45, 46). After absorption of
the blood a scar may form.

MICROANEURYSMS.   These are punctate red dots that resemble
deep hemorrhages; they are usually indicative of diabetes, especially
when they occur around the macula.

EXUDATES.   White or slightly yellowish patches of variable size
may be seen along the course of one or more of the retinal vessels. They
may appear to be somewhat fluffy ("cotton wool exudates") (Fig. 47)
or dense and waxy. The former are more common with hypertensive and
arteriosclerotic changes; the latter are seen with diabetes.

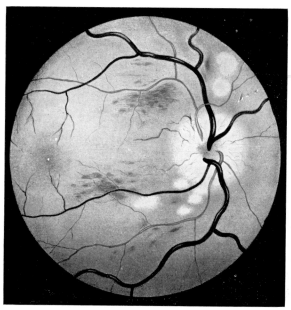

Fig. 47.   Grade IV hypertensive changes, with no sclerosis. In addition to extreme narrowing of the arteries, note flame-shaped hemorrhages, cotton-wool patches
and edema of disk. (Courtesy of H. G. Scheie, M.D., in Adler, F. H.: Textbook of
Ophthalmology. 7th ed. Philadelphia, W. B. Saunders Co., 1962.)

VISUAL ACUITY

Determination of visual acuity may provide clues to local ocular disturbances, to neurologic disorders or to systemic disease. Each eye is tested individually; the other eye is covered with a card or the palm of the hand. If the person normally wears glasses, vision should be tested with and without them.

Whenever possible, the Snellen[12] chart or a modification of it should be used for testing distant vision; this is placed at a distance of 6 meters (20 feet). Have the patient cover one eye; determine the smallest type that he can read. Then check the other eye. The results are recorded as fractions. If the letters on the "6" line can be read at 6 meters, the visual acuity is 6/6 (normal). If nothing smaller than the "12" line can be seen the acuity is recorded as 6/12.

For near vision the Jaeger[13] card is used; this has lines of print of various type sizes. Hold the card at the normal reading distance (30 to 35 cm.; 12 to 14 inches) and determine the smallest type that can be read. Record the appropriate number; if the smallest line can be read (J-1) the near vision is normal.

If the patient is not ambulatory and if there are no other ocular abnormalities, it may be acceptable to perform crude checks of visual acuity by asking him to read newsprint or other small type (if he can read) and to identify small objects at a distance from his bed. If he wears glasses they should be examined to determine whether he is farsighted (*hyperopic*), nearsighted (*myopic*) or has astigmatism. A rough estimate of the degree of abnormality should be recorded.

VISUAL FIELDS

Alterations in the visual fields may be due to disease of the eye itself, or can be produced by a lesion in the optic nerve, the visual pathways or the occipital lobe of the brain. Figure 48 shows the common sites for such processes and the abnormality produced by each. A normal eye does not see everything within the field of vision; the optic disk produces a blind spot. However, in a person with binocular vision the two blind spots do not coincide, so one eye will see objects missed at the blind spot of the other eye.

Confrontation.   Accurate plotting of the visual field requires special equipment, but a rough estimate can be made by confrontation.

[12] Hermann Snellen, Dutch ophthalmologist, 1834–1908.
[13] Edward Jaeger von Jastthal, Austrian oculist, 1818–84.

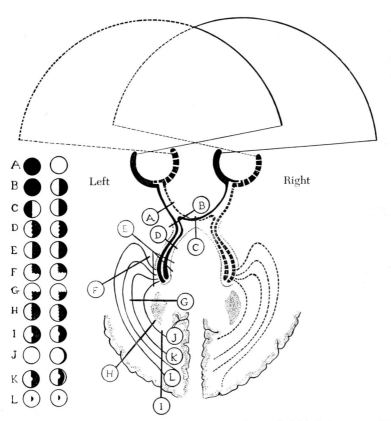

Fig. 48. Composite diagram showing type of visual field defect caused by lesions affecting the optic pathways. The solid black lines represent the nasal retina of the right eye and the temporal retina of the left eye. The crossed-hatch lines represent the temporal retina of the right eye and the nasal retina of the left eye. On the left are represented the visual field changes, with the site of the lesion indicated in the diagram corresponding to the letters as follows: A, lesion behind eyeball, anterior to the chiasm; B, commencement of optic nerve just anterior to the chiasm—ipsilateral blindness with contralateral temporal hemianopia; C, chiasmal lesion—bitemporal hemianopia; D, optic tract—markedly incongruous homonymous hemianopia; E, beginning of optic tract—clear-cut homonymous hemianopia without sparing of the macula; F, anterior loop of optic radiations—slightly incongruous superior quadrantopia (right superior hemianopia); G, inner part of optic radiations—slightly incongruous inferior quadrantopia; H, middle of optic radiations—slightly incongruous homonymous hemianopia without macular sparing; I, posterior part of optic radiations with macular sparing; J, anterior part of calcarine cortex—contralateral blindness in temporal crescent; K, middle part of calcarine cortex—congruous homonymous hemianopia with sparing of the macula and contralateral sparing of temporal crescent; L, occipital pole—congruous homonymous hemianopic central scotoma.

Sometimes a bilateral thrombosis of the posterior calcarine arteries will cause complete blindness, or there may be sparing of a small island of vision slightly excentric to the macular areas.

Tubular fields of vision are frequently seen in the later stages of glaucoma. The examiner should always make certain that the intraocular tension is normal and that there is no evidence of glaucoma before attempting to interpret the visual fields. (Modification of Sir Stewart Duke-Elder's drawings by Paton. From Cecil, R. L., and Conn, H. F. (eds.): The Specialties in General Practice. 3rd ed. Philadelphia, W. B. Saunders Co., 1964.)

Sit facing the patient at a distance of about two feet. Cover your right eye and have him cover his left eye; each then looks directly at the other person's uncovered eye. Hold a cotton-tipped applicator stick, a pencil or other object in your left hand midway between you and the patient; bring it slowly toward his eye. Have the patient tell you as soon as the sees the test object. Repeat the procedure at various points around the periphery of the visual field; then check the other eye in a similar manner. If you and the patient both have normal visual fields the test object should be visible to each at about the same point.

OCULAR SIGNS IN THYROTOXICOSIS

Although a large number of eye signs occurring with thyrotoxicosis have been described, certain ones are so characteristic that inspection alone may be enough to suggest the diagnosis. Usually the first to appear is widening of the palpebral fissures caused by retraction of the upper lids, and to a lesser extent of the lower lids (Dalrymple's[14] sign). Spasm of the smooth muscles of Müller[15] and Landström[16] is believed to produce this widening. A lag or failure of the upper lids to move downward normally as the gaze is directed downward is von Graefe's[17] sign. Infrequent or incomplete blinking (Stellwag's[18] sign), inability to maintain convergence (Möbius'[19] sign) and diminution or absence of wrinkling of the forehead when the gaze is directed upward (Joffroy's[20] sign) may also be observed in these patients but are more frequently found in examination questions.

Exophthalmos develops in about 50 per cent of persons who have toxic diffuse goiter, but is seen infrequently with toxic nodular goiter. The widened palpebral fissure and the lid lag give rise to the typical appearance of apprehension or fright; they also make the eyeballs seem more prominent. The actual amount of proptosis is usually less than one would expect; it can be determined accurately only by measurement with an exophthalmometer.

THE EARS

Auricles.   Congenital malformation of the auricles is not rare; occasionally there is congenital absence of one or both. A difference in

[14] John Dalrymple, English oculist, 1804–52.
[15] Heinrich Müller, German anatomist, 1820–64.
[16] John Landström, Swedish surgeon, 1869–1910.
[17] Albrecht von Graefe, German ophthalmologist, 1828–70.
[18] Carl Stellwag von Carion, Austrian oculist, 1823–1904.
[19] Paul Julius Möbius, German neurologist, 1853–1907.
[20] Alexis Joffroy, French physician, 1844–1908.

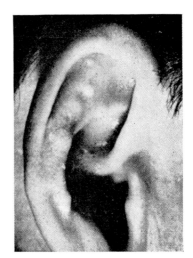

Fig. 49. Gouty tophi in the anthelix of the auricle. (Courtesy of E. P. Pendergrass, M.D.)

size, in the angle of attachment or in the relative position of the two auricles is frequently seen but is of no otologic importance; however, this may give rise to emotional problems. Severe or repeated injuries with perichondrial hemorrhage can lead to destruction of cartilage; fibrosis and scarring then help to produce the "cauliflower ear" often seen in pugilists and wrestlers. Cyanosis may be conspicuous in the auricle, especially in the lobule. With gout there may be small hard nodules (*tophi*) in the helix or anthelix, formed by deposition of crystals of sodium urate (Fig. 49). A tophus should not be confused with the darwinian[21] tubercle, a small projection sometimes seen in the edge of the helix and attributed by some to our arboreal ancestry. Sebaceous cysts may also be present, particularly in the lobule and on the posterior surface of the auricle.

When one auricle appears to be displaced forward, make sure that this is not due to edema of the mastoid region. Always inspect this area; the scar of a forgotten mastoidectomy may be found. With mumps, the lower portion of the auricle is displaced outward; the upper portion retains its normal position.

Auditory Canals. The outer portion has a cartilaginous wall and is relatively insensitive. The inner portion has a bony wall and is very sensitive. Usually the canal is slightly angled; it can be straightened by gently pulling the auricle upward and backward.

To inspect the canal, proper illumination is essential. Either a head mirror or an electric otoscope may be used; the latter has a magnifying lens that aids in the examination. Use the largest speculum that will fit into the canal, but insert it only a few millimeters to avoid touching the

[21] Charles Robert Darwin, English naturalist, 1809–82.

bony meatus. To visualize the canal easily it is usually necessary to tip the patient's head slightly away from you.

The healthy canal will have a pale pink, slightly glistening surface. Look for roughness or oozing of the skin due to eczema or fungus infection, and for inflammation. Purulent secretions may come from an infection of the canal; more commonly they are due to acute or chronic infection of the middle ear (*otitis media*). Blood may be present from local trauma or a lesion of the canal, from otitis media with rupture of the drum, or as a result of fracture of the middle fossa of the skull. Cerumen ("wax") is frequently present; there may be enough to obstruct the canal completely. This must be removed so that the eardrum can be visualized.

Tympanic Membrane.   The normal drum is a pearly gray, translucent membrane. It is somewhat diagonally situated; the posterior superior portion is closer to your eye than is the anterior inferior portion. The surface is slightly concave, and the outline of the malleus is visible. The light reflex fans downward and forward from the tip of the umbo. At the periphery is the annulus, a ring of fibrous tissue that appears whiter than the rest of the membrane.

The most commonly seen abnormalities are changes in color, alteration of the light reflex, excessive retraction, bulging or perforation. An inflamed eardrum will be pink or red; a scarred or thickened drum will be whiter than normal. A distorted or absent light reflex usually indicates acute or chronic disease. Excessive retraction occurs when the eustachian[22] tube is obstructed. Bulging is produced by serous or purulent effusion behind the drum; the normal landmarks are indistinct or absent. A perforation appears as a dark area; sometimes it is obscured by secretions. With chronic otitis media a shiny red polypoid mass may partially or completely fill the perforation.

Tests for Hearing.   An audiometer must be used to determine accurately changes in auditory acuity, but one of the simpler tests should be performed as a part of every physical examination. Whenever possible the ability to recognize words should be tested. A quiet room is essential. Have the patient stand at a distance of 20 feet with his right ear toward you, covering his left ear with his left hand. He should be able to recognize whispered words at that distance. If not, walk slowly toward him until he does hear them. With marked impairment of hearing, spoken words may be required. Determine the distance; then test the other ear in the same manner. Often it is necessary to use even cruder methods such as a tuning fork or watch. Determine the distance at which you hear the sound; compare the patient's hearing with yours.

Tuning Fork Tests.   If the hearing seems somewhat diminished special tuning fork tests may help to establish the type of deafness. To

[22] Bartolomeo Eustachio, Italian anatomist, 1520–74.

test for air conduction, hold the vibrating fork as close to the ear as possible, without actually touching the auricle. For bone conduction, place the base of the fork behind the ear on the mastoid area. If the hearing is normal, air conduction will be better than bone conduction (AC>BC). To verify this, test bone conduction and have the patient signal or tell you when the sound stops. Quickly shift the fork to test air conduction; he should again hear the note faintly (Rinne's[23] test). If air conduction is poorer than bone conduction there may be obstruction of the auditory canal, damage to the eardrum or middle ear disease. If there is disease of the labyrinth or neural pathways, air and bone conduction may both be decreased but the normal relationship is preserved.

For Weber's[24] test, hold the handle of the vibrating tuning fork against the forehead or vertex of the skull in the midline, and ask the patient if he hears the sound. If he does, ask him in which ear he hears it. That should confuse him because normally there is no difference; he may hesitate or be unable to tell you. If he immediately says that he hears it in one ear, the answer is reliable. With nerve deafness of one ear, the sound seems louder in the other ear; with otitis media or an occluded auditory canal the sound is louder in the affected ear.

THE NOSE

External Examination. The size and contour of the nose are the concern primarily of the artist or the lover, not the physician; he is interested only when gross abnormalities are present. In men, a crooked nose is not rare; often it is considered a badge of honor, due to a fracture incurred in sports. Chronic nasal obstruction, especially if it occurs in early childhood, may produce narrowing of the nose and result in mouth breathing, giving the adenoid facies. A saddle-shaped nose results from destruction of the nasal bones, often by syphilis but occasionally by some other disease. The bulbous nose (*rhinophyma*) is produced by hypertrophy of the skin and sebaceous glands in the late stages of acne rosacea. Abnormal redness with dilated venules may occur with chronic alcoholism but it is also seen in total abstainers. With severe dyspnea and with emotional stress the alae nasi may alternately dilate (flare) and then contract, synchronous with inspiration and expiration.

Intranasal Examination. A head mirror to focus artificial light is the preferred type of illumination for an adequate examination; a flashlight is a poor substitute and for emergency use only. Place the mirror as close as possible to your eye and adjust the angle so that the light shines

[23] Friedrich Heinrich Rinne, German otologist, 1819–68.
[24] Friedrich Eugen Weber, German otologist, 1832–91.

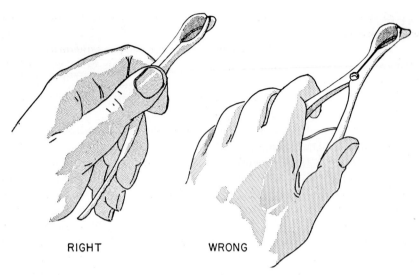

RIGHT   WRONG

Fig. 50.   Proper and improper way to hold nasal speculum (From Proetz, A. W., *in* Cecil, R. L., and Conn, H. F.: The Specialties in General Practice. 2nd ed. Philadelphia, W. B. Saunders Co., 1957.)

on the patient's nose; then move your head forward or backward until the light is sharply focused. A nasal speculum is also needed; this should be held in the left hand if you are right-handed (Fig. 50). The right hand is used to change the position of the head as various areas are inspected, or for handling instruments.

The vestibule is covered by skin that has hairs (*vibrissae*); this is the usual site of furuncles of the nose. Beyond that point the nose is lined by a mucous membrane that is moderately red in color. On the lateral wall directly beyond the vestibule the inferior turbinate can be seen; above this is the middle turbinate. At or near the midline is the nasal septum, formed by cartilage anteriorly and bone farther back.

THE SEPTUM.   The nasal septum is rarely straight and seldom exactly in the midline; minor aberrations are to be expected. A marked displacement, gross irregularity or angulation and large projections (ridges or spurs) should be recorded. If a perforation is present it is often in the anterior (cartilaginous) portion; this may appear more striking if light is directed into one nostril while you look into the other one. A history of an intranasal operation (submucous resection) may be obtained; syphilis or exposure to chromic acid or chromates are two other common causes for this. At a point about one centimeter from the vestibule and one centimeter upward from the floor of the nose there is a plexus of vessels (Kiesselbach's[25] area). This is the most common

[25] Wilhelm Kiesselbach, German otolaryngologist, 1839–1902.

site of nasal bleeding (*epistaxis*), which may result from trauma but which also occurs in various diseases.

THE TURBINATES. To examine the turbinates satisfactorily a local vasoconstrictor is generally applied to shrink the tissues. Without this, you will probably be able to see no more than the anterior two-thirds of the inferior turbinate and the anterior half of the middle turbinate; the superior turbinate will rarely be visible.

With inflammation the turbinates become swollen, especially the inferior ones, and acquire a deeper red color. In vasomotor or allergic rhinitis ("rose cold"; "hay fever") the turbinates are very pale, glistening and water-logged. Occasionally nasal polyps may be seen; these are round or ovoid pale gelatinous masses that look somewhat like white currants or peeled grapes. They are usually associated with nasal allergy.

SECRETIONS. The amount and character of nasal discharge is important. In a healthy nose there is a small amount of mucus only. In allergic rhinitis the discharge is profuse and watery. With the common cold (*coryza*) there is a tremendous outpouring of clear watery mucus in the early or viral stage; later the secretions become much thicker and yellow (*mucopurulent* or *purulent*) if bacterial infection supervenes. With chronic infection of the paranasal sinuses the discharge is variable in amount and character but usually it is rather viscid. Often this tends to flow backward into the nasopharynx (*postnasal drip*).

Paranasal Sinuses. Only the frontal and maxillary sinuses can be examined without special procedures. Look for swelling or redness above one or both eyebrows, or in the malar region. To detect tenderness in the maxillary sinuses, apply pressure to both cheeks simultaneously; for the frontal sinuses, press upward on the floor of the sinuses just below and behind the eyebrows.

TRANSILLUMINATION OF THE SINUSES. This can be done only in a darkened room; a small flashlight can be used to provide illumination if a transilluminator is not available. Have the patient remove his upper denture, if he has one. Place the flashlight in his mouth with the bulb in the midline and pointed toward the palate. Have him close his mouth; cover the lips with your free hand. Compare the relative pinkness of the two pupils and of the two malar areas; look for crescents of light just below the lower eyelids. A marked difference in the two sides often indicates disease on the darker side. To examine the frontal sinuses place the bulb near the naso-orbital angle so that the light shines upward through the roof of the orbit; shield the light with your other hand. Test each side alternately, comparing the size of the sinuses and the intensity of illumination.

Developmental differences are common and are often misinterpreted as pathologic changes. When disease of the sinuses is known to be present or is suspected, x-ray studies are indicated.

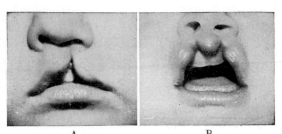

Fig. 51. Harelip. *A*, Unilateral; *B*, bilateral. (From Thoma, K. H., and Robinson, H. B. G.: Oral and Dental Diagnosis. 5th ed. Philadelphia, W. B. Saunders Co., 1960.)

A   B

THE LIPS

The examination of the mouth begins with the lips. Abnormal color may occur with anemia, polycythemia or cyanosis; cosmetics may simulate, alter or conceal this. Numerous small dots of brown pigment resembling freckles may be clustered around the mouth, on the lips and in the oral mucosa; these are seen in persons with multiple polyposis of the intestines (Peutz[26] syndrome). Abnormal contour can result from edema or from scars of disease or injury such as those that result from congenital syphilis or from accidents. Harelip is due to failure of union of the frontonasal and maxillary processes during fetal life. It may be unilateral or bilateral, partial or complete (Fig. 51). Surgical repair is usually performed early in infancy; in adults only a faint scar may remain. Congenital syphilis may produce linear scars radiating outward from the borders and angles of the lips (*rhagades*) (Fig. 52). Enlargement of the lips is seen in acromegaly, cretinism and myxedema. Abnormal dryness with cracks and fissures occurs in prolonged febrile states, with dehydration or from excessive heat such as sunburn. Inflammation (*cheilitis*) results from trauma or infection. Fissuring and dry scaling of the vermilion, especially at the angles of the mouth (*cheilosis*), often indicates riboflavin deficiency. Thickening and desquamation, and sometimes fissures, are seen in perlèche, a monilial infection. Tremor of the lips accompanies certain neurologic diseases or emotional disturbances.

Herpes Simplex. The common "fever blister" or "cold sore" is due to a viral infection; it produces an acute vesicular eruption chiefly on or around the lips, but other areas of the face may also be involved (Fig. 53). Although it occurs with pneumococcal pneumonia, meningococcal meningitis and malaria, the common cold or excessive exposure to ultraviolet light more often seems to be the precipitating factor. Recurrent episodes may accompany menstruation. This lesion should be differentiated from herpes zoster, a similar but more serious eruption that may occur in the distribution of one or more branches of the fifth cranial nerve.

[26] John Law Augustine Peutz, Dutch internist, 1886–1957.

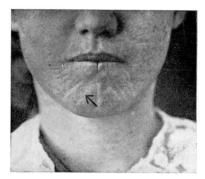

Fig. 52.   Rhagades and hacking (scars) produced by infiltrative and erosive syphilids about the mouth and chin in infancy. (From Stokes, J. H., Beerman, H., and Ingraham, N. R., Jr.: Modern Clinical Syphilology. 3rd ed. Philadelphia, W. B. Saunders Co., 1944.)

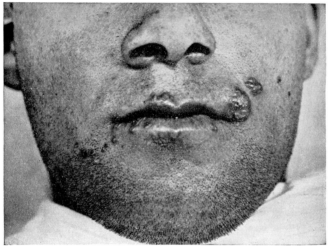

Fig. 53.   Herpes simplex. (From Andrews, G. C.: Diseases of the Skin. 3rd ed. Philadelphia, W. B. Saunders Co., 1946.)

Fig. 54.   Chancre of lip proved by darkfield examination. (From Lewis, G. M., *in* Cecil, R. L., and Conn, H. F. (eds.): The Specialties in General Practice. 3rd ed. Philadelphia, W. B. Saunders Co., 1964.)

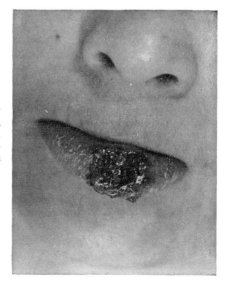

Ulcers.   A primary syphilitic lesion (*chancre*) may mimic herpes at first, but it persists and enlarges (Fig. 54). Usually it is a solitary lesion; the regional lymph nodes become enlarged soon after it appears.

Epidermoid carcinoma may resemble a chancre. It occurs almost invariably on the lower lip, particularly at the site of chronic irritation, and usually in males past middle life. The regional lymph nodes enlarge slowly and are small and hard. Any "sore" that persists two weeks or longer must not be ignored; darkfield examinations, serologic studies and diagnostic biopsy should be performed. White patches of thickened epithelium (*leukoplakia*) are occasionally seen on the lips; they must be considered potentially malignant.

THE TONGUE

When a patient is asked to open his mouth, the odds are good that he will immediately stick his tongue out. If he does, you may as well examine it at once. Our predecessors often seemed to make astute diagnoses after looking at the tongue; even today it sometimes has a silent message.

Size.   The size and shape of the tongue are variable. Enlargement (*macroglossia*) may be present with Mongolian idiocy, cretinism, myxedema or acromegaly. Such a tongue may have deeply serrated lateral borders from pressure against the teeth. Occasionally the tongue may be so large that the patient cannot close his mouth completely. Severe dehydration will produce a small wrinkled tongue (*microglossia*).

Movement.   Since the tongue is pushed forward by contraction of the intrinsic muscles, it should protrude in the midline. If the hypoglossal nerve supply to one side of the tongue is injured or destroyed, the tongue will deviate toward that side when it is protruded; hemiatrophy may develop later. Scars or other intrinsic or destructive lesions can also produce deviation by limiting muscular contractions. With facial palsy the tongue may seem to deviate because of facial asymmetry. Tremor of the tongue may be present with organic disease of the nervous system or with various other conditions such as thyrotoxicosis, alcoholism, old age or generalized muscular weakness. It can also be due to fatigue from keeping the tongue protruded while you examine it. Easy fatigability, with or without tremor, may occur in myasthenia gravis.

General Appearance.   The mucosa covering the tongue should be moist and glistening. Dryness of the mouth is often indicative of generalized dehydration, regardless of the specific cause; it can also be due to breathing through the mouth. Papillae should be visible on the upper surface and sides. The filiform papillae are most numerous and give the tongue its velvety appearance. The fungiform papillae appear as small red dots scattered irregularly on the surface; they are most numerous laterally and at the tip. The circumvallate papillae, usually about ten in number, form a "V" near the back of the tongue, with the apex posteriorly.

A coated tongue is rarely of clinical significance, but to many patients it is an infallible sign of "stomach trouble" of some sort. The coating is composed of desquamated epithelial cells, food particles, saliva and other foreign substances such as tobacco tars. A small amount of white or grayish material is physiologic; large amounts indicate poor oral hygiene.

ABNORMALITIES. Fungus infection occasionally occurs; this may produce a black shaggy coating (Fig. 55) or small, white, firmly adherent patches (*thrush*) if *C. albicans* is responsible. Prolonged administration of broad-spectrum antibiotics may suppress the normal bacterial flora and thus permit overgrowth of various fungi.

Abnormal smoothness of the tongue is due to atrophy of the papillae. This is a characteristic finding in pernicious anemia; it may also occur with secondary anemia or with gastrointestinal diseases (Fig. 56). Such a tongue is usually abnormally sensitive or actually sore. A furrowed tongue (Fig. 57) (*scrotal tongue*) has a number of deep and superficial grooves on the dorsal surface; this is often a congenital or familial variant, interesting but of no diagnostic significance. Another innocuous abnormality is the geographic tongue (Fig. 58). Here one sees areas with atrophic epithelium that are surrounded by elevations of thickened epithelium. From month to month these areas change in shape and position as they wander over the surface of the tongue. The "strawberry" tongue has enlarged, inflamed fungiform papillae that are very con-

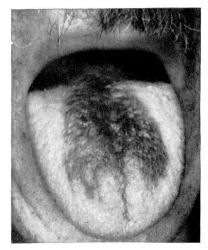

Fig. 55. Black hairy tongue. (From Thoma, K. H., and Robinson, H. B. G.: Oral and Dental Diagnosis. 5th ed. Philadelphia, W. B. Saunders Co., 1960.)

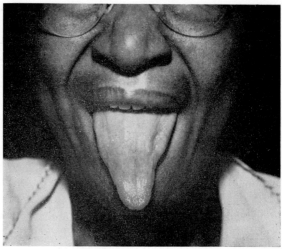

Fig. 56.   Thin, smooth tongue in primary pernicious anemia.

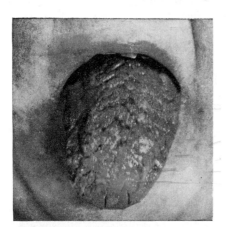

Fig. 57.   Furrowed tongue. (From
Andrews, G. C., and Domonkos, A. N.:
Diseases of the Skin. 5th ed. Philadelphia,
W. B. Saunders Co., 1963.)

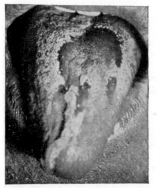

Fig. 58.   Geographic tongue (lingua geograph-
ica). (From Andrews, G. C.: Diseases of the Skin.
3rd ed. Philadelphia, W. B. Saunders Co., 1946.)

spicuous. It is usually associated with scarlet fever, but it may also be seen in other types of glossitis. Scars may be present as a result of injury; occasionally they are seen in an epileptic who has bitten his tongue during a convulsion. Leukoplakia similar to that seen on the lips may occur on the tongue and has the same significance; it is more common in heavy smokers (Figs. 59, 60).

ULCERS.   Whenever a persistent ulcer or "sore" develops on the tongue syphilis, tuberculosis and carcinoma are the three conditions that must be considered first. To establish a diagnosis, a biopsy is usually required. Twenty per cent of patients with cancer of the tongue are said to have syphilis, and many of them have x-ray evidence of pulmonary tuberculosis. A positive serologic test for syphilis or sputum that shows *M. tuberculosis* is no guarantee that carcinoma is not present.

Syphilis of the tongue may develop during any stage of the disease. The primary syphilitic lesion (chancre) is similar to that seen on the lip. In the secondary stage of syphilis the characteristic lesion is the *mucous patch*, single or multiple. This is a flat or slightly elevated, grayish, rounded area with superficial erosion, from 5 to 10 mm. in diameter,

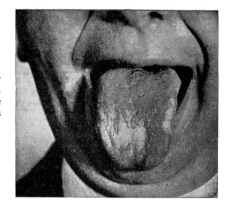

Fig. 59. Leukoplakia of upper surface and lateral margin of the tongue. (From Andrews, G. C.: Diseases of the Skin. 3rd ed. Philadelphia, W. B. Saunders Co., 1946.)

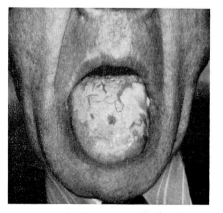

Fig. 60. Extensive leukoplakia of the tongue in a syphilitic patient. (Courtesy of E. P. Pendergrass, M.D.)

and covered by a delicate soggy membrane. Ulceration of a nodular lesion (*gumma*) may occur in late syphilis. Tuberculosis of the tongue is becoming less common; almost invariably it is secondary to active pulmonary tuberculosis. One or more indolent irregular ulcers develop; pain is a prominent feature. Carcinoma is usually epidermoid in type; the lateral margins and tip of the tongue are the common sites.

Sublingual Area.   Having examined the protruded portion and the upper surface of the tongue, next inspect the under surface. Ask the patient to touch his palate with the tip of the tongue, first in the midline and then on either side. The mucosa should be smooth, and the ridge of the frenum in the midline. On either side of the frenum there is a fairly large sinuous superficial vein; smaller veins are visible in other areas. Occasionally there are numerous small varicosities that are almost black; "caviar tongue" has been applied to this anomaly.

To inspect the extreme posterior portion of the tongue a laryngeal mirror must be used (p. 115).

THE ORAL MUCOSA

A tongue blade should be used to secure adequate exposure of all areas. Normally the mucosa is pale pink. In Addison's disease, bluish or brownish patches of melanin pigmentation may be present on the buccal mucosa and on the palate. Small bluish white spots surrounded by a red areola (Koplik[27] spots) appear in the prodromal stage of measles, before the skin eruption develops. Petechiae are occasionally seen; they should not be confused with small red areas that result from accidental biting of the cheek or from irritation due to a rough or carious tooth.

A mucous retention cyst may occur at any point; most frequently it is found on the labial mucosa, especially of the lower lip. It may be several millimeters in diameter and does not empty readily on pressure. A venous cavernous hemangioma presents as a small rounded blue protuberance; if pressed with a glass slide it can be seen to empty promptly. A papilloma is usually due to chronic irritation from dentures or a rough tooth. Leukoplakia may also develop on the buccal mucosa.

Salivary Ducts.   The orifices of the salivary ducts should be identified. Stensen's[28] ducts open opposite the second upper molar teeth, and Wharton's[29] ducts open under the tongue near the frenum. The sublingual gland usually has a number of small ducts (Rivinus'[30] ducts)

---

[27] Henry Koplik, New York pediatrician, 1858–1927.

[28] Niels Stensen, Dutch anatomist, physiologist and physician, who abandoned medicine for a nobler field and became first a priest and later a bishop, 1638–86.

[29] Thomas Wharton, English physician and anatomist, 1614–73.

[30] August Quirinus Rivinus, German anatomist and botanist, 1652–1723.

that open on the floor of the mouth. With disease of a salivary gland there may be increased redness of the orifice of the duct, and abnormal secretions may be visible with or without pressure on the involved gland. Cystic degeneration of a sublingual or submental salivary gland produces a bulge under the tongue; this was described by Hippocrates[31] who named it *ranula* because of its supposed resemblance to a "little frog belly."

THE TEETH

A sufficient number of healthy teeth, or adequate comfortable dentures, are essential for proper mastication. Mild ill-defined gastrointestinal symptoms may be due to inadequate grinding surfaces. The number of teeth present and their integrity or state of repair should be recorded.

Time of Eruption. The deciduous teeth, twenty in number, should be erupted by the time a child is 2½ years old; delayed dentition occurs with rickets, cretinism and other developmental defects. The time for eruption of the 32 permanent teeth is variable; approximate figures would be: central incisors, age 6 to 8 years; lateral incisors, age 7 to 9; cuspids ("eyeteeth"), 9 to 12; first premolars, 10 to 12; second premolars, 12 to 13; first molars, 6 to 7; second molars, 12 to 13; third molars ("wisdom teeth"), 17 to 30.

Color. The color of the teeth is variable. Few people normally have pearly or porcelain-white teeth; a faint tinge of yellow or brown is much more common. With poor dental hygiene, stains appear; broken or carious teeth are often brown or almost black. Pitting and brown spots may be seen in the teeth of persons who have used water with an excessively high fluoride content during the years when the teeth were developing. A tooth that has lost its nerve supply (devitalized) usually darkens slowly.

Abnormalities. If some of the teeth seem to be missing, ask when and why they were removed. Occasionally a person never has the expected number because of developmental defects or anomalies. Often one or more of the third molars will grow in an abnormal direction, become impacted and fail to erupt. Pressure on the adjacent tooth may cause pain at that point or referred pain elsewhere along the facial nerve. Malposition is not uncommon; the teeth erupt at an angle or are crowded together and jostled out of normal alignment. This may interfere with chewing or may cause chronic irritation of the tongue or buc-

[31] Hippocrates, Greek physician, born on the island of Cos about 460 B.C.; died circa 375 B.C. The famous Hippocratic Oath is usually attributed to him, although some scholars doubt that he wrote it.

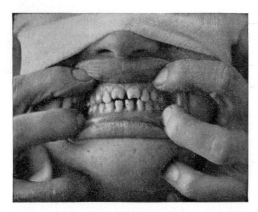

Fig. 61. Typical hutchinsonian teeth. (From Stokes, J. H., Beerman, H., and Ingraham, N. R., Jr.: Modern Clinical Syphilology. 3rd ed. Philadelphia, W. B. Saunders Co., 1944.)

cal mucosa. Correction may be undertaken for cosmetic reasons also; the orthodontist applies suitable "braces" until the alignment is satisfactory. Wandering may be seen following an extraction; the teeth adjacent to the gap slowly shift to partially bridge this space.

A loose tooth is usually the result of infection, either of the gums (*gingivitis*) or of the periodontal tissues (*pyorrhea alveolaris*). Loosening may also occur in metabolic disturbances such as hyperparathyroidism, in which there is generalized loss of the supporting bony structures. Wearing away of the biting surface (*attrition*) may be excessive and may advance to such a point that there is little or none of the tooth visible above the gingival margin.

Dental Caries.   Cavities may be present, or fillings may mark the site of previous trouble. When a cavity extends inward to the tooth pulp, pain results. This may be experienced only intermittently, as when hot, cold or sweet substances come in contact with the area, or it may be continuous. Infection may develop in such a tooth and spread to the root and adjacent bone to produce a localized alveolar abscess, or a more widespread cellulitis with edema and inflammation of the adjacent areas. Tapping the suspected tooth with a tongue blade or other hard object may cause pain, but a definite diagnosis cannot be made without dental roentgenograms.

Hutchinson's Teeth.   In 1861 Hutchinson[32] described certain abnormalities of the permanent upper central incisors that he correctly attributed to congenital syphilis. "The teeth are short and narrow. Instead of becoming wider as they descend from the gum, they are narrower at their free edge than at their crowns, their angles having been as if rounded off. In the center of their free edge is a deep vertical notch made by the breaking away or nondevelopment of the middle lobe of the tooth crown." In other words, these teeth are small, short, widely spaced, peg-shaped and notched (Fig. 61). This deformity should

[32] Sir Jonathan Hutchinson, English surgeon, 1828–1913.

not be confused with the notching sometimes seen in teeth otherwise
normal in size and shape; the latter occurs not infrequently and is often
seen in women who persistently use the upper incisors to help them
spread open their bobby pins. With syphilis, the first permanent molars
may also be abnormal in shape ("mulberry molars").

THE GINGIVAE

Normally the gums are pink, firm and in close apposition to the
teeth. Inflammation (gingivitis) may be localized or it may involve a
large area. There is abnormal redness, swelling and discomfort or pain;
slight bleeding may follow minor trauma such as brushing the teeth or
chewing hard foods. Infection may be limited to the gingivae, but not
infrequently it also involves other areas of the oral cavity. Vincent's[33]
infection ("trench mouth") due to *B. vincenti* and *F. plauti vincenti*
may involve the tonsils and pharynx also; necrosis frequently develops
(Fig. 62).

Atrophy is often present in elderly persons; it may also result from
chronic infection or improper brushing. Hypertrophy, if localized, is
usually the result of chronic irritation from a carious tooth or an improperly fitting prosthesis. Generalized hypertrophy may occur in pregnancy or with prolonged use of diphenylhydantoin (Dilantin) to control
epilepsy (Fig. 63). In leukemia the gingivae may be swollen, bleed
easily and have a reddish blue color (Fig. 64).

Dentures.   If dentures are worn the patient should remove them
so that adequate inspection of the gums is possible. An ulcer may develop if there is undue pressure at any point, or chronic irritation may
lead to the formation of a firm, pink, relatively insensitive granuloma.

[33] Henri Vincent, Paris physician, 1862–1950.

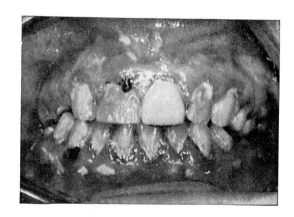

Fig. 62.   Acute Vin-
cent's infection. (From Pullen, R. L.: Medical Diag-
nosis. 2nd ed. Philadelphia,
W. B. Saunders Co., 1950.)

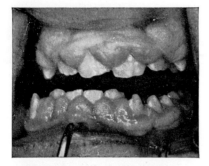

Fig. 63. Dilantin gingivitis. (From Thoma, K. H., and Robinson, H. B. G.: Oral and Dental Diagnosis. 5th ed. Philadelphia, W. B. Saunders Co., 1960.)

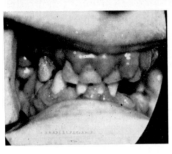

Fig. 64. Marked swelling of gums in a patient with acute leukemia.

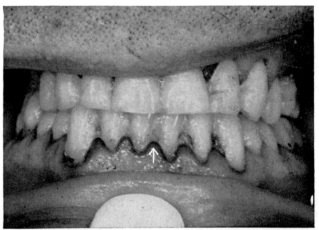

Fig. 65. Bismuth line along gingival margin. (From Thoma, K. H.: Oral Diagnosis. 3rd ed. Philadelphia, W. B. Saunders Co., 1946.)

Epulis. This is a tumor arising from the alveolar periosteum or from the periodontal membrane; it may develop between two teeth and spread them apart. Growth is very slow but often the lesion is malignant.

Pigmentation. With lead poisoning a narrow blue line may appear near the gingival margin. This is formed by microscopic dots of lead sulfide produced by bacterial action and occurs only when oral hygiene is neglected. A similar line can be produced by bismuth or mercury, formerly used extensively for treating syphilis (Fig. 65). This line is most easily recognized if a small wedge of paper is inserted between a tooth and the gingival margin. It should not be confused with a wider area of deep blue pigmentation seen occasionally in Negroes.

THE PALATE AND UVULA

Unless the tongue is abnormally large, these structures can usually be seen easily and adequately if the patient opens his mouth without protruding his tongue, and then breathes through his mouth. The anterior portion or hard palate has a somewhat irregular surface with rugae running transversely. Behind this is the soft palate, which is pinker in color; small superficial vessels are often visible there. The uvula projects downward from the posterior margin of the soft palate. It varies greatly in size and length; it may be partially or completely divided (*bifid*). If it is excessively long, surgical removal (staphylectomy) may be indicated.

Malformation.   Abnormalities of the palate are occasionally seen. Cleft palate results from failure of the palatal processes to unite; there is an abnormal communication in the midline between the buccal and nasal cavities. Harelip is frequently associated with this. A high, narrow palatal arch may result from prolonged nasal obstruction during infancy or early childhood due to hypertrophy of the adenoids or to marked irregularity of the nasal septum. It is also seen occasionally in a person with congenital syphilis.

A bony protuberance (*torus palatinus*) may be present at the point of union of the intermaxillary and palatomaxillary sutures (Fig. 66). It is somewhat irregular in outline, with one or more crypts that can become the site of inflammation; the patient often fears that he has cancer

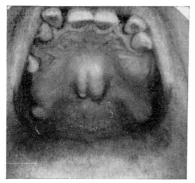 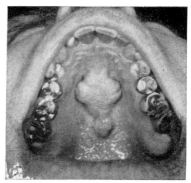

Fig. 66.   Torus palatinus. (From Thoma, K. H., and Robinson, H. B. G.: Oral and Dental Diagnosis. 5th ed. Philadelphia, W. B. Saunders Co., 1960.)

of the mouth. This malformation is of no medical significance, but it can interfere with proper fitting of an upper denture.

Perforation of either the hard or the soft palate may result from trauma, from infection or from gummatous destruction of the tissues in congenital or acquired syphilis.

Mobility.   The soft palate rises during swallowing, to close off the nasopharynx; it also moves with phonation. An attempt should be made to elicit the gag reflex by touching the posterior portion of the tongue or the pharyngeal wall with a tongue blade. This should be followed by elevation of the soft palate, gagging or cough, lacrimation, and contraction of the facial and abdominal muscles. If the reflex is hyperactive, regurgitation or vomiting may occur. A diminished or absent gag reflex is not always abnormal, but it suggests a lesion of the ninth (sensory) or tenth (motor) cranial nerve, either unilateral or bilateral.

THE TONSILS

The faucial tonsils, commonly called merely "the tonsils," are masses of lymphoid tissue and constitute a part of Waldeyer's[34] ring, which includes the faucial tonsils, the lingual tonsils, the pharyngeal masses or adenoids and the lateral bands. The tonsils lie just anterior to the pharynx, in fossae formed by the anterior and posterior tonsillar pillars. The mesial surface can usually be seen without difficulty, but for adequate examination of the entire anterior surface a retractor must be used to displace the anterior pillar laterally.

In an adult the tonsils usually project mesially slightly beyond the anterior pillars, but the size is variable. Marked enlargement or protrusion suggests infection or infiltration. The color is essentially the same as that of the oral mucosa. The surface may be relatively smooth or it may show deep indentations (*crypts*); these are often filled with desquamated epithelial cells and present as white spots or plugs. A red zone surrounding a plug suggests infection in the crypt.

A history of tonsillectomy does not mean that inspection of these areas can be omitted. It is often difficult to remove a tonsil completely; a small tonsillar tag may remain and be the site of disease. Occasionally these remnants of lymphoid tissue gradually hypertrophy; you may find what seems to be small or even normal-sized tonsils.

Infection.   In acute tonsillitis the entire tonsil is usually red and swollen. The surface may be studded with white or yellow dots of exudate; these may coalesce to form a membrane. In diphtheria a dull

[34] Wilhelm von Waldeyer, Berlin anatomist, 1836–1921.

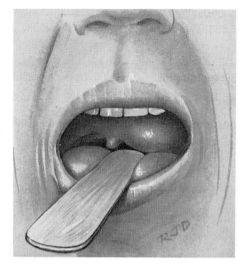

Fig. 67. Peritonsillar abscess (quinsy), left.

grayish membrane is present and is firmly adherent; if forcibly removed it leaves a raw or bleeding surface. A tonsil may also be the site of a tuberculous ulcer, a syphilitic lesion, a carcinoma or a lymphoma.

A peritonsillar abscess (quinsy) develops in the capsule, between the tonsil and the pharyngeal muscles. This tends to spread upward and may produce a bulge in the soft palate (Fig. 67).

THE PHARYNX

The oropharynx extends from the soft palate to the lingual surface of the epiglottis; the portion above the soft palate is called the nasopharynx.

Oropharynx. To examine the oropharynx a good light is essential, and a tongue blade is usually required. If a very active gag reflex is present it may be difficult to obtain more than a brief glimpse of this area without a local anesthetic.

PROCEDURE. When the patient sees the tongue blade he will probably open his mouth and protrude his tongue. Have him close his mouth and then open it again without putting his tongue out; it may be necessary to repeat this several times before he relaxes. Then have him breathe fairly rapidly through his mouth while you inspect the visible portion. Have him say "ah-h-h"; this will expose additional areas. Then gently place the tongue blade on the anterior two-thirds of the tongue and slowly depress it; sudden pressure will usually evoke a contraction of the tongue or a gag reflex and ruin the view.

The mucosa of the pharynx has a number of small vessels that are easily visible; this vascularity should not be mistaken for hyperemia or pharyngitis. Small rounded or irregular collections of lymphoid tissue are frequently seen; these are slightly elevated and paler than the adjacent mucosa.

A thin coat of clear mucus is normal; large amounts, in the absence of pharyngitis, usually have come from the nasopharynx or nose. Often this postnasal discharge is mucopurulent or even frankly purulent in character, indicating chronic rhinitis or sinusitis.

INFECTION. Acute pharyngitis is characterized by edema and hyperemia of the mucosa; exudate is occasionally present. Acute or chronic infection of one or more of the lymphoid follicles may occur; in such cases the nodules are moderately swollen and red, contrasting sharply with the paler mucosa. Localized bulging of the pharyngeal wall may be produced by a retropharyngeal abscess. Usually this is secondary to acute pharyngitis, but a more chronic form secondary to tuberculosis of the cervical spine or lymph nodes is occasionally seen. Benign or malignant tumors are uncommon, but can occur in the pharynx.

Nasopharynx. To examine this area completely a nasopharyngoscope is desirable. However, valuable information may be obtained by the proper use of a small postnasal mirror. Have the patient open his mouth but breathe through his nose, to relax the palate; this may seem difficult at first and may require a little practice. Warm the mirror, to prevent fogging, and focus the source of light on the plane of the uvula. Depress the tongue as much as possible and insert the mirror; avoid touching the uvula or the pharyngeal wall. Then rotate the mirror slowly until the entire oropharynx has been seen.

Locate first the posterior edge of the nasal septum. Then inspect the posterior nares (*choanae*) and the posterior portions of the turbinates. Rotate the mirror to bring into view the lateral wall of the pharynx. This allows you to see a depression (*fossa of Rosenmüller*[35]), a cartilaginous ridge (*torus tubaris*) and the internal opening of the eustachian tube. Variable amounts of lymphoid tissue will also be seen; this is the adenoid or pharyngeal tonsil. If excessive in amount, it may obstruct the nasopharynx and lead to mouth breathing, or it may cause occlusion of the eustachian tubes, thus impairing the hearing and predisposing to infection of the middle ear. Finally, the posterior aspect of the soft palate and uvula should be inspected.

THE BREATH

Offensive breath ("halitosis") is designated *fetor oris*. In most in-

[35] Johann Christian Rosenmüller, German anatomist, 1771–1820.

stances this is due to improper oral hygiene, particularly the failure to remove decomposing food particles from between the teeth or from under dentures. Less common causes are chronic gingivitis or pyorrhea alveolaris, infection of the tonsils or of the lymphoid tissue in the throat, infection of the nasal mucosa with resulting atrophic rhinitis (*ozena*), or other inflammatory or neoplastic lesions in the buccal cavity. Pyloric obstruction leading to retention and putrefaction of gastric contents may cause the breath to become unspeakably fetid. Retention of secretions in bronchiectasis, particularly if infection results in a gangrenous lesion of the lung, may produce fetor oris of such overpowering intensity that the presence of gangrene may be suspected as one approaches the patient.

Acetone imparts a characteristic sweetish, fruity odor to the breath. The presence of acetone is frequently due to uncontrolled diabetes, but acidosis can also occur in conditions such as dehydration or uremia. More commonly the breath of the uremic patient has an odor resembling that of ammonia or urine. Detection of alcohol on the breath should never lead you to assume that the staggering gait, mental confusion, coma or other neurologic disturbance is due to intoxication; an autopsy may show a fractured skull, intracranial hemorrhage or other lesion that should have been diagnosed and treated. In severe liver failure there is often a peculiar musty or mousy odor. Paraldehyde and certain other drugs impart characteristic odors to the breath, as does the inhalation of illuminating gas.

THE LARYNX

Inspection of the larynx is not a part of the routine physical examination but is mandatory if there are symptoms such as hoarseness, croup or a "croupy cough," or partial or complete aphonia. Direct laryngoscopy is the most satisfactory method but this requires special equipment and training. However, every physician should be able to do mirror laryngoscopy.

Procedure. If the gag reflex is very active an anesthetic lozenge will diminish it; occasionally spraying the throat with a small amount of a local anesthetic solution will be necessary. Allow sufficient time for this to be effective before starting the examination. Have the patient open his mouth, protrude his tongue and breathe through his mouth. Wrap a piece of gauze around the tip of the tongue and grasp this with your left hand, or have the patient hold it. Focus the light on the uvula. Warm a mirror of suitable size (to prevent fogging) and insert it carefully; avoid touching the tongue or pharynx unless they are well anesthetized. Gently displace the uvula and soft palate upward and backward, and rotate the mirror so that the epiglottis and larynx can be seen. Remember that in the laryngeal mirror the anterior structures of the larynx appear in the upper portion of the mirror, and the posterior (aretynoid) region is seen lower down.

THE EPIGLOTTIS.   This is of variable size, shape, color and contour; the free edge is usually thin and slightly curled. When at rest it may obscure the anterior portion of the vocal cords.

THE VOCAL CORDS.   The false cords lie just above the true cords; these appear as two bands of tissue that converge from below (posteriorly). They are dull pink and look thicker than the true cords. Although capable of closing the larynx, they usually do not move during the examination. The true vocal cords are seen below the false cords and look almost white. Anteriorly (at the top of the mirror) they meet in the midline; posteriorly they are attached to the vocal processes of the aretynoid cartilages. The latter move with phonation and respiration, widening and narrowing the space between the cords.

MOTILITY.   To test motility, have the patient sing a high-pitched "e-e-e-e-e." The cords should come together and appear taut; vibration may be visible. At the same time the epiglottis should tense slightly, thus providing a better view of the anterior commissure.

LESIONS.   In acute laryngitis the entire area including the cords will appear red and edematous. In chronic laryngitis slight congestion and thickening of the cords is commonly seen. This may be present when there is chronic infection elsewhere in the respiratory tract, such as sinusitis or bronchitis. It also occurs in singers, public speakers and others who continually use or strain their vocal cords.

Paralysis may be unilateral or bilateral, partial or complete. Partial paralysis of one cord may be asymptomatic. Complete unilateral paralysis causes hoarseness; bilateral paralysis produces aphonia. Unilateral paralysis is due to injury or destruction of one laryngeal nerve. This may be caused by compression in the neck by a goiter or other tumor, or by an intrathoracic lesion such as a mediastinal tumor, an aneurysm of the aortic arch or a tremendously dilated left atrium, which develops occasionally with mitral stenosis. In rare instances paralysis is a complication of an operation on the thyroid or other structures in the neck. Bilateral paralysis may be due to the same causes, but more commonly it is a sequel of disease of the tenth nerve nuclei in the medulla.

A tumor of the vocal cord may be benign or malignant. Benign vocal nodules are sometimes seen in singers or public speakers. Papilloma, polyps and carcinoma can also occur. Laryngeal tuberculosis is now rarely seen; it is a complication of uncontrolled pulmonary tuberculosis. Biopsy is necessary to establish the etiology of any vocal cord lesion.

Before withdrawing the mirror, examine the posterior surface of the tongue; unsuspected disease may be present there.

PALPATION OF THE ORAL CAVITY

In certain instances palpation will provide additional information to supplement the findings on inspection; it may also be the only simple way to discover an abnormality. A glove should always be worn; this should be moistened to remove any powder present and to provide lubrication. A mouth gag of some sort is almost mandatory if the patient is a child or an unconscious or uncooperative adult.

A sore or tender tongue may appear normal on the surface, but a nodule or inflammatory swelling may be palpable in the deeper tissues. A swollen salivary gland may be due to a calculus in the duct. Minor degrees of motor weakness or atrophy may also be felt before they are noticeable on inspection. Any ulcer, nodule or other abnormality should be palpated to determine its consistency and true extent. In a child, the size of the adenoids can be determined by the palpating finger; rhinoscopy is often difficult or unsatisfactory in young children.

An internal carotid artery can be felt in the lateral wall of the pharynx at the pharyngopalatine muscle, especially if pressure is also exerted externally in the carotid fossa. Decreased or absent pulsations in one of these vessels may precede or accompany transient or permanent contralateral cerebral symptoms such as hemiparesis or hemianesthesia. If the pulsations in one carotid artery are diminished, and if compatible neurologic signs and symptoms are present, cerebral arteriography may be advisable. Surgical procedures can often restore adequate circulation.

VI

The Neck

For examination of the neck, inspection and palpation are most important; auscultation is occasionally used. Certain general features should be observed first; specific structures are then studied.

PRELIMINARY OBSERVATIONS

Size and Shape.   The size and shape depend largely upon the habitus of the person and therefore are variable in health; disease may also produce alterations. The neck may appear gracile and swanlike in a small-boned asthenic person with a long flat chest and sloping shoulders; the same appearance may be simulated by severe malnutrition or cachexia. The stocky, barrel-chested, broad-shouldered person has a relatively large neck that appears short; severe pulmonary emphysema may produce the same picture.

Scars.   If a scar is present, the history should have mentioned the reason for it. In older persons tuberculosis of the cervical lymph nodes (scrofula; the king's evil) may have led to spontaneous rupture with drainage, or to surgical incision or excision of the diseased nodes. This is now a rare disease in young people. The scar of a skillfully performed thyroidectomy is easily overlooked if it is concealed in one of the natural transverse creases in the skin at the base of the neck. Have the patient tip his head backward to tense the skin, or raise the rolls of fat as you look.

Symmetry.   Asymmetry may be due to disease of the vertebrae, but more often it is produced by enlargement of one or more of the normal structures in the neck; some of these will be considered later.

Movement.   An abnormal position of the head and neck is apparent immediately; this may be temporary or permanent. Limitation

118

of motion is less obvious; this is considered in Chapter XXI. Muscle spasm is a frequent cause of limitation of motion; usually this is unilateral. It may follow chilling, acute or chronic strain, trauma or infection in the tissues adjacent to the muscle. Occasionally it is congenital or a sequel of birth injury.

Vertebral column disease may also cause limitation of motion or stiffness of the neck. Arthritis is the most common; fracture, dislocation, "whiplash" injury, tuberculosis, malignancy or an injury of the intervertebral disk must also be considered.

Abnormal movements of the head may be seen in elderly persons or as a manifestation of chorea. In myasthenia gravis or other diseases causing severe muscular weakness the patient may be unable to hold his head in any one position for more than a short time. Rhythmic nodding of the head, synchronous with the pulse, may be seen in a person with insufficiency of the aortic valve (p. 277).

Meningeal Irritation.   Meningeal irritation, acute or chronic, will affect flexion and extension; this may range from slight limitation of motion to complete fixation. To test for this, have the patient lie on his back. Ask him to attempt to bend his neck until his chin touches his chest. If he cannot do this, or if he is too ill to cooperate, place one hand under the head and attempt to flex the neck passively; repeat this maneuver several times to rule out voluntary resistance. If flexion is limited, watch the legs; involuntary flexion of the thighs and legs may occur while the head is being raised (Brudzinski's[1] neck sign). Occasionally the spasm of the paravertebral muscles is so intense that the neck is hyperextended, the entire trunk is bowed forward, and the patient rests on his occiput and heels; this is called *opisthotonos* and is rarely seen except with tetanus.

Meningeal irritation may be the result of actual infection of the meninges (*meningitis*). It can also be caused by certain toxins such as lead (*acute lead encephalopathy*), or by the presence of blood in the subarachnoid space or over the cerebral cortex. In infancy and childhood particularly, certain systemic febrile illnesses are accompanied by increased intracranial pressure and irritation of the meninges without demonstrable invasion by the causative organism; this gives rise to a similar condition, called *meningismus*.

A sensation of tightness in the posterior cervical muscles is not uncommon in persons working under tension. This often appears during the afternoon and becomes progressively more annoying; headache may accompany it. Limitation of motion is not present, but often the muscles feel firm or tense and sometimes they are moderately sensitive to palpation.

[1] Josef von Brudzinski, Polish physician, 1874–1917.

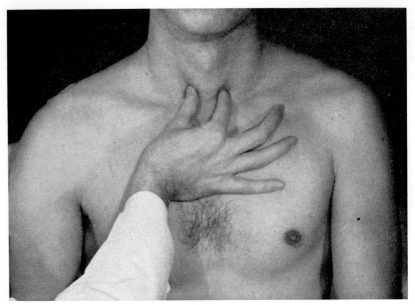

Fig. 68. Palpating the position of the trachea.

THE TRACHEA

Position.   The trachea should lie in the midline. In a very thin neck it is easily seen, especially in men, in whom the thyroid cartilages are large and protrude (Adam's[2] apple). Sometimes these cartilages are asymmetrical or slightly rotated, giving a false impression of tracheal deviation. Unless the entire trachea can be seen, the position must be determined by palpating it just above the sternal notch with the thumb and index finger (Fig. 68).

Displacement.   Lateral displacement may be due to pressure from a visible or palpable mass in the neck such as a large thyroid, or it may be produced by intrathoracic disease. The trachea can be pushed to one side by an intrathoracic mass of any type, or it can be pulled laterally by fibrosis or some other contracting process; some of these will be discussed later (Chapter XIII).

Other Signs.   Certain historic signs are worthy of brief mention. *Tracheal tug* (Oliver's[3] sign) was described by Oliver in 1878 as follows: "Place the patient in the erect position and direct him to close his mouth and elevate his chin to the fullest extent, then grasp the cricoid cartilage between the thumb and finger and use gentle upward pressure on it; when a dilatation or aneurysm exists, the pulsations of the aorta will

[2] Adam, a renowned agrarian who sustained a disastrous loss following a venture into the fruit market.

[3] Sir Thomas Oliver, English physician, 1853–1932.

be distinctly felt transmitted through the trachea to the hand." In 1879 Cardarelli[4] described the physical sign of aortic aneurysm that bears his name; it is a visible and palpable transverse pulsation of the laryngo-tracheal tube synchronous with the pulse. It is elicited by displacing the larynx to the left by pressure on the thyroid cartilage.

CERVICAL VEINS

Prominence. The jugular veins should not be prominent on in-spection when a person is erect and breathing quietly. Coughing, strain-ing or even talking may cause brief fluctuating filling and emptying of these veins. Persistent distention, best seen in the external jugulars, is most commonly due to right-sided heart failure. It may also be produced by compression or thrombosis of the superior vena cava, or by any other process that interferes with normal venous circulation in this area.

When a person is recumbent the veins fill and frequently are very prominent. To differentiate this from pathologic distention, gradually elevate the head of the bed, or have the patient change position slowly from supine to upright. In a normal person the visible portions of the veins will empty at once. With a moderate increase in venous pressure the meniscus will be seen fluctuating somewhere between the clavicle and the angle of the jaw. If the pressure is extremely high the veins will remain filled to the angle of the jaw even when the person is upright (Fig. 69).

Pulsations. If the veins are visible, look for pulsations in the column of blood; these must not be confused with impulses transmitted

[4] Antonio Cardarelli, Italian physician, 1831–1926.

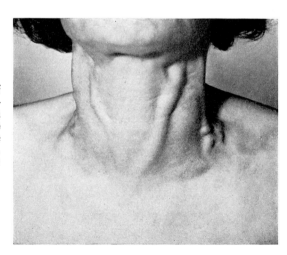

Fig. 69. Distention of veins of the neck in right-sided cardiac failure. (From Leaman, W. G., Jr.: The Management of the Cardiac Patient. Philadelphia, J. B. Lippincott Company, 1940.)

from the carotid arteries. In tricuspid regurgitation the fluctuation in the column may be very marked; in congestive failure or with obstruction of the return flow of blood, movement may be slight or absent. Abnormalities of cardiac rhythm may also be reflected in the jugular pulsations.

ARTERIES

Pulsations.   The pulsations of the common carotid artery should not be visible except in a very thin person, but should be palpable when the finger tips are pressed inward and backward along the anterior border of the sternomastoid muscle. Normally the artery can be felt from the sternal notch to the angle of the jaw. Palpation of the internal carotid artery has already been described (p. 117). Visible pulsations may appear after strenuous exercise or with emotional stress. They may also indicate the presence of disease states such as thyrotoxicosis, anemia, hypertension or aortic regurgitation. With arteriosclerosis, the innominate or the common carotid artery may become elongated, tortuous and easily felt or seen writhing under the skin. Even the arch of the aorta may participate in this vascular dance in the suprasternal notch. An aneurysm of the aortic arch can give rise to a similar picture; an aneurysm of the innominate artery or of either carotid artery will produce a visible bulge that is definitely pulsatile on palpation (Fig. 70).

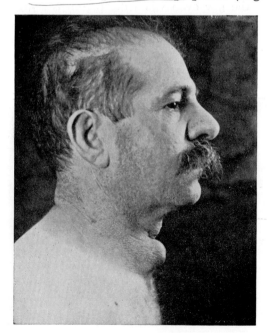

Fig. 70.   Aneurysm of the innominate artery.

Auscultation. Whenever an abnormality of an artery is seen or felt, auscultation is indicated. A murmur or bruit may be heard in systole, in diastole or in both. The bell of the stethoscope should rest lightly on the surface; firm pressure will indent or flatten the artery and may give rise to a factitial but similar sound.

THE THYROID

Anatomy. The thyroid is composed of two lateral lobes and the isthmus that connects them. The lateral lobes are roughly pyramidal in shape, and from 3 to 6 cm. high. The isthmus is rarely more than 1 cm. high, and crosses the trachea in the region of the second to the fourth tracheal rings. The thyroid is adherent to the trachea; therefore it rises and falls with swallowing unless it is fixed to other structures by malignancy or by surrounding infection.

Except in a very thin person, a normal thyroid is not definitely visible. In a very well nourished person a pad of fat is sometimes present in the suprasternal region; this may look like an enlarged isthmus, but it does not move with deglutition.

Palpation. One method of palpating the thyroid is shown in Figures 71 and 72. Others prefer to stand behind the seated patient and examine the isthmus and both lateral lobes with the finger tips (Fig. 73). Palpation should be performed with the patient's head in a normal position, and with his neck flexed and then hyperextended. Determine the size, shape, position, contour and consistency of each portion of the gland.

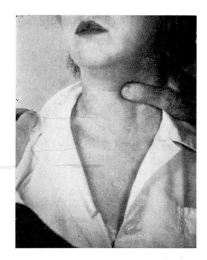

Fig. 71. Method of dislocating the larynx out of its bed to permit palpation of the lobe of the thyroid through and through. The finger pressing the larynx out of its position is applied against the thyroid cartilage where it will not produce coughing or choking. Note how definitely the right thyroid lobe can be dislocated outward for through and through palpation. (From Lahey, F. H., and Hare, H. F.: J.A.M.A., 145:689, 1951.)

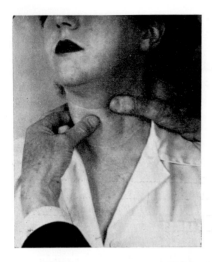

Fig. 72. Method of palpating the dislocated right lobe of the thyroid. Note the index finger behind the right sternocleidomastoid muscle, which has been relaxed by turning the chin to the right. The examining thumb is applied over the thyroid lobe in front as the larynx is dislocated to the right by the thumb of the other hand. When the patient is asked to swallow, the thyroid lobe to be palpated ascends and descends between the index finger and the thumb so that it can be thoroughly palpated for a nodule, the consistency that goes with hyperplasia characteristic of hyperthyroidism, or the ligneous type of infiltration characteristic of thyroiditis. (From Lahey, F. H., and Hare, H. F.: J.A.M.A., *145*:689, 1951.)

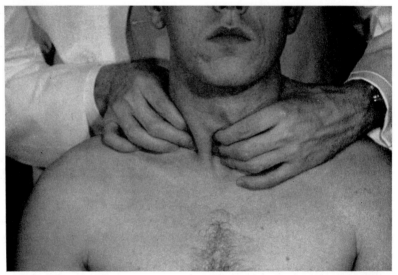

Fig. 73. Palpation of thyroid with examiner behind patient.

Goiter. Enlargement of the thyroid (goiter) may be minimal or massive. One lobe alone may be enlarged or the entire gland may be involved. The consistency may be soft, firm or hard; the latter suggests inflammation (*thyroiditis*) or carcinoma. The enlargement may be diffuse, or there may be one or more nodules present; record the size, shape and consistency of each nodule, and its position in the gland. Attempt to determine the lower border of an enlarged gland by having the patient tip his head far backward. Sometimes this border cannot be felt; the thyroid extends downward behind the sternum (*substernal* or *intrathoracic goiter*) (**Fig. 74**).

If the thyroid is enlarged, palpate lightly for a vascular thrill; this is the vibration produced by the flow of blood through the gland. Then listen for the audible component or *bruit,* a continuous humming sound with accentuation during cardiac systole.

TYPES OF GOITER.   Enlargement of the thyroid, whether diffuse or nodular, may be accompanied by normal thyroid activity or by overactivity (*hyperthyroidism*). Thus there are four general types of goiter.

Nontoxic Diffuse Goiter (Colloid Goiter).   This may develop during childhood or adolescence as a result of iodine deficiency; it is more common in females. It may also appear later in life, especially during pregnancy (Fig. 75); iodine deficiency does not seem to be the major factor here. If large enough, the thyroid may displace or compress the trachea or esophagus, giving rise to cough or to difficulty in swallowing (*dysphagia*); surgical intervention may be necessary to relieve the pressure. Occasionally partial excision is performed for cosmetic reasons alone.

Nontoxic Nodular Goiter.   This may be the end result of colloid goiter, or it may develop as a result of local hyperplasia of thyroid tissue (Figs. 76, 77). Occasionally the nodules are large enough to cause pressure symptoms.

Toxic Diffuse Goiter (Graves' Disease; Basedow's Disease; Parry's Disease[5]). This may develop slowly or very rapidly. Overproduction of thyroid hormone occurs; this leads to various eye signs (p. 94), tachycardia, nervousness, tremor, weight loss and other manifestations of increased metabolic activity.

Toxic Nodular Goiter.   This rarely produces the typical eye signs, and usually does not lead to as marked symptoms of toxicity as does a toxic diffuse goiter.

Thyroiditis.   Inflammation of the thyroid is occasionally seen; this may begin acutely with chills, fever and leukocytosis, together with local redness and tenderness of the gland. In most instances the infection is due to streptococci, staphylococci or pneumococci. Chronic thyroiditis of two types is also recognized; the gland becomes firm or hard and mild hypothyroidism may develop. The Hashimoto[6] type is currently attributed to autosensitization to thyroglobulin, with subsequent antigen-antibody reaction occurring in the gland. Slow enlargement occurs, with little or no tenderness. The etiology of the Riedel[7] type is still unknown. Differentiation usually depends upon microscopic study of the tissue.

---

[5] Robert James Graves, Irish physician, 1796–1853; Carl Adolph von Basedow, German physician, 1790–1854; Caleb Hillier Parry, English physician, 1755–1822. Although Parry's description (1786) antedated the papers of Graves (1835) and of Basedow (1840), his name is rarely seen in connection with this disease.

[6] Hakaru Hashimoto, Japanese surgeon, 1881–1934.

[7] Bernard Moritz Carl Ludwig Riedel, German surgeon, 1846–1916.

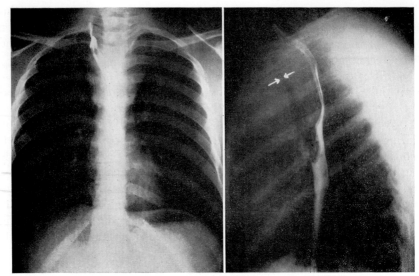

Fig. 74. *A*, Substernal enlargement of the thyroid. Note the supracardiac shadow and displacement of the barium-filled esophagus and air-filled trachea. *B*, Lateral roentgenographic view showing narrowing of the trachea (arrows) and the separation of the trachea and esophagus caused by pressure from the enlarged thyroid. (This tumor at operation was malignant.) (Courtesy of E. P. Pendergrass, M.D.)

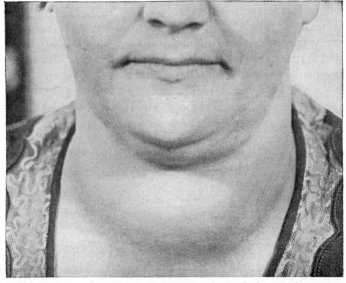

Fig. 75. Diffuse enlargement of the thyroid gland that is characteristic of a parenchymatous goiter. The enlargement developed about the time of the birth of the patient's first child. (From Pullen, R. L.: Medical Diagnosis. 2nd ed. Philadelphia, W. B. Saunders Co., 1950.)

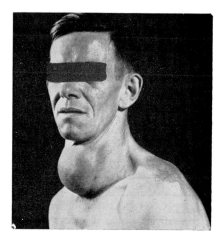

Fig. 76.   Huge nontoxic nodular goiter.

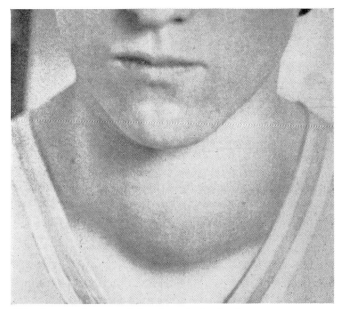

Fig. 77.   Large adenoma of the thyroid gland. The new process extended beneath the sternum and displaced the trachea. (From Pullen, R. L.: Medical Diagnosis. 2nd ed. Philadelphia, W. B. Saunders Co., 1950.)

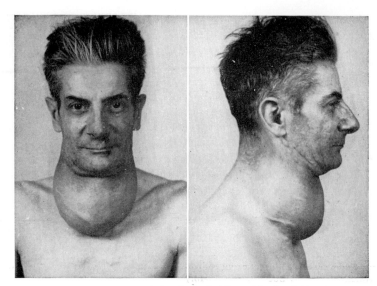

Fig. 78.   Malignant tumor of the thyroid. (From Hardy, J. D.: Surgery and the Endocrine System. Philadelphia, W. B. Saunders Co., 1952.)

Carcinoma.   This may develop in a pre-existing nodule, or it may occur in a previously normal gland. The gland itself may be nodular or smooth, but the malignant area is usually hard or stony on palpation, and feels firmly fixed. The nearby lymph nodes may also be invaded and become large and firm (Fig. 78).

LYMPH NODES

Location.   As shown in Figure 79 there are a number of lymph nodes in the neck. Also, there are nodes in the suboccipital region, not shown in this diagram. When healthy, these are small enough so that they are rarely palpable or visible; if diseased, they may enlarge tremendously. It is essential to look at each side of the neck, and to compare the two sides; asymmetry may indicate enlargement of one or more of these nodes.

Palpation.   This is best performed with the patient seated; nodes in the supraclavicular region may drop down behind the clavicle and not be felt if the patient is lying down. Stand behind him, and with gentle pressure of the finger tips go over the entire area, comparing the two sides. Then have him tilt his head to the right so that you can feel for nodes under the relaxed sternomastoid muscle; repeat this procedure on the left (Fig. 80). Whenever a node is felt, determine its size, shape,

129

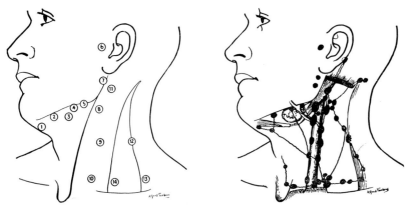

Fig. 79. Deep lymphatics of the neck. *Submaxillary group:* 1, submental; 2, preglandular; 3, intraglandular; 4, prevascular; 5, retrovascular. *Parotid group:* 6, preauricular; 7, infra-auricular. *Internal jugular chain:* 8, subdigastric; 9, midcervical; 10, lower cervical. *Spiral accessory chain:* 11, upper; 12, middle; 13, lower. 14, *Transverse cervical chain.* (From Martin, H.: Cancer of the Head and Neck. New York, American Cancer Society, Inc., 1949.)

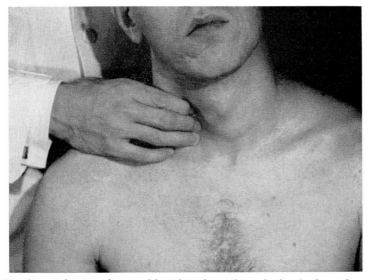

Fig. 80. Palpation of cervical lymph nodes. Tilting the head relaxes the sternocleidomastoid muscle and facilitates adequate examination.

consistency and sensitivity, and whether it is freely movable or fixed to the skin or deeper structures.

Bimanual Palpation.   If enlargement of submaxillary or submental nodes is suspected, bimanual palpation is desirable. With a gloved finger, press downward on the floor of the mouth and make upward pressure externally with the other hand. At the same time you can palpate the salivary glands, which should not be mistaken for enlarged lymph nodes.

Enlarged Nodes.   These may result from local infection, may be a manifestation of a generalized systemic infection or disease, or may occur with conditions involving primarily the lymphoid tissues. The most common cause is infection in the region drained by the enlarged node. Acute tonsillitis and pharyngitis head the list; one or more of the nodes in the anterior triangle will become enlarged and tender. The swelling may persist for some days after the acute process has subsided. Other acute infections such as a dental alveolar abscess, gingivitis or stomatitis will also produce enlargement. Infection of the scalp and also pediculi must be remembered when there is enlargement of the suboccipital nodes. With repeated infections, there may be fibrosis and permanent enlargement of a node, which is then moderately firm, freely movable and not tender.

SYPHILIS.   Enlargement may be due to a local syphilitic lesion in the mouth, which has already been noted, or it may be a part of the generalized lymphadenitis that can occur in this disease.

TUBERCULOUS ADENITIS.   This is rarely seen now; formerly it was not uncommon (Fig. 81). Raw milk from infected cows was probably

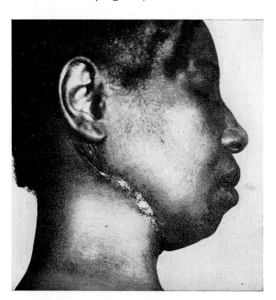

Fig. 81.   Tuberculous cervical lymphadenitis.

the source of infection. The submaxillary, anterior cervical or supra-clavicular nodes are involved; they enlarge slowly, become fused and may suppurate and drain. Initially these nodes are usually firm and may be fixed to the skin or underlying tissues. Gradually they soften, and if several nodes are involved, different stages of the process may be present at any one time. Sarcoidosis can also cause enlargement of the nodes that is indistinguishable on physical examination from that seen with tuberculous involvement, but suppuration is rare.

INFECTIOUS MONONUCLEOSIS.   This is a systemic disease, probably of viral etiology, with fever, sore throat, an abnormal blood picture and enlargement of the lymph nodes and spleen. Usually the occipital nodes are involved; this should suggest that the "sore throat" may be something more serious than a localized acute pharyngitis.

EXANTHEMS.   Measles (*rubeola*) may also produce cervical adenitis. In German measles (*rubella*) one of the diagnostic features is enlargement of the posterior cervical and postauricular lymph nodes; this may occur before the rash appears.

HODGKIN'S DISEASE.   Enlargement of the cervical nodes may be the first visible sign of this disease. Initially it is unilateral; later both sides are involved. The nodes are firm but not tender. As they enlarge they tend to fuse, and eventually they present as a large irregular mass fixed to the underlying structures and occasionally to the overlying skin; suppuration is rare. Other lymphomas such as lymphosarcoma or reticulum cell sarcoma present a similar picture. In leukemia the enlargement is slow and the nodes usually remain discrete.

CARCINOMA.   Invasion of the cervical nodes by carcinoma is usually secondary to cancer of the lip, tongue, mouth or other structures in the head or neck. Occasionally it represents metastasis from a distant organ such as the stomach or lung. A firm node just above the left clavicle, behind the insertion of the sternomastoid muscle, may be present with carcinoma of the stomach. This *sentinel node* is also called Virchow's node, Ewald's node or Trosier's sign.[8]

A definitive diagnosis cannot be made by inspection and palpation of cervical nodes; whenever there is reason to suspect any serious disease, biopsy with microscopic study is essential.

SALIVARY GLANDS

Normal parotid glands are not visible and are rarely felt on palpating the neck or angle of the jaw. Normal submaxillary and submental glands can often be felt on bimanual palpation, with one finger in the patient's

[8] Rudolph Virchow, German pathologist, 1821–1902; Carl Anton Ewald, German gastroenterologist, 1845–1905; Charles Emile Trosier, French pathologist, 1844–1919.

mouth. Enlargement of a parotid gland will produce swelling anterior to the ear and lateral displacement of the lobe. An enlarged submaxillary gland will be seen or felt about 2 cm. anterior to the angle of the jaw just below the mandible. A sublingual gland will be felt just below the chin or within the curve of the bone.

Parotitis. Mumps (epidemic parotitis), a virus disease, is the most common cause of rapid enlargement of the salivary glands, especially of the parotids. Although primarily a disease of childhood, it may occur in adults. The swelling is usually bilateral but often it predominates on one side; that is why a person may say that he had mumps "on one side only." With parotid involvement, the swelling is visible under the angle of the jaw, and behind and in front of the lobe of the ear, which is displaced laterally. The lower border can usually be determined; the other margins tend to be indistinct. The gland itself feels firm or hard and is tender. The swelling subsides spontaneously; suppuration does not occur. The other salivary glands may be similarly involved.

Acute parotitis of bacterial origin can follow oral infection that ascends through Stensen's duct. This produces swelling, redness and marked tenderness, and may progress to suppuration or abscess formation. On gentle massage of the gland a drop of pus may appear at the orifice of the duct, thus differentiating this condition from mumps. Occasionally partial stenosis or a calculus in the duct predisposes to repeated infections; chronic parotitis may then develop.

Stone. A *sialolith* may be present in the salivary duct without infection of the gland; initially this will cause partial obstruction. The amount of pain and swelling may be greater shortly after eating if the gland is still forming saliva. A nodule may be palpable along the course of the duct, or a stone may be seen on a suitable roentgenogram.

Sarcoidosis (Boeck's[9] Sarcoid). This disease can produce slow painless enlargement, especially of the parotid gland. When there is involvement of the uveal tract and lachrymal glands also, the term uveoparotid fever or Mikulicz's[10] syndrome is sometimes applied.

Tumors. These may be benign or malignant; the parotid gland is most commonly involved. A mixed tumor may appear in the third or fourth decade and grow slowly. It is a firm or hard, well defined and relatively insensitive mass. It is commonly regarded as benign at first, but unless widely excised, recurrence with malignant degeneration is not uncommon. Carcinoma tends to develop later in life; the gland is hard and fixed. Metastasis to the cervical lymph nodes may occur before the primary lesion becomes apparent or symptomatic.

[9] Caesar P. M. Boeck, Norwegian dermatologist, 1845–1917.
[10] Johann von Mikulicz-Radecki, Polish surgeon, 1850–1905.

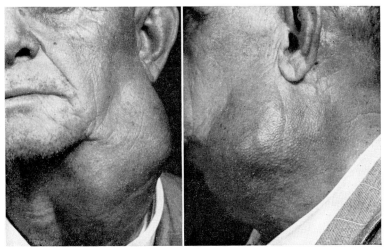

Fig. 82.   Recurrent carotid body tumor. (From Ochsner, A., and DeBakey, M. E. (eds.): Christopher's Minor Surgery. 8th ed. Philadelphia, W. B. Saunders Co., 1959.)

CAROTID BODY

The carotid body (carotid sinus) is situated at the bifurcation of the common carotid artery. It is composed of special sensory end plates surrounded by a plexus of nerves. Overactivity of this structure can slow the cardiac rate and lead to dizziness, syncope or convulsions; denervation may be indicated to control these symptoms. The carotid body can be stimulated by pressure directed mesially and slightly posteriorly at the bifurcation; bilateral compression can cause cardiac arrest (*asystole*). Occasionally an endothelial tumor develops; this usually grows slowly (Fig. 82). Although it may metastasize to the adjacent lymph nodes, widespread metastasis has not been observed.

CONGENITAL ANOMALIES

Thyroglossal Duct Cyst.   This may present in the midline at any point between the hyoid bone and the thyroid. It may be mistaken for an enlarged thyroid isthmus; transillumination can be helpful, since fluid in a cyst is less opaque than is thyroid tissue.

Branchial Cyst.   This results from incomplete closure of one of the branchial clefts, and occurs along the anterior border of the sterno-mastoid muscle. Such a cyst is usually symmetrical in outline and softer in consistency than an enlarged lymph node. It may discharge clear mucoid material intermittently, either into the pharynx or through a small cutaneous fistula.

Cervical Rib.   Ribs arising from the seventh cervical vertebra are occasionally present; often they are not felt until mentioned by the radiologist. They may be entirely asymptomatic, but they can cause pressure on nerves or vessels in the neck. This will produce paresthesias or circulatory disturbances in one or both upper extremities, especially when the arm is in some certain position. A similar clinical picture can be produced by pressure from an abnormal scalenus anticus muscle (*scalenus anticus syndrome*); this will be discussed as part of the neurologic examination.

VII

The Breasts

Every physical examination of a woman should include systematic and careful inspection and palpation of the breasts. Since the breast is the commonest site of carcinoma in women of every age, any abnormal mass that is discovered should be considered malignant until proved otherwise.

INSPECTION

The patient should sit facing you on the examining table or edge of the bed with her arms at her sides (Fig. 83). Compare the size, shape, symmetry, contour and position of the two breasts, and the relative position of the areolae and nipples. Minor differences are very common and are usually of no clinical significance if other abnormalities are not found; even a considerable difference may be physiologic. Then look carefully at the skin. One or more surgical scars may be visible; the history should have specified why the operation was performed. An area of redness suggests inflammation. Edema will cause bulging of the skin lying between the hair follicles, giving an illusion of scattered indentations and an appearance like that of orange peel ("peau d'orange"; "pigskin"); this is usually due to underlying carcinoma.

The areola may be large and deeply pigmented as a result of pregnancy, past or present. Enlargement or infection of the sebaceous glands of Montgomery[1] in the outer portion of the areola may be present. Nipples are of various sizes and shapes. One or both may be inverted, but this must be differentiated from retraction due to underlying disease. An inverted nipple lies in a crease or sulcus and can be everted by gentle manipulation; retraction tends to be irregular and the nipple is usually fixed. A fissure may be present, especially post partum; this can lead to

[1] William Fetherstone Montgomery, Irish obstetrician, 1797–1859.

135

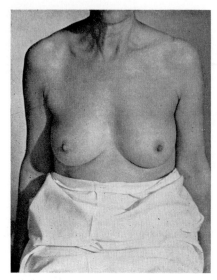

Fig. 83. Inspection of the breasts with arms at the sides.

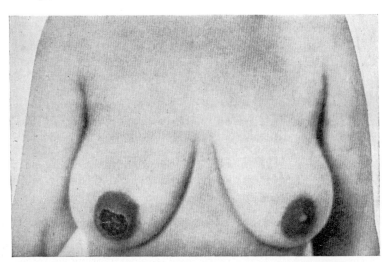

Fig. 84. Paget's disease of the nipple. This is a far-advanced stage; the nipple has completely disappeared. Paget's disease is a nipple duct carcinoma that spreads slowly in the epidermis, and in and along the ducts. (From Auchincloss, H., *in* Pullen, R. L.: Medical Diagnosis. 2nd ed. Philadelphia, W. B. Saunders Co., 1950.)

infection of the breast or abscess formation. An eczematoid appearance should be considered as evidence of a form of intraductal carcinoma (Paget's disease of the breast, Figure 84) until proved otherwise. The character of any discharge should also be noted.

The patient should then raise her arms above her head (Fig. 85). This tends to tense the pectoral muscles and may result in unilateral appearance or increase of altered contour, suggesting abnormal fixation of the breast to the fascia (Fig. 86). Another method of tensing the muscles is to have the patient place her hands on her hips and press in toward the midline (Fig. 87).

Finally, the patient should lean forward with the arms horizontal.

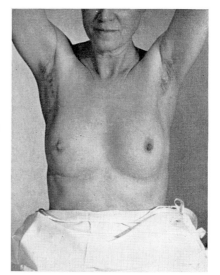

Fig. 85. Inspection of the breasts with the arms raised above the head.

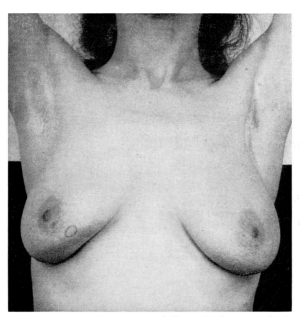

Fig. 86.   Indentation in the contour of the right breast with the arms raised (circled). This was due to carcinoma of the lower inner quadrant. (From Haagensen, C. D.: Carcinoma of the Breast. New York, American Cancer Society, Inc., 1950.)

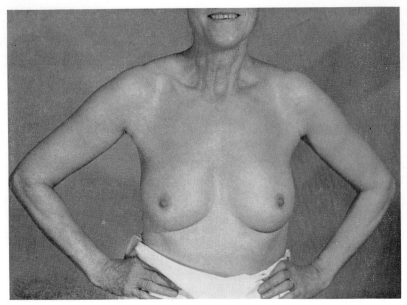

Fig. 87. Tensing the pectoral muscles by pressing inward on the hips.

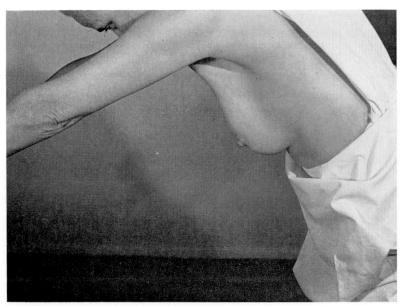

Fig. 88. Inspection as the patient leans forward. The relative mobility of each breast should be noted and any inequality recorded.

Both breasts should swing away from the thoracic wall; inequality of movement or unilateral changes in contour are important (Fig. 88).

Accessory breast tissue or accessory nipples may be present in the milk line, which runs in a gentle curve from the axilla to the groin and down the medial aspect of the upper thigh. Accessory nipples are fairly common both in men and in women, and often are thought to be "moles."

PALPATION

Lymph nodes should be sought in the supraclavicular and axillary regions (Figs. 89, 90A, 90B). To relax the pectoral muscles the arm should be supported during palpation.

The patient should then lie with a small pillow under her shoulders. Her arm should be raised above her head during palpation of the inner half of the breast, and rest at her side when the lateral half is examined. If the breasts are very large and sag laterally, it may be preferable to place the pillow under the shoulder of the side which is being examined, to rotate the trunk slightly and bring the breast back over the chest wall.

With the fingers extended and approximated, gently compress all areas of breast tissue against the chest wall. Heavy pressure, pinching or squeezing are unwarranted and often traumatic; bimanual palpation is rarely indicated. Then press on the tissue around the areola and look for secretion at the nipple. If this appears, attempt to determine the duct

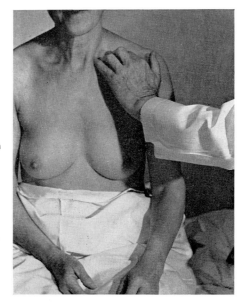

Fig. 89. Palpation for lymph nodes in the supraclavicular area.

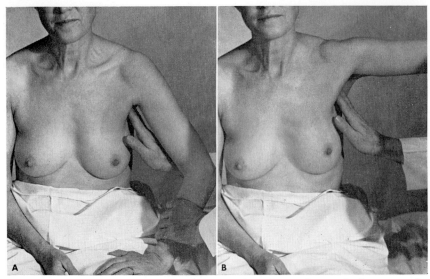

Fig. 90. Palpation for axillary lymph nodes. This is done with the arm at the side (*A*) and with the arm raised (*B*) to tense the axillary fascia.

or portion of the breast from which this is coming, and search for a small mass (*intraductal papilloma*), which may be very superficial.

PHYSIOLOGIC VARIATIONS

The normal breast is composed largely of strands of glandular tissue radiating from the nipple and surrounded by fat. The consistency of these tissues is variable. In some individuals the strands are firm and easily distinguished; in others they may be palpable centrally but gradually lose their identity peripherally, especially in the lateral half.

Slight increase in size of the breasts, accompanied by discomfort or tenderness, is common in the premenstrual period; this soon reverts to normal. Similar changes that are progressive occur during pregnancy; the areola also enlarges and becomes darker. When lactation ceases or is suppressed, the breasts tend to revert to their former size but are usually more flabby and pendulous. A variable degree of atrophy occurs during and after the menopause.

Fairly rapid growth of the breasts may precede the menarche by several months. At times one breast enlarges much more rapidly than the other, causing embarrassment to the girl and apprehension to her parents; Nature soon corrects this. The eventual size is unpredictable;

the breasts may never be more than small nubbins on the thoracic wall, or they may weigh several pounds apiece.

PATHOLOGIC CHANGES

Carcinoma.   Although the incidence of cancer of the breast increases with advancing age, and especially during and after the menopause, it can occur at any age. A solitary nodule that is firm or hard but usually not tender, or a mass that seems to differ in size and consistency from other palpable portions of the breast tissue (*dominant mass*), should immediately suggest malignancy. Fixation to the pectoral fascia is usually a late sign. In rare instances the first sign may be discharge from the nipple, enlargement of axillary nodes or inflammatory changes in the skin with no mass palpable in the breast itself (Figs. 91, 92, 93).

Chronic Cystic Mastitis.   This may be found at any age after puberty, but is usually less frequently present and less pronounced after the menopause, when carcinoma is more prone to develop. The name encompasses many different forms of benign lesions, ranging from a single large cyst to multiple small ones, or areas of fibrosis with little or no true cyst formation.

The physical findings will depend upon the nature of the changes

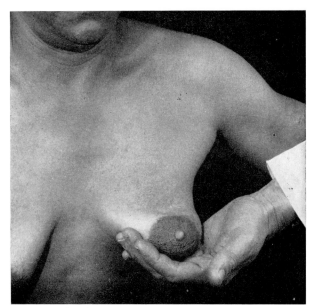

Fig. 91.   When this breast was lifted, a dimple appeared above the areola. This marks the site of a carcinoma. (From Haagensen, C. D.: Carcinoma of the Breast. New York, American Cancer Society, Inc., 1950.)

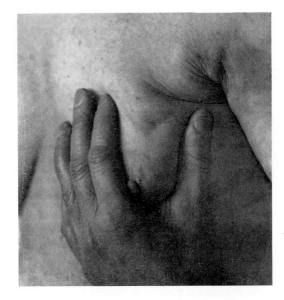

Fig. 92. Gentle compression produced a dimple in the surface of the upper outer quadrant of the left breast; this was due to underlying carcinoma. (From Haagensen, C. D.: Carcinoma of the Breast. New York, American Cancer Society, Inc., 1950.)

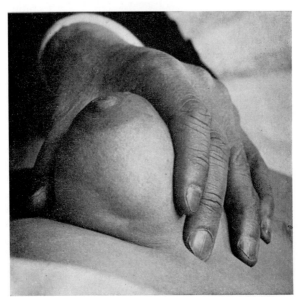

Fig. 93. With gentle compression a dimple became apparent in the lower half of this carcinomatous breast. (From Haagensen, C. D.: Carcinoma of the Breast. New York, American Cancer Society, Inc., 1950.)

present, but ordinarily the breasts are symmetrical and no retraction can be demonstrated. On palpation the involved area is often tender; this is accentuated in the premenstrual period and may be associated with definite enlargement at that time. A large cyst is usually regular in outline and somewhat rubbery in consistency. Smaller cysts may be present in any or all of the ducts; the upper outer quadrant is the most common site. These are of variable size and consistency; they may be firm, but they are never stony hard. Sometimes the entire breast feels like a bag partially filled with small nodules and lumps formed by cysts and fibrous tissue; they are "shotty" to palpation. Occasionally it is impossible to differentiate a cyst from a carcinoma, especially when the cyst seems to resemble a dominant mass; surgical exploration is necessary. However, if there are diffuse changes in both breasts and no dominant mass, and if the nodules increase and decrease in size during the menstrual cycle, the diagnosis of cystic disease is most probable. The examination should be repeated at regular intervals and at various times during the menstrual cycle; a carcinoma may develop in such a nodule or elsewhere in the breast at any time.

Fibroadenoma.   One or more firm, discrete, smooth, round or slightly ovoid masses may be felt, most commonly in a young woman. A distinguishing feature is the apparent lack of fixation to the breast tissue; these nodules have been called "slippable." When first discovered, such a mass may range in size from a few millimeters in diameter to many centimeters. Rapid growth, especially in an older woman, suggests the possibility of sarcomatous changes and the development of cysto-sarcoma phylloides.

Fat Necrosis.   An injury, either remembered or long-forgotten, may result in replacement of traumatized fat and extravasated blood by scar tissue. Eventually this may form a hard ill-defined mass with fixation, skin retraction or other signs suggesting carcinoma. Unless the history of injury is definite and the mass developed rapidly thereafter. surgical exploration is indicated.

Acute Mastitis.   This rarely develops except post partum or during lactation and is preceded by "caking" due to partial obstruction of one or more of the ducts by inspissated milk. Organisms enter through the nipple and spread outward to the congested area; local swelling, tenderness and redness appear. This cellulitis may subside within a few days with appropriate antimicrobial therapy, or it may progress to tissue destruction and abscess formation. The local signs increase, fluctuation can be detected, and fever, leukocytosis and other systemic signs develop or increase. Incision and drainage is then needed to prevent widespread destruction of breast tissue.

Tuberculosis.   This may be primary in the breast, or secondary to tuberculosis of the chest wall. A slowly enlarging ill-defined mass with minimal inflammatory changes develops; this is easily confused with carcinoma. The axillary nodes are also involved and become enlarged or tender. Later, this cold abscess may rupture through the skin and give rise to intermittent or persistent drainage through one or more sinus tracts. The diagnosis is established by finding *M. tuberculosis* in the discharge, or by biopsy of the involved tissue.

Other Tumors.   Lipoma, fibroma, metastatic carcinoma and other unusual lesions may be found in the breast, but these are rare.

SELF-EXAMINATION

Every young woman should be taught to examine her own breasts,

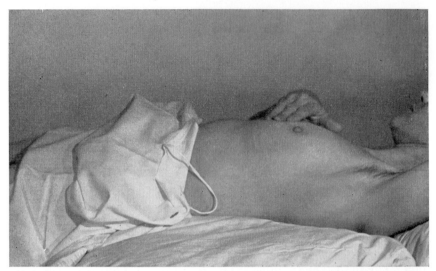

Fig. 94.   Self-examination of the inner half of the breast; arm raised above head.

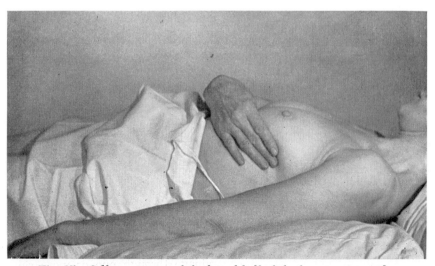

Fig. 95.   Self-examination of the lateral half of the breast; arm at side.

and she should be urged to do this every two months shortly after the completion of a menstrual period. Only when this becomes a routine procedure will early malignancy be discovered. Obviously, it should be stressed that most lumps are not cancer but that a medical opinion should be obtained at once if any abnormality is found. The procedure for this examination is essentially the same as that described above. For palpation, the hand on the opposite side is used (Figs. 94, 95).

THE MALE BREAST

Although carcinoma of the breast is mainly a disease of women, from 1 to 2 per cent of such tumors develop in men. Often this is overlooked or ignored until the mass become large and annoying, or metastatic enlargement of the axillary nodes is discovered.

In overweight boys and men localized collections of subcutaneous fat may simulate enlargement of the breasts. These masses are soft and uniform in consistency; no glandular tissue can be felt.

In boys, a tender firm mass lying beneath the nipple may appear during or soon after puberty. This condition is self-limiting and does not require therapy; it is attributed to hormone imbalance.

In older men there may be a similar enlargement of the rudimentary breast tissue, either unilateral or bilateral; this is called gynecomastia (Fig. 96). It may appear without obvious cause, but more commonly it is seen in the late stage of portal cirrhosis; the damaged liver no longer inactivates the circulating estrogens that are normally present in small

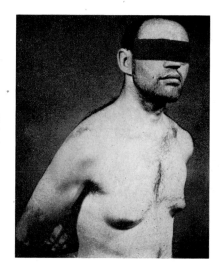

Fig. 96. Gynecomastia due to an estrogen-secreting tumor of the adrenal cortex. (Courtesy of F. Curtis Dohan, M.D.)

amounts. It also develops when large amounts of estrogens (with or without castration) are used for palliation of prostatic carcinoma. In rare instances it is due to a testicular tumor or appears as a manifestation of Cushing's syndrome.

VIII

Sounds from the Thorax

Final

The perception of vibrations by palpation or by auscultation plays an important role in physical diagnosis, especially in the examination of the heart and lungs. Vibrations are produced physiologically by such factors as movement of air or flow of blood; they can also be induced by phonation or percussion. If these vibrations reach the ear, they may be perceived as sound. If the vibrations are constant in frequency they will give rise to a musical note (Fig. 97). If they are inconstant in frequency, or if vibrations of conflicting frequencies are superimposed, the result is noise.

Sounds heard over the thorax may arise in the heart or lungs; they may also be produced in adjacent organs and be transmitted by the tissues of the thoracic wall. Peristaltic sounds, for example, are sometimes loud enough to interfere with auscultation of the heart or lungs.

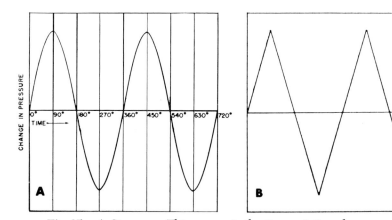

Fig. 97. *A*, Sine wave. This represents the time variation of pressure in the air through which a pure sound is being propagated. (From Miller, D. C.: Science of Musical Sounds. New York, The Macmillan Company, 1916.) *B*, For simplicity, this modification of sine waves will be used in subsequent drawings.

Although various types of sound may be present, it is usually possible to concentrate on one and to determine its characteristics. In the analysis of sounds heard during the examination certain fundamental principles of acoustics must be remembered. The most important characteristics of any sound are the pitch, duration, quality or timbre, and the intensity.

FUNDAMENTAL CHARACTERISTICS OF SOUNDS

Pitch

Pitch is determined by the frequency of vibrations per second. Low tones have relatively few vibrations; very frequent vibrations produce a high-pitched note (Fig. 98). In the examination of the lungs two factors are important. A dense (solid) tissue or organ produces a high-pitched note. As the density decreases and the amount of air increases, the note becomes progressively lower in pitch. Also, the pitch varies with the size of the resonator. The large thoracic cage of a man will have a much lower fundamental note than that found in a young child. Pitch does not change as one moves away from the source of the sound; intensity does. The music may be louder when you sit near the orchestra, but it will have the same pitch wherever you sit.

The ability to recognize changes in pitch is extremely variable. One

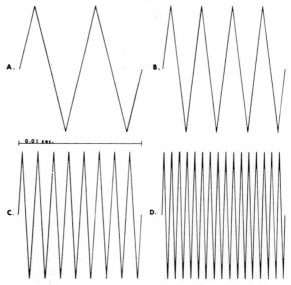

Fig. 98. Low-pitched note (A) to high-pitched (D). A, 200 cycles per second (cps); B, 400 cps; C, 800 cps; D, 1600 cps.

person can recognize a change of relatively few vibrations per second. Another may be "tone-deaf" and unable to differentiate two notes that are half an octave apart; he will find that this is a handicap in physical diagnosis.

Duration

The duration of the vibrations depends upon both the mass of tissue present and the amount of force used to displace it. Light percussion over an area of normal lung tissue will yield a short note, while heavy percussion at the same spot will produce a sound that will persist for an appreciably longer time (Fig. 99). Percussion over the region of the liver, which is dense, will give rise to a very short high-pitched note. As a general rule, sounds of low pitch tend to persist longer than those of high pitch.

Heart & lung low pitch sounds Normally.

Timbre

Timbre or quality is difficult to describe but it is easily recognized. The fundamental note, overtones and harmonics all play a part. A violin

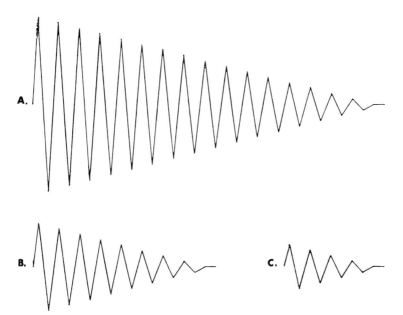

Fig. 99. Duration. Vibrations of the same frequency (pitch) but of varying amplitude. *A*, Forceful percussion produces a prolonged note. *B*, Normal percussion, normal duration. *C*, Light percussion, very short sound.

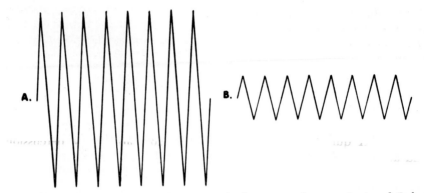

Fig. 100.   Intensity. The frequency of vibrations is the same in *A* and *B*, but the amplitude of the vibrations in *A* is four times as great as in *B*. Thus, under similar conditions, *A* will be "louder" than *B*.

and a trumpet may each sound a note of the same pitch and intensity, but one soon learns to differentiate the timbre and to identify the instrument.

Intensity

The intensity of a sound depends upon the amplitude of the vibrations at the site of their production; this is a physical measurement. If more force is applied the displacement is greater and the waves have greater amplitude (Fig. 100), but the frequency (pitch) is unchanged. With percussion, a more forceful blow will produce a sound of greater intensity. Deep rapid breathing will move more air and produce more powerful vibrations or "louder" breath sounds. Exercise will accelerate the rate of blood flow and thus accentuate a murmur. However, density again plays a part. A solid structure will be displaced much less than an air-containing one, if forces of the same magnitude are used. Percussion of the muscles of the thigh cannot produce a sound equal in intensity to that elicited when the thorax is similarly percussed. Also, as the pitch rises the amplitude of vibrations decreases; a telephone bell can never produce as "loud" a note as does the booming bass drum.

Loudness

Loudness is the subjective interpretation of the intensity of sound; it is extremely variable since the human element plays an important part. Auditory acuity varies somewhat even in persons with "normal" hearing and decreases with advancing age. There may be a slight loss of hearing for all sounds, or a person may have a moderate loss primarily for low, medium or high-pitched sounds. Since most of the physiologic sounds from the heart and lungs are comparatively low-pitched, a loss of hearing in that range may be a serious handicap. You must hear the sound before you can attempt to interpret it.

Another problem is extraneous or ambient sounds that may mask what you are attempting to hear. When a low-flying jet roars overhead, even the loudest murmur may be inaudible, yet its intensity has not changed. A quiet environment is essential for satisfactory percussion and auscultation.

Attenuation

Attenuation of energy also plays an important part. Whenever sound

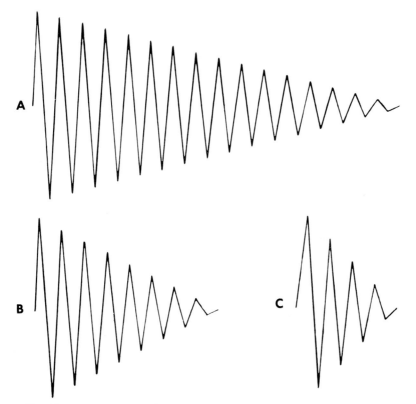

Fig. 101. Attenuation. Vibrations initially of the same frequency and intensity, but transmitted through different media. A, Prolonged note; B, moderate attenuation; C, rapid attenuation.

waves pass through any medium, friction converts some of the energy into heat, thus reducing the amplitude of the vibrations and decreasing the intensity and loudness of the sound (Fig. 101). The greater the distance from the source, the fainter the sound will be.

Reflection

At a boundary between two different media some of the energy is transmitted across the barrier, but much of it is reflected back toward the source. Sound waves originating in the lung have to overcome many such boundaries (alveolar air; alveolar walls) before they hurdle the two layers of pleura, traverse the chest wall, reach the skin and finally set up waves in the surrounding air. It has been calculated that only a fraction of 1 per cent of the sounds originating in the lung will be transmitted to the air. The same is true of heart sounds; normally they are inaudible a few millimeters from the chest wall.

THE STETHOSCOPE

To localize and study sounds of various types, you will need to use a stethoscope. Laennec made out very well with a hollow wooden tube, and many important observations were made by him and others who used similar instruments. Now you can choose from a wide variety of simple or complicated modifications, but the chest piece is basically either a funnel or open bell (Ford type) or a shallow cup covered by a diaphragm (Bowles type). The bell is often preferred for relatively low-pitched sounds; it can also be applied more easily to small areas such as sunken supraclavicular fossae or the interspaces of an emaciated chest. Diaphragm chest pieces are available in various diameters, but most of them are larger than the bell. They tend to attenuate low-pitched sounds and thus accentuate the high-pitched element. Double, triple and quadruple chest pieces have been designed and promoted, ostensibly to enable the physician to have the exact equipment for each particular phase of the examination.

The novice should start with a bell, or a diaphragm of medium size, and learn to use that properly; later he may wish to experiment with more expensive but clumsier equipment. For comfort, the ear plugs must fit snugly to exclude ambient noises, but should not be too small. The tension in the spring should be sufficient to hold the ear pieces in place, yet not cause discomfort even after prolonged use. The tubing should be firm and relatively short, to minimize loss of sound due to friction.

SOUNDS FROM THE THORAX

Respiratory Sounds

The frequency or pitch of the most important sounds produced by breathing ranges from about 400 to 1700 cycles per second (cps). However, the higher pitched sounds are markedly attenuated by normal lung tissue and are usually inaudible. With consolidation of the lung, transmission is considerably improved and they become more prominent.

Circulatory System Sounds

Vibrations can be produced by muscular contraction, movement of the heart valves and flow of blood. Their frequencies range from a few cycles per second to several thousand. Components with frequencies above 1500 cps are so greatly attenuated that they are rarely audible; the stethoscope covers primarily the range from 80 cps to 500 cps.

Vocal Sounds

These can be very intense as compared to respiratory or circulatory sounds. Even though the attenuation in the thorax and in the stethoscope is high, sounds ranging from 80 or 100 cps to 2000 or 3000 cps may be heard.

SUMMARY

Recognition of certain principles of the physics of sound can aid in the interpretation of sounds from the thorax. These sounds are extremely complex; they vary in pitch, timbre, duration and intensity. They are attenuated by physiologic and pathologic processes, and the degree of attenuation varies with the pitch. Any stethoscope acts as an acoustic filter; it transmits sounds in a certain frequency range much better than others outside this range. The human ear is not infallible; it responds differently to variations of pitch and intensity. Even the mental attitude can play a part. The person who is tense, worried or otherwise distracted will be unable to devote his full attention to the sounds that are present, and may miss some important abnormality.

In the analysis of physiologic and pathologic sounds, experience and memory are also important. The trained clinician can listen for a few seconds and correctly appraise the various characteristics of the sound he hears; the novice must start by concentrating on one factor at a time.

IX

Inspection of the Thorax

According to reliable records Hippocrates, who was born about 460 B.C., described the succussion splash and certain other signs of lung disease; hence it may be assumed that for over 2,400 years physicians might have known about examination of the chest. During the first twenty-two centuries little of permanent value was recorded, but in 1761 Leopold Auenbrugger[1] wrote his extraordinary book on immediate percussion of the chest. However, this book of ninety-five pages, which had the impressive Latin title *Inventum Novum ex Percussione Thoracis Humani ut Signo Abstrusos Interni Pectoris Morbos Detegendi* (*New Invention by Means of Percussing the Human Chest as a Sign of Detecting Obscure Disease in the Interior of the Chest*), was neglected by the medical profession for almost half a century.

In 1808, when Auenbrugger was eighty-six years old, Corvisart[2] translated *Inventum Novum* into French and established Auenbrugger's fame. When one considers that all of Auenbrugger's observations were based on immediate percussion performed by striking directly with the bare or gloved finger tips through clothing drawn tightly across the patient's chest, the accuracy of his interpretation of the sounds that he produced as indicative of underlying pulmonary and pleural disease is almost incredible.

In 1816 Laennec[3] began to use a new device that he called a stethoscope (*stethos,* chest). Three years later he published his immortal *Traité de l'Auscultation Médiate*. Despite the fact that his original monaural stethoscope was a crude instrument, he described in detail physical signs of disease of the lungs, the pleura and the heart which, with few exceptions, are recognized and accepted today. Even his

[1] Leopold Auenbrugger, Austrian physician, musician and composer, 1722–1809.

[2] Jean-Nicholas Corvisart Des Marest, French physician, 1755–1821. He was the favorite physician of Napoleon.

[3] René Théophile Hyacinthe Laennec, French physician, 1781–1826. He probably died of pulmonary tuberculosis, contracted during his studies.

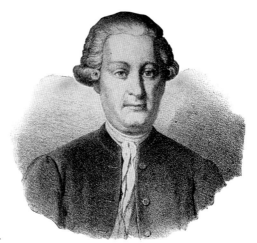

Fig. 102. Leopold Auen-
brugger and the frontispiece of
Inventum Novum. (From the collection of Dr. William G. Leaman,
Jr.)

LEOPOLDI AUENBRUGGER

MEDICINÆ DOCTORIS
IN CÆSAREO REGIO NOSOCOMIO NATIONUM
HISPANICO MEDICI ORDINARII.

INVENTUM NOVUM

EX
PERCUSSIONE THORACIS HUMANI
UT SIGNO

ABSTRUSOS INTERNI
PECTORIS MORBOS
DETEGENDI.

VINDOBONÆ,
TYPIS JOANNIS THOMÆ TRATTNER, CÆS. REG.
MAJEST. AULÆ TYPOGRAPHI.

MDCCLXI.

original terminology descriptive of these auscultatory signs has come
down to us essentially unchanged.

In 1895 Röntgen[4] discovered the "X" ray, but several decades elapsed
before fluoroscopy and roentgenography began to be widely used for
diagnosis of pulmonary disease. In recent years there has been an increasing tendency to minimize the importance of physical examination
of the chest, and to rely mainly on the radiologist. It is true that a
roentgen examination of the chest should be an essential part of *every
initial complete examination* of a patient. It can show abnormalities that
may not be demonstrable on physical examination such as enlarged hilar

[4] Wilhelm Conrad Röntgen, German physicist, 1845–1922.

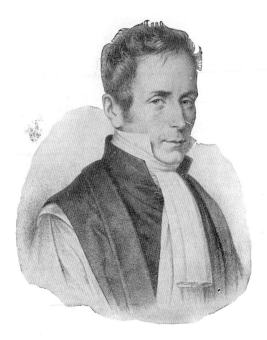

Fig. 103. René Théophile Hyacinthe Laennec.

nodes, a small tuberculous lesion, a centrally located pneumonic consolidation, a deeply placed cavity or cyst, miliary tuberculosis, metastatic malignancy, silicosis and other diseases.

Then why spend time doing a careful physical examination? Unfortunately, neither method alone is adequate; the two procedures should be considered supplemental. For example, the human ear can hear a friction rub; the roentgenogram cannot record this. An area of density may be apparent on the film, but one cannot always say unequivocally whether this represents consolidation, fluid, or both. In asthma the physical signs may be diagnostic; the x-ray may appear normal.

After you have completed the examination, study the films to see where you have erred. Then go back to the patient and try again. Only in this way will you acquire the proficiency that will be essential when you are called to see a patient in the middle of the night. You will have to rely on the history and your physical examination; there will be no radiologist to help you. You alone will have to make the diagnosis and institute proper treatment. As Waring[5] aptly wrote: "The roentgen-ray should be used not merely for diagnosis but as a teacher of physical diagnosis."

Although examination of the thorax is often divided into two separate sections—the lungs and the heart—there seems to be little to justify this artificial partition. For inspection, palpation and percussion this dichotomy will be disregarded; only when auscultation is discussed will the two organs be considered separately.

[5] James J. Waring, American physician, 1883–1962.

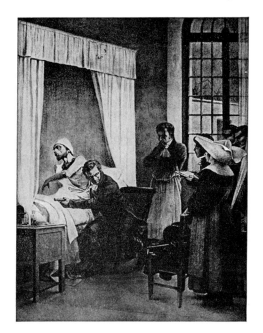

Fig. 104. Laennec examining a patient at the Necker Hospital.

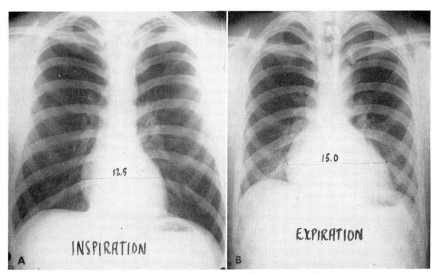

Fig. 105. Films of the same individual, taken during full inspiration and forced expiration. The diaphragmatic excursion is about two interspaces. Note also the change in position and contour and the apparent change in size of the heart.

ANATOMIC CONSIDERATIONS

Before beginning the actual examination of the chest it would be well to review the anatomy of the thorax and its contents. This includes the position and normal range of excursion of the diaphragm (Fig. 105); the area occupied by the heart, great vessels and mediastinal structures; and the location of the lobes and interlobar fissures of the lungs (Fig. 106). For more accurate localization of a pulmonary lesion, the lung lobules are utilized (Fig. 107).

Landmarks.   Two important landmarks anteriorly are the supra-sternal notch and the tip of the ensiform or xiphoid process; the *mid-sternal line* connects these points. The costal cartilages of the second ribs are attached to the sternum at the junction of the manubrium and the gladiolus (*angulus sterni; angle of Ludwig* or of *Louis*[6]). The other ribs can be identified by counting downward from this point. The clavicles should be easily recognized. The depressed area above the clavicle is the *supraclavicular fossa;* a similar depression below the clavicle is the *infraclavicular fossa* (Fig. 108).

Posteriorly, certain bony landmarks are also important (Fig. 109). The spinous process of the seventh cervical vertebra (*vertebra prominens;* C 7) can usually be seen and should be easily palpable. The spinous processes of the thoracic vertebrae may be conspicuous in a thin person but invisible in a very obese person; however, they can be identified by palpation and counted with C 7 as the starting point. The *midspinal line* is the line drawn through the tips of the spinous processes. It should be remembered that the spinous processes slope backward and downward about one interspace; the tip of T 5, for example, is at the level of the sixth vertebral body.

The scapulae are next identified. Normally they are of equal size and fit closely against the thoracic wall. The spine of the scapula lies at the level of the third or fourth thoracic vertebra; the lower angle is over the eighth rib. Using the scapulae as reference points, there are the suprascapular areas, the scapular areas, the infrascapular areas and the interscapular region.

In addition to the midsternal and midspinal lines, certain other vague perpendiculars are sometimes used by those who disdain accuracy. The anterior axillary line is described as the downward projection of the anterior axillary fold; the posterior axillary line, of the posterior muscle group. The midaxillary line lies midway between these two. Obviously the exact location of these lines depends largely upon the judgment of the examiner. The "midclavicular line" is even more vague; no two texts

---

[6] Daniel Ludwig, German anatomist, 1625–80; Antoine Louis, French surgeon, 1723–92.

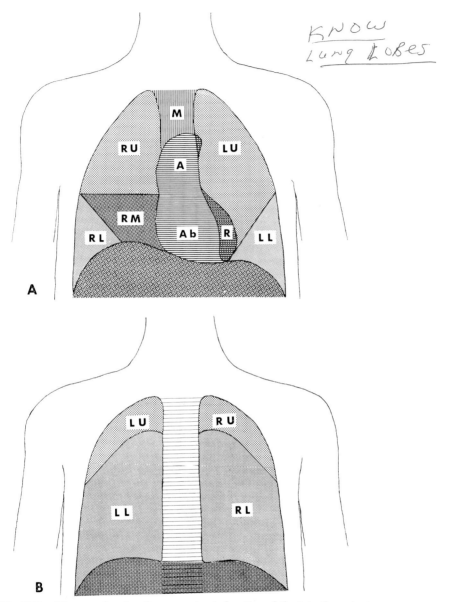

KNOW
Lung Lobes

Fig. 106. Diagram showing the approximate location of the intrathoracic structures anteriorly (A) and posteriorly (B).

    A, All five lobes of the lungs present anteriorly: right upper (RU); right middle
(RM); right lower (RL); left upper (LU); left lower (LL). The superior mediastinum
(M), the aorta (A) and the areas of relative (R) and absolute (Ab) cardiac dullness
are also shown.

    B, Only the upper and lower lobes present posteriorly.

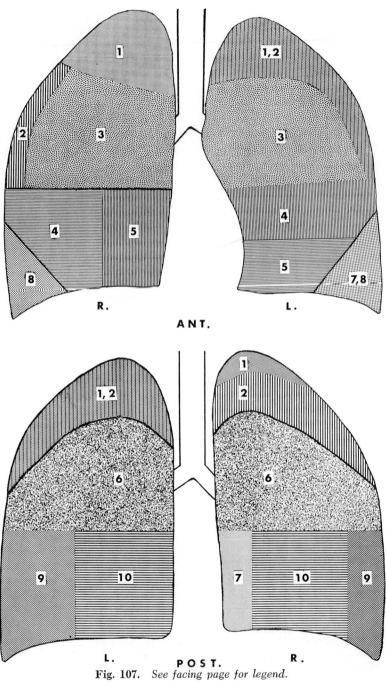

Fig. 107.   *See facing page for legend.*

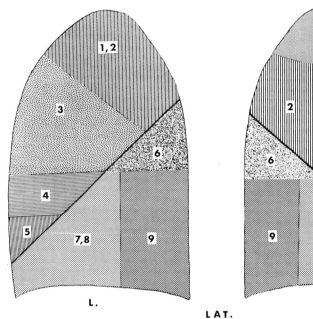

Fig. 107. Diagrams illustrating the lobular or segmental divisions of the lungs. The exact anatomic borders are somewhat variable; each is supplied by a major branch bronchus. The common designations are:

RIGHT LUNG
Upper Lobe
   1. Apical
   2. Posterior
   3. Anterior
Middle Lobe
   4. Lateral
   5. Medial
Lower Lobe
   6. Superior
   7. Medial basal*
   8. Anterior basal
   9. Lateral basal
 10. Posterior basal

LEFT LUNG
Upper Lobe
   1, 2. Apical-posterior

   3. Anterior

   4. Superior lingular
   5. Inferior lingular
Lower Lobe
   6. Superior
   7, 8. Anteromedial basal

   9. Lateral basal
 10. Posterior basal

   * Medial basal rarely touches posterior chest wall.

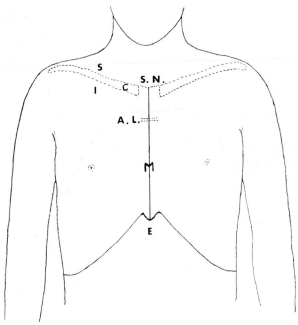

Fig. 108. Landmarks, anterior chest. Clavicles (C); supraclavicular fossa (S); infraclavicular fossa (I); angle of Ludwig or Louis (A.L.); suprasternal notch (S.N.); ensiform (E); midsternal line (M).

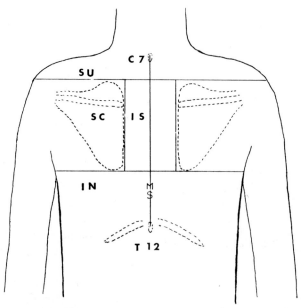

Fig. 109. Landmarks, posterior chest. Suprascapular area (SU); scapular area (SC); infrascapular area (IN); interscapular area (IS) bisected by midspinal line (MS), which connects the spinous processes of the seventh cervical vertebra (C 7) and the twelfth thoracic vertebra (T 12).

illustrate it in the same place, and as it is commonly indicated it has no relation to the middle of the clavicle. And the mammary or "nipple line," especially in women, may occasionally leave one in doubt as to what part or which side of the chest in involved.

Localization. When an abnormality is discovered, its location should be described accurately. For large lesions it may suffice to use one of the lobes of the lung as the area of reference, such as the right middle lobe. More commonly one will have to depend upon certain fixed points; these are the ribs and intercostal spaces, the sternum and the spinous processes. If bronchial breath sounds are said to be present in the fourth right intercostal space 6 cm. from the midsternal line, anyone else can determine exactly where the examiner heard them.

PROCEDURE

The room must be comfortably warm and the light should be adequate; shadows may mask minor abnormalities. Examination of the chest should invariably begin with inspection. Any attempt to examine the chest through clothing is fraught with frustration and often is worse than no examination at all; the chest must be *bared*. With men, this usually presents no problem. For women an examining cape or gown must be provided; this can be maneuvered tactfully so that eventually all parts of the anterior chest wall can be studied. The back can be exposed to the waist without objection.

Whenever possible, the patient should be sitting in a comfortable position, on a revolving stool if available. Initially you should also be seated at the same level or lower, preferably with your head level with his thorax. The front, back and both sides of the chest should be scrutinized. Then stand behind the patient and look downward over his shoulders so that you can see the upper anterior portion of the thorax.

THE NORMAL THORAX

Points to be noted on inspection of the chest include the general configuration, size, shape, symmetry and movement. The examination of the skin and of the breasts is discussed elsewhere; one should focus attention on the thorax itself.

With experience you will learn to decide whether the general conformation, size and shape are normal for a given individual. The tall thin ectomorph should have a thin flat chest, prominent clavicles and

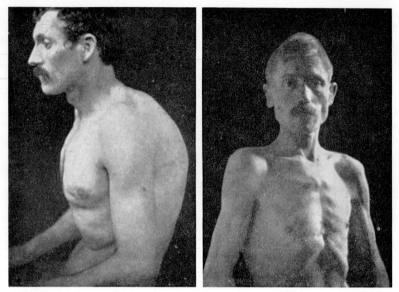

Fig. 110.   Barrel-shaped chest due to long-standing pulmonary emphysema.

ribs and an acute subcostal angle; the mesomorph, a short thick chest with an obtuse subcostal angle. A considerable degree of deviation from this may be within normal limits. However, a marked increase in the anteroposterior (A-P) diameter of the thorax of an ectomorph suggests overinflation of the lungs (*pulmonary emphysema*) (Fig. 110). An unexpected decrease may be caused by fibrosis with retraction of the ribs (Fig. 111); chronic tuberculosis is one of the diseases that can produce this, but there are others. Occasionally in a very elderly person the thoracic spine becomes bowed forward (*kyphotic*) to an extreme degree. This will produce a very definite increase in the A-P diameter of the thorax even in the absence of underlying lung disease.

Symmetry.   Theoretically, the normal chest is symmetrical; actually this is rarely true. The right shoulder is frequently lower than the left. The pectoral muscles may bulge on the right if the person is right-handed and uses those muscles frequently. The shoulder girdle muscles are often larger on one side as a result of the person's occupation or avocation, as in a carpenter or tennis player.

Clavicles.   The clavicles are more prominent in men than in women. Look for abnormal swelling or a bulge that may represent an old fracture. Compare the supraclavicular fossae on the two sides; they should be equal. This applies also to the infraclavicular fossae. If the fossa on one side is more prominent than the corresponding one, it suggests disease of the underlying lung tissue; less commonly a neurologic disorder may cause this.

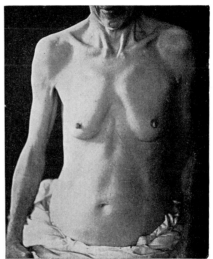

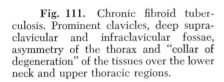

Fig. 111. Chronic fibroid tuber-culosis. Prominent clavicles, deep supra-clavicular and infraclavicular fossae, asymmetry of the thorax and "collar of degeneration" of the tissues over the lower neck and upper thoracic regions.

Sternum.   The sternum should not protrude anteriorly beyond the ribs; usually it is slightly depressed (1 to 2 cm.). Minor elevations and depressions are not uncommon; the major ones will be considered later.

Ribs.   Then look at the ribs. When the patient is upright they should slope downward from the spine to the costal cartilages at an angle of about 45 degrees. In the long flat chest the angle will be greater; in the short chest the ribs will be more nearly horizontal. Make sure that the angle is the same on the two sides; a difference is more important than the exact angle itself. Any disease, acute or chronic, that decreases the volume of the underlying lung will tend to pull the chest wall inward and increase the angle of the overlying ribs. Overdistention of one lung will push the ribs outward and decrease the angle. If the two sides are not equal, other procedures in the examination may help you to decide which side is normal.

Costal Angle.   The subcostal angle is then noted; this too should be essentially the same on the two sides. Inequality here is usually asso-ciated with changes in the lung as mentioned above.

The Back.   Posteriorly, compare the two sides with especial ref-erence to the size, shape and position of the two scapulae, and of the various muscles in those areas. With a long thin chest the mesial border and angle of the scapulae may protrude slightly; in muscular or neuro-logic disorders this may become marked, producing a "winged" scapula.

Thoracic Movement.   Motion of the thorax is now determined. The ribs are hinged at the spine; with inspiration they swing outward and upward. The range of motion should be the same on the two sides. After watching while the patient breathes quietly, have him inhale

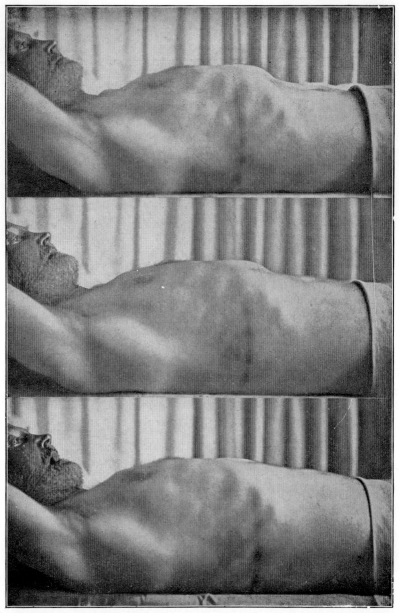

Fig. 112. Litten's diaphragmatic phenomenon (phrenic wave). The linear shadow has been emphasized in the reproduction of the photographs.

Upper, Full expiration. Note the height of the shadow and the slight concavity of the abdomen, corresponding to this phase of respiration.

Middle, Medium inspiration. The linear shadow has descended somewhat; there has also been a slight change in the contour of the abdomen.

Lower, Deep inspiration. There has been further descent of the shadow; the abdomen in now flat, not concave.

forcibly; minor inequalities or a slight lag on one side become more prominent. Inequality of expansion can usually be attributed to some disease within the chest which restricts movement on one side; these will be discussed later. Occasionally it may be due to a neurologic disorder, with muscular weakness or paralysis on one side.

Always try to estimate the degree of expansion or vital capacity of every patient. If pulmonary disease is present or suspected it is advisable to measure this also. In quiet respiration the thoracic excursion is usually slight in men; diaphragmatic movement is the major component. In women the diaphragm plays a less important role in respiration and thoracic expansion is much more prominent.

Intercostal Spaces.   The intercostal spaces should then be examined; they become more prominent during inspiration, because the negative intrathoracic pressure retards these tissues as the ribs move outward. The degree of apparent retraction varies with the thickness of the chest wall and overlying tissues, but it should be equal on the two sides.

This negative pressure gives rise to *Litten's*[7] *diaphragmatic phenom-* *Read* *enon* or *phrenic wave.* This is most easily demonstrable in a moderately thin person lying on his back with his feet toward a bright light (Fig. 112). As he take a slow, deep "abdominal" breath, watch the anterolateral chest wall. The diaphragm peels away from the chest wall; the intercostal tissues are temporarily pulled inward and fall in the shadow of the next lower rib. This "shadow" moves downward from the fifth to the eighth or ninth interspace. Equally valuable information can often be obtained without all these formalities. Retraction of the intercostal tissues can be observed in the same areas, even though the "shadow" is not seen.

If the intercostal areas are not symmetrical in corresponding interspaces, one must decide whether there is abnormal retraction on one side or lack of retraction on the opposite side. Abnormal retraction indicates increased negative pressure in that hemithorax. Increased positive pressure, as from pleural effusion or tension pneumothorax, will result in loss of retraction or actual bulging of the intercostal tissues in the area involved. Thickened pleura will mechanically restrict movement of the tissues in the interspaces.

THE PRECORDIAL AREA

As a final step, look for pulsations over the precordial area. In many persons one can see an outward thrust synchronous with cardiac

[7] Moritz Litten, German physician, 1845–1907.

systole; this is usually in the fifth intercostal space 8 to 10 cm. from the midsternal line. There may also be some retraction of the tissues mesial to this as the right ventricle contracts and tends to fall away from the chest wall. If the right ventricle is markedly hypertrophied this may be much more prominent than the systolic thrust of the left ventricle.

Physiologically, the exact location of this impulse depends largely upon the contour of the thorax and the position of the patient. The ectomorph will have a "vertical" heart, with the apex nearer the sternum; the endomorph will have a more transverse or horizontal heart. When the patient is lying on his left side the impulse may shift several centimeters to the left. In the right lateral decubitus the shift is less marked.

Pathologically the position of the pulsations may be shifted by cardiac enlargement, by a right-sided pleural effusion, hemothorax or pneumothorax, by pulmonary fibrosis, by atelectasis of one lung or by pressure upward from the abdomen with elevation of the diaphragm due to such things as gaseous distention, ascites or pregnancy.

Physiologically the impulse will be more prominent if the patient is very thin or emaciated. It will be less prominent or absent when the patient lies on his back and in an obese person or in a woman with large breasts. Pathologically this decrease may be produced by conditions such as a left-sided pleural effusion, hemothorax or pneumothorax, by pericardial effusion or by pulmonary emphysema.

THE BEDFAST PATIENT

If the patient is very sick, bedside inspection is occasionally necessary. If he is not too ill it may be possible to have him sit on the edge of the bed for a short time while you examine his back. Do not ask him to *sit up in bed;* this is very uncomfortable unless there is a third party to lend support. If the patient must remain recumbent try to have him lie *flat,* unless dyspnea prevents this. The anterior and lateral portions of the thorax should first be studied *completely*—inspection, palpation, percussion and auscultation. It may then be possible to have the patient sit up, supported by an assistant, while the back is examined, or he may be able to lie face downward for this. When neither of these positions can be tolerated it will be necessary to examine the back one side at a time. Help the patient roll over on his right side; inspect, palpate, percuss and auscultate the left side. Then help him roll on his left side and repeat the procedures over the right hemithorax.

Direct comparison of the "up" side with the "down" side is unreliable. Some of the distorting factors are: (1) pressure on the dependent side due to the weight of the thoracic viscera; (2) curvature of the spine with narrowing of the intercostal spaces on the upper side; (3) a confusing damping or resonating element introduced by the mattress and bedding; (4) elevation of the diaphragm on the lower side due to pressure by the abdominal viscera.

ABNORMALITIES

Spinal Deformity.   Certain abnormalities of the thorax are not uncommon. Minor degrees of spinal curvature are present in many persons and explain the frequency with which slight asymmetry is seen. Gross spinal deformities such as scoliosis, kyphosis, lordosis or a combination of these may produce such marked thoracic deformity and asymmetry that physical examination becomes unsatisfactory, deceptive and frustrating (Fig. 113). Even a roentgenogram may fail to reveal the truth.

Rickets.   This may be responsible for a variety of thoracic deformities. Vitamin D deficiency prevents proper mineralization of the bones; deformities begin to appear in the infant between the sixth and eighteenth month. Congenital abnormalities of the diaphragm or of the respiratory tract may alter respiratory dynamics and facilitate the development of these deformities.

The costochondral junctions may become enlarged; these bulges

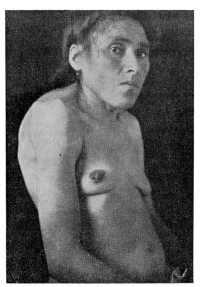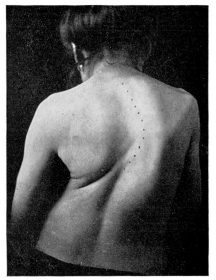

Fig. 113.   Chest deformity resulting from kyphoscoliosis. Abnormal physical signs must be construed with great caution in such a person

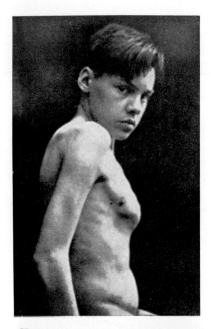

Fig. 114.   Pigeon breast (rachitic) in a boy of 12.

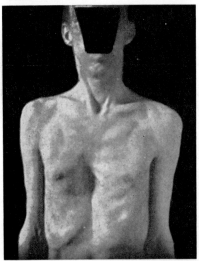

Fig. 115.   Funnel breast due to rickets. The man now has pulmonary tuberculosis also, but this was not related to the deformity.

constitute the *rachitic rosary*. A transverse depression known as *Harrison's*[8] *groove* may develop at the level of the fifth to seventh rib anteriorly; the cause is debatable. The sternum may protrude excessively (*pigeon breast,* keel breast, pectus carinatum [Fig. 114]), or it may be unduly retracted (*funnel breast,* cobbler's breast, pectus excavatum, "trichterbrust" [Fig. 115]). As the infant grows older, mineralization of

8 Edward Harrison, English physician, 1766–1838.

the bones occurs and the deformities become permanent. The rachitic rosary and Harrison's groove are of no clinical significance in an adult; they are of historical interest only, supplying a clue to nutrition and development during infancy. Pigeon breast and, more especially, funnel breast deformity may in rare instances lead to alterations in cardiac function. In such instances surgical intervention may be indicated; occasionally this is done for cosmetic reasons only.

Abnormal Contour.   A long flat chest (pterygoid chest; alar chest) may be normal in the ectomorph, but in others it should raise the suspicion of pleural or pulmonary disease with fibrosis and contraction of lung volume, such as that which occurs with pulmonary tuberculosis.

The emphysematous or barrel-shaped chest is an exaggeration of the contour seen at the end of a full inspiration. The ribs are elevated and everted; the sternum is arched and the angle of Ludwig is prominent. The anteroposterior diameter of the chest is increased; it may exceed the transverse diameter. The spine is bowed forward, the shoulders are thrown forward and the head and neck are held forward. The neck appears short because the thorax is drawn upward; it may also be enlarged by hypertrophy of the sternomastoid and other accessory muscles of respiration. The supraclavicular fossae may become obliterated or actually seem to protrude.

Localized Abnormalities.   A definite bulge may be present in the precordial area (Fig. 116). This is often a clue suggesting the presence

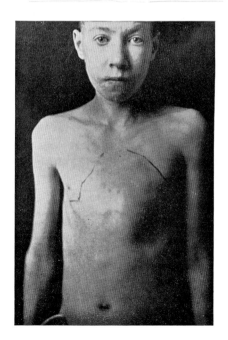

Fig. 116. Bulging of the precordial area caused by cardiac hypertrophy secondary to rheumatic heart disease in a boy of 14. Poor nutrition and underdevelopment often accompany cardiac disease of this severity occurring in childhood.

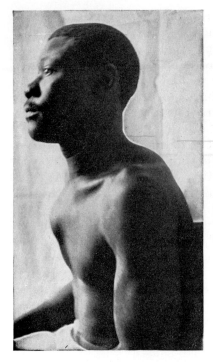

Fig. 117. Chest deformity due to thoracic aneurysm.

of congenital heart disease or of severe rheumatic carditis occurring early in childhood. The enlarged heart is able to displace the soft and yielding thoracic cage, and when calcification is more complete, usually early in puberty, the asymmetry becomes permanent.

Localized areas of bulging, retraction or pulsation can sometimes be seen over other areas of the thorax. A collection of pus in the pleural cavity may produce a pronounced protrusion of one interspace anteriorly or laterally (*empyema necessitatis*); without treatment, this may actually rupture through the chest wall.

An aneurysm of the ascending arch of the aorta, the "aneurysm of physical signs," may exert pressure on the second and third ribs and costal cartilages, usually to the right of the sternum; eventually it may protrude in this area. In that case, pulsations will be visible and palpable (Figs. 117, 118).

Tumors of the anterior mediastinum rarely produce deformity of the thoracic wall. They tend to extend backward, compressing more yielding tissues such as the trachea, esophagus and superior mediastinum. A sarcoma will occasionally produce a localized bulge, as will a superior sulcus tumor (Pancoast[9] tumor).

[9] Henry K. Pancoast, Professor of Roentgenology, University of Pennsylvania, 1875–1939.

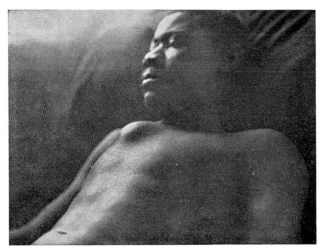

Fig. 118. Aneurysm of ascending and transverse portions of the arch of the aorta.

A localized deformity of one or more of the ribs may be the result of injury or fracture; occasionally it is due to a tumor of the bone. With Tietze's[10] syndrome there may be painful nonsuppurative swelling of the costal cartilages.

[10] Alexander Tietze, Breslau surgeon, 1864–1927.

X

Palpation of the Thorax

In examining the chest, palpation is used to confirm and amplify the points already noted on inspection, particularly the extent and equality or inequality of thoracic movements.

PROCEDURE

If the patient is a male the entire chest can be bared. A woman should wear a gown which can be adjusted to permit visualization and palpation of the entire back, the lateral chest walls and the upper anterior areas.

Have the patient sit with his back toward you; his thorax should be no lower than yours. Place your hands on the ribs posteriorly and postero-laterally with the fingers slightly spread and parallel to the ribs and the thumbs extended so that they are roughly parallel to the spinous processes (Fig. 119 A). Have the patient breathe normally and then more deeply. Compare the movement of the two hands and the amplitude of thoracic excursion as he breathes. Repeat this maneuver with the hands laterally and in the axillae (Fig. 119 B). Then place the hands over the upper anterior thorax with the finger tips extending down to the second or third ribs, and finally over the lower ribs anteriorly.

ALTERED EXPANSION

In time you will learn to judge whether expansion is within normal limits or is definitely decreased for the general body build, age and activity of the patient; it is rarely increased. Conditions such as emphysema or diffuse pulmonary fibrosis will limit thoracic expansion.

174

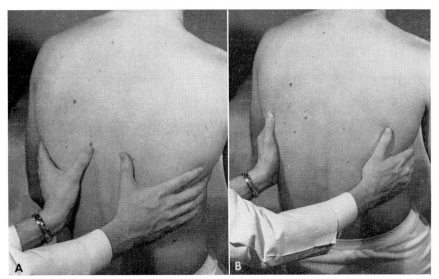

Fig. 119.   Proper position of hands to determine degree of expansion posteriorly (*A*) and laterally (*B*). The same procedure is repeated over the apical regions and upper thorax anteriorly, and over the lower ribs.

Unilateral or localized limitation of expansion is more easily perceived. When present over the upper portion of the thorax, fibrosis secondary to tuberculosis should be your first thought unless the patient is acutely ill with pneumonia. Over the lower ribs pleural effusion must be considered, as well as acute or chronic lung disease. Pleurisy or broken ribs will also limit expansion over the region involved.

FREMITUS

Palpation is also used to perceive vibrations or *fremitus*. If the lungs are healthy there is no palpable fremitus with respiration, but it can be produced by having the person talk (*vocal fremitus*).

Production of Vocal Fremitus.   When the vocal cords are approximated, they can be thrown into vibration by the passage of air between them. These vibrations are modified by structures such as the lips, teeth, tongue and nasal passages; they are reinforced by the thorax, which acts as a large resonator.

Certain requirements must be met if these vibrations are to be produced and become palpable. The patient must be conscious and able to talk. A stroke may have paralyzed the speech center; extreme dyspnea may limit or prohibit adequate phonation; a tracheostomy tube will divert the current of air away from the vocal cords. The cords must be

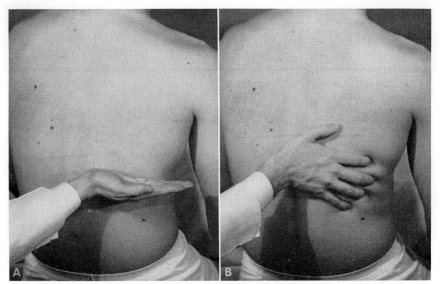

Fig. 120. Palpation for tactile fremitus using the ulnar surface of the hand (*A*) or the finger tips (*B*).

functionally efficient; paralysis will prevent approximation and proper vibration. The vibrations must be of sufficient force or amplitude; a very feeble voice may not produce vibrations great enough to be palpable when they are transmitted to the chest wall.

Testing Vocal Fremitus. To elicit vocal fremitus, have the patient repeat slowly some word such as "one, one, one" or "ninety-nine, ninety-nine" loudly and in as low a pitch as possible. Usually it is necessary to coach him before he does this properly; then start palpating.

To feel these vibrations you can use the ulnar surface of the hand and fifth finger (Fig. 120 *A*), the finger tips, or the spread-finger method (Fig. 120 *B*), but until you acquire some skill it is preferable to use one method only, usually the ulnar surface.

Compare the intensity of vibrations in the intercostal spaces at corresponding areas of the chest, palpating first one side, then the other. Go from apex to base posteriorly, laterally and anteriorly.

Physiologic Variations. Fremitus is normally more intense in the interspaces than over the ribs; the soft tissues respond more readily than do the relatively fixed and rigid bones.

Fremitus is more readily perceived if the vibrations are low in pitch; therefore it is normally less intense in women and children.

Fremitus is normally more intense over the right apical region than over the left. The trachea lies in immediate contact with the apex of the right lung, whereas on the left side it is separated a distance of about 3 cm. by the interposition of the aorta, carotid artery, esophagus and areolar tissue.

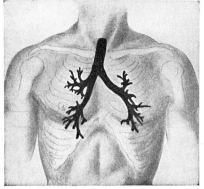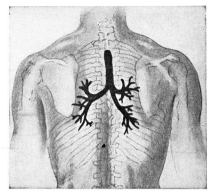

Fig. 121. Diagrams showing the relation of the bronchi to the chest wall. The right bronchus is larger and a more direct continuation of the trachea, which slopes slightly to the right. The trachea bifurcates at the level of Ludwig's angle slightly to the right of the midsternal line. In this region vocal and tactile fremitus are increased, and breath sounds are bronchovesicular in character.

Fremitus is normally increased in the second right interspace anteriorly because of the proximity of the bronchial bifurcation, and posteriorly between the scapulae because of the proximity of large bronchi (Fig. 121).

Fremitus is normally decreased or absent if the voice is not sufficiently forceful or resonant. It is also diminished by a thick layer of fat in the thoracic wall, by large pectoral muscles and especially by large breasts.

Pathologic Variations. Fremitus is pathologically increased wherever the ratio of lung tissue or solid matter to air is *increased,* if the bronchus to that area is patulous (patent). For example, it will be increased with fibrosis as from pulmonary tuberculosis, over superficially situated thick-walled cavities, or over a solid mass lesion such as a primary or metastatic tumor. It will also be increased if the lung is consolidated by a pneumonic process of any type.

Fremitus is pathologically decreased whenever the ratio of lung tissue to air is decreased. This occurs over thin-walled cavities, with generalized emphysema, over giant bullae, or in the late stage of asthma with emphysema.

Fremitus will be decreased or absent when the bronchus supplying that segment is occluded by compression, endobronchial tumor, foreign body or retained secretions, regardless of the status of the lung tissue distal to that point.

Air in the pleural cavity (*pneumothorax*) or fluid of any type (*hydrothorax, hemothorax, pyothorax*) tends to block the transmission of vibrations from the lung to the chest wall; fremitus will be diminished or abolished. In rare instances a massive effusion will produce so much compression of the underlying lung tissue that the dulling effect of the fluid is outweighed by the increased vibrations in the solid lung tissue; in that case fremitus may be normal or increased. Fremitus will be decreased if the pleura is markedly thickened.

Pathologic Types of Fremitus.   Partial obstruction of a bronchus, especially when produced by secretions, may set up vibrations in the bronchus and lung tissue during normal respiration. Probably everyone has experienced this "rattle" during some stage of a chest cold. These vibrations may give rise to palpable *rhonchal fremitus*. A cough may also be palpable (*tussive fremitus*).

PATHOLOGIC VIBRATIONS

Vibrations of other types may occasionally be felt over the thorax and must not be confused with fremitus. Flowing blood may produce a *thrill*, which is the palpable component of a murmur. Fluid plus air can give rise to a *succussion splash* (p. 201), first described by Hippocrates. *Friction fremitus* denotes palpable vibrations produced by movement and rubbing of altered endothelial surfaces; they may be pleural, pleuropericardial, pericardial or, rarely, peritoneal (splenic or hepatic) in origin.

Crepitation is a peculiar sensation perceived when pressure is made over a collection of interstitial air. When felt over the thorax it usually indicates that air has escaped from the lung and pleural cavity or mediastinum into the adjacent tissues. It may occur with pneumothorax, with fractured ribs and laceration of the lung, or following penetrating wounds, accidental or surgical. In rare instances it is due to gas gangrene.

PALPATION OF THE PRECORDIAL AREA

Place one hand lightly on the chest wall to determine the general characteristics of the cardiac impulse (Fig. 122); then use the finger tips for more definite localization (Fig. 123). It is customary to determine two points. One is the point of *maximum* impulse (P.M.I.). The other is the apex beat or apical impulse (A.I.), the point *farthest downward and outward* at which definite pulsations can still be felt. In some persons there may be a distance of several centimeters between these; in others the two areas seem to coincide.

In an adult of average build the apex beat will usually be found in the fifth left interspace about 8 or 9 cm. from the midsternal line. Normally its position will change slightly with respiration. On deep inspir-

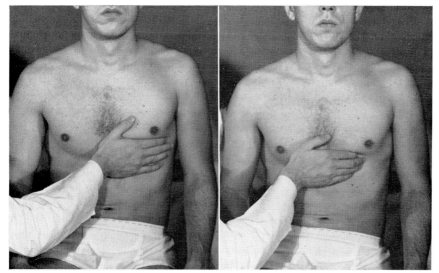

Fig. 122　　　　　　　　　　　　Fig. 123

Fig. 122. Palpation of precordium to determine the general characteristics of the cardiac impulse.

Fig. 123. Finger tips used to localize the site of the point of maximum impulse (P.M.I.) and of the apical impulse (A.I.).

ation it may move downward to the sixth interspace, or it may disappear as inflated lung tissue is interposed between the heart and the chest wall. With forced expiration it moves upward and somewhat laterally. Other causes for variations in position and force of the cardiac impulse have already been considered (p. 168). It should be remembered that a feeble cardiac impulse is not necessarily or even usually indicative of weak cardiac contractions.

Precordial Thrill. A thrill felt over the precordium is usually due to vibrations produced in the heart or large vessels. Light palpation is required; firm pressure may damp the vibrations or completely obliterate them. Rest the hand very lightly on the chest wall; then slowly increase the pressure. If a thrill is present it will impart a vibratory sensation very similar to that felt when one touches a purring cat.

A thrill may occur either during systole or during diastole; determine the exact time by observing or palpating the apex beat or the pulsations of a carotid artery. The location, intensity and extent should be noted. The most intense thrills are systolic in time and are felt over the base of the heart, either to the right or to the left of the sternum; they are encountered with narrowing (*stenosis*) of the aortic or pulmonic valve. Aortic insufficiency (regurgitation) may give rise to a diastolic thrill; mitral stenosis sometimes produces a late diastolic thrill. These conditions will be discussed in Chapter XV.

XI

Percussion of the Thorax

In Chapter IX brief reference was made to Leopold Auenbrugger, the discoverer of the value of percussion in physical diagnosis, and to his method of immediate percussion, which involved striking the chest with the finger tips. In 1828 Piorry[1] published his work *De la Percussion Médiate,* in which he described the use of a narrow piece of ivory (*pleximeter*) pressed firmly against the chest to transmit the blow struck by the finger (*plexor*). Later modifications included the use of a small rubber hammer to strike the blow, and the substitution of a finger as the pleximeter. Eventually the modern method became universal; fingers are now used both as plexor and as pleximeter.

TECHNIQUE OF PERCUSSION

For a right-handed examiner, the middle finger of the left hand usually serves as pleximeter; it is placed firmly against the chest wall in an intercostal space (Fig. 125). The plexor is the tip of the middle finger of the right hand; the finger nail should be short. With wrist motion, the left finger is struck sharply between the nail and the distal interphalangeal joint.

Skill in percussion is acquired only by prolonged practice. Certain common faults must be overcome: (1) The novice has difficulty in striking the left finger at the proper point; coordination will come with practice. (2) The pleximeter finger is not pressed firmly against the chest wall; this alters and muffles the note. (3) The whole hand is allowed to rest on the chest; this also renders percussion unreliable. Learn to keep the hand and other fingers away from the chest wall. (4) The beginner is too tense; the fingers are apposed, the wrist is held fixed

[1] Pierre-Adolphe Piorry, French physician, 1794–1879.

180

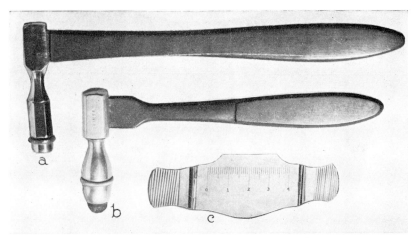

Fig. 124. Plexors and pleximeter formerly used for percussion. *a*, Skoda model; *b*, Seitz model; *c*, metal pleximeter with centimeter scale (Traube's model). (Courtesy of Mütter Museum, Philadelphia College of Physicians.)

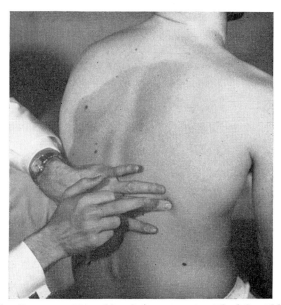

Fig. 125. Correct position of hands for percussion. The left middle finger makes firm pressure in an intercostal space; the other fingers are slightly raised so that they do not touch the chest wall. The right middle finger is poised to strike a short, sharp blow.

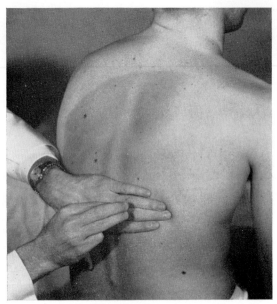

Fig. 126. Incorrect. The whole hand is pressed against the chest wall, thus damping the vibrations produced by the blow of the plexor. The fingers of the right hand are apposed, the wrist is rigid and the fingers are ready to deliver a sledge hammer blow. These are the most common faults of the novice.

and the blow is delivered with the forearm, as with a sledge (Fig. 126). The expert strikes a short, sharp blow and allows the finger to rebound, just as the hammer in a piano does; this avoids muffling of the vibrations by pressure of the plexor. (5) The amateur thumps repeatedly, like a woodpecker. One or two properly delivered blows will be sufficient when the mechanics of the procedure have become automatic; full attention can then be devoted to listening to the note produced. Learn to slow up; strike—listen; strike—listen.

The percussion blow may be light or forceful. Light percussion is essential for demonstrating small superficial lesions or for outlining organs. More forceful percussion is needed to detect large lesions deeper in the chest; it may also be required to elicit a satisfactory percussion note if the subcutaneous tissues are thick. For practical purposes it may be assumed that the penetration of the percussion wave is no more than 6 cm. inward from the skin. Even in an emaciated adult this will fail to demonstrate a deeply situated mass that is covered by aerated lung (Fig. 127).

Generally the novice uses too forceful a blow; he thinks that the harder he strikes, the easier it will be to discover what he should find. He tends to concentrate on the loudness of the sound, which is often the least important factor. Eventually he learns to recognize and evaluate

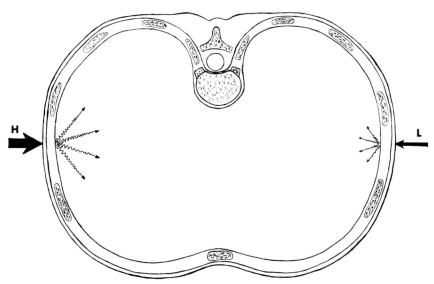

Fig. 127. Penetration of percussion wave with moderately forceful percussion (H) and with light percussion (L). A deeply situated lesion surrounded by normal lung tissue would not alter the percussion note.

the other characteristics—pitch, duration and timbre; then he will find that light percussion is much more rewarding.

Sense of Resistance. With experience, the sense of touch can become as important as the percussion note actually heard, or even more helpful. The character, duration and relative pitch of the vibrations can be felt as well as heard. Moreover, there is a sense of resistance over solid tissues which contrasts with the elasticity felt over air-containing areas. The development of this tactile recognition will enable you to detect percussion changes even in a relatively noisy area where distracting sounds hamper the usual auditory interpretation of the percussion note.

TYPES OF PERCUSSION SOUNDS

On percussing various areas, several different types of sound can be produced; the characteristics of these depend upon the nature of the tissue percussed. Over the thorax the note is determined largely by the ratio of air to solid tissue. A relative increase in the amount of air will give a more booming note; a relative decrease results in a duller or deader sound. If there were nothing but air inside the thoracic cage, the note would be drum-like. Any solid tissue gives a dead or flat sound.

Between these two there are various gradations, and sometimes it is difficult to classify the sound exactly.

By convention, the sounds produced by percussion are called: (1) tympany; (2) hyperresonance; (3) resonance; (4) impaired resonance; (5) dullness; (6) flatness. Each of these will now be described and discussed but not in this same order.

Resonance.   Since this is the sound produced by percussing the thorax over healthy lung tissue it will be considered first. Resonance is a fairly sustained note of moderate pitch. The lung supplies a relatively low-pitched element and also acts as a resonator. The combination of these produces resonance. It should be obvious that there can be considerable variation in pitch and in amplitude of this "normal" sound, which is influenced by factors such as the general contour of the thorax, the amount of muscle and subcutaneous tissue and the elasticity of the underlying lung. To recognize such alterations as physiologic and to decide whether or not the percussion note can be considered resonant for a given individual requires judgment; this will come with practice and experience.

Tympany.   This derives its name from the tympanum or kettle drum. It is a musical note of somewhat higher pitch than resonance. It is elicited when air in a closed chamber vibrates in unison with its elastic wall; it occurs over an air-filled hollow viscus such as the stomach or the intestine. If such an air-filled organ lies under the costal cage it will give rise to tympany in that area.

Except with transposition of the viscera, tympany is not normally present over the right hemithorax; on the left it may be physiologic in certain areas. The upper portion of the stomach lies beneath the lower ribs; if it contains a moderate amount of air, as it often does, this will give rise to a tympanitic note to the left of the ensiform and extending a few centimeters lateral to that point. This is known at *Traube's*[2] *semilunar space.* If the stomach is distended with gas a tympanitic note will be elicited over the left upper abdomen and much of the lower portion of the left hemithorax anteriorly. If the stomach contains no gas, but is filled with fluid or solid material, this area will be dull or flat on percussion. Traube's space will be reduced or obliterated by enlargement of the left lobe of the liver, by a large pericardial or left pleural effusion, or by massive enlargement of the spleen. It will not be altered by consolidation of the lung. It will decrease in size or disappear when the person lies down; gastric contents fill the upper portion of the stomach and the air is displaced caudad below the costal margin.

Tympany can be the result of a pocket of gas in the splenic flexure of the colon; this lies lateral to the stomach. Unless the bowel is markedly

2 Ludwig Traube, German physician, 1818–76.

dilated this note will be higher in pitch than gastric tympany, since the resonating chamber is smaller in diameter.

When tympany is present over other areas of the thorax it is abnormal. Collapse of the lung due to the presence of air in the pleural cavity (*pneumothorax*) will give rise to such a note; so will a large superficial cavity or an emphysematous bulla.

Hyperresonance. This sound lies between resonance and tympany. It is indicative of an increased amount of air, a decreased amount of tissue, or both. It may occasionally be produced physiologically at the base of the left lung by the combination of lung resonance plus tympany from a small amount of air in the stomach or splenic flexure. Pathologically, it is present with pulmonary emphysema. It may also be present if there is a small pneumothorax with only minimal collapse of the lung; here again resonance and tympany combine to produce this note.

Flatness. This is a very short, high-pitched sound. It is the normal note produced by percussing over tissue which contains no air, such as the muscles of the thigh. It is never present normally over the lungs. Pathologically, it usually denotes the presence of a massive pleural effusion; the air-containing lung has been displaced mesially beyond the range of the percussion stroke. Occasionally it is elicited over a completely airless lung.

Dullness. This is a short, high-pitched sound with very little resonance and with limited carrying power. It represents the composite sound produced by resonance from the lung plus a more pronounced element from solid airless tissue. It is normally present over the borders of the heart, the mediastinum, the upper portion of the liver and spleen —organs which are solid but which are adjacent to air-containing lung.

Liver Dullness. This is normally demonstrable on the right side anteriorly below the fourth rib; the note becomes flat below the sixth rib. These same changes are present laterally and posteriorly, where the level of dullness is opposite the tenth thoracic spinous process.

Splenic Dullness. This is more difficult to demonstrate. If the spleen is of normal size it will give rise to an oval area of dullness on the left in the region of the ninth to eleventh ribs laterally. This may be obscured by tympany produced by air in the stomach or colon, or by flatness if those viscera contain solids or liquids. When the spleen is markedly enlarged it is much easier to demonstrate the area of dullness, but palpation of the abdomen is more helpful in such cases.

Abnormal Dullness. When dullness is found over normally resonant areas of the chest it indicates a pathologic change in the underlying tissues. This alteration may be in the lung tissue itself or in the pleural space. If in the lung, either much of the air has been absorbed (*atelectasis*, p. 214) or it has been replaced by solid material. The latter may be fluid in the alveoli, as in pneumonia or in cardiac failure with severe passive congestion, or it may represent cellular proliferation such as a primary or metastatic tumor. In the pleural space a moderate amount of fluid will result in percussion dullness; a primary or secondary malignant process will give a similar note.

Impaired Resonance.　This term refers to a slight decrease in resonance, but not enough to constitute dullness. It can result from a decreased amount of air in the lung; more commonly it is due to diffuse fibrosis or an infiltrative process in the lung parenchyma such as tuberculosis, or to thickening of the pleura.

MODIFIED PERCUSSION SOUNDS

Various modifications of the percussion note can be the result of certain pathologic changes in the underlying tissues.

Metallic Ring.　This is a sound heard on percussing over a large superficially situated and relatively empty pulmonary cavity with tense walls, over a high-pressure pneumothorax (tension pneumothorax) or over a markedly distended and relatively empty hollow viscus.

Cracked-pot Sound.　This note has a peculiar character which is more easily demonstrated than described. Percussion of a fully inflated cheek with the mouth closed produces a tympanitic note. Open the mouth very slightly and repeat the percussion; this simulates the cracked-pot sound. It is produced by suddenly forcing air through a small or slit-like opening. Percussion of the chest of a crying child may produce such a sound as air is suddenly forced through the glottis. A large superficial cavity with a small opening into a bronchus may also produce this note. Sometimes it can be heard best with the aid of a stethoscope; have the patient hold the chest piece close to his opened mouth while you percuss.

Skodaic Resonance.　This sound was mentioned by Auenbrugger but apparently it was not until Josef Skoda[3] published his treatise in 1839 that this sign became widely known, and by Skoda's name. A translation of his observation is: "When the lower portion of a lung is entirely compressed by any pleuritic effusion, and its upper portion reduced in volume, the percussion note at the upper part of the thorax is distinctly tympanitic." The explanation of this sound is not well established; apparently it is produced by relaxed lung near the upper limit of effusion. Even Skoda himself, an expert physicist also, was baffled; he commented: "That the lungs partially deprived of air, should yield

---

[3] Josef Skoda, Austrian physician, 1805–81.

a tympanitic, and when the quantity of air in them is increased, a non-tympanitic sound appears opposed to the laws of physics."

DEMONSTRATION OF PERCUSSION SOUNDS

A simple way to learn to recognize some of these alterations is to select a healthy adult with a thin chest wall and percuss in the right anterior third, fourth, fifth, sixth and seventh interspaces. In the third interspace the note will be resonant. In the fourth it will be resonant or slightly impaired by the dome of the underlying liver. In the fifth, dullness will be found; there is little lung overlying the liver. The sixth or seventh interspace will yield a flat note because liver alone is present.

To demonstrate a moderate degree of impaired resonance and of hyperresonance, percuss again in the third interspace. Then have the subject exhale as completely as possible.* Percuss the same area; the note will have lost some of its resonance and would be classified as impaired resonance. Then have him take a deep breath; the percussion note will become more resonant than before, or slightly hyperresonant. In this example the amount of lung tissue has remained constant but the amount of air has been altered. In various disease states it is common to find that both factors have been altered.

PROCEDURE FOR PERCUSSION

The most satisfactory results will be achieved if both you and the patient are comfortable, and preferably are seated. If possible, have the patient's thorax as high as or higher than yours. You will find it easier to reach upward and percuss accurately than to bend forward or reach down to examine the lower portions of his thorax. Needless to say, the room should be comfortably warm, and so should your hands.

Whenever possible, examine the back first; this is especially important if lung disease is suspected. Before you start, get the patient into a comfortable position. He should fold his arms or drop his hands on his lap; this relaxes the shoulder girdle muscles and moves the scapulae laterally. He should not try to sit upright with the spine rigid; let him slump forward a little while you examine his back.

Until you gain experience, it is advisable to attempt to establish

---

* Whenever you say something like "Stop breathing" or "Take a deep breath," do the same thing yourself. Then you will not forget to tell the patient to breathe again before he becomes cyanotic or unconscious.

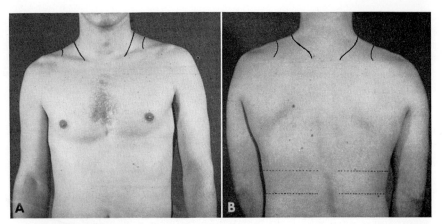

Fig. 128. Krönig's isthmus. *A*, Normal anterior view; *B*, normal posterior view. One isthmus may be narrow if there is unilateral tuberculosis or other fibrotic disease producing retraction of the apex; both will be narrowed if the disease is bilateral.

Diaphragmatic excursion posteriorly is also indicated. Normally this should be at least two interspaces.

a "normal" note for each patient. Select an area that is probably not diseased, and that has a minimal amount of subcutaneous tissue and muscle. The seventh or eighth posterolateral interspace fairly well out toward the axilla is often suitable. Determine the characteristics of the note here, and use that as the standard for describing the findings elsewhere.

Now start at the apex and outline Krönig's[4] isthmus (Fig. 128). This is a band or "shoulder strap" of resonance over the apex of the lung, which lies between the neck and the shoulder girdle muscles. In mapping out the isthmus it is well to begin the percussion well up the side of the neck and gradually come downward until a change from nonresonance to resonance is noted. The outer line is mapped out similarly by approaching the resonant area from the point of the shoulder. This isthmus will be narrowed by fibrotic contraction of the apex of the lung or by infiltration of any type; occasionally resonance is completely lost in this area.

Then percuss downward, comparing corresponding areas in each interspace on the two sides. As you approach the lower margin of the thorax the percussion note will change in character; if no disease is present, this marks the position of the diaphragm during quiet respiration. The extent of diaphragmatic excursion should now be determined. Have the patient exhale completely; percuss the lower level of pulmonary resonance. Then have him take a deep breath and hold it; again check the limit of resonance. The distance between these two points represents the diaphragmatic excursion; in a healthy adult it should be at least

[4] George Krönig, German physician, 1856–1911.

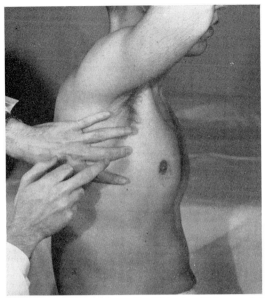

Fig. 129. Percussion of chest laterally. This should be carried as high as possible into the axilla.

two interspaces. The same procedure should be repeated when examining the sides and front of the chest.

When you have finished percussing the back, have the patient place his hands on or behind his head while you percuss each lateral aspect, starting high in the axilla and proceeding downward to the base (Fig. 129).

When examining the front of the chest it is advisable to have the patient seated at one side, rather than directly in front of you. If this is not possible, make sure that he turns his head away from you; thus you can minimize the risk of inhaling potentially dangerous droplets if he coughs. He should now sit upright, with his arms hanging loosely at his sides; this widens the interspaces and makes percussion easier. Again you should percuss each interspace from apex to base, and determine the excursion of the diaphragm.

CARDIAC DULLNESS

The area of cardiac dullness often seems difficult to delineate, but with practice one can become fairly proficient. It is true that emphysema, obesity, heavy pectoral muscles or large breasts make percussion more difficult and less reliable, but no examination of the thorax is adequate

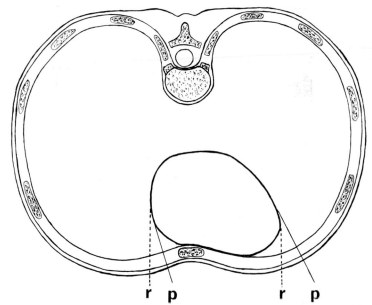

r p   r p

Fig. 130. In the usual PA chest x-ray, the tube is located at some distance behind the chest; the film is placed in front. Since the roentgen rays are practically parallel at this distance, they delineate the cardiac borders as indicated (r, r). The percussion vibrations (p, p) are propagated at right angles to the thoracic wall at the point of impact; the normal contour of the chest results in an apparent shift of the heart to the left. The degree of displacement will depend upon the contour of the thorax and the skill of the examiner; very light percussion will demonstrate changes farther to the right than those shown in the drawing.

unless an attempt is made to determine and record the apparent size of the heart.

To outline the heart, it is essential that light percussion be used; with too forceful a stroke the borders will not be picked up accurately. To determine the left border, start percussing in the third left interspace well out toward the axilla and gradually move the pleximeter finger toward the sternum until a slight but definite change is noted. Mark that spot, or measure its distance from the midsternal line. Repeat this performance in the fourth and fifth interspaces, and in the sixth if the diaphragm has been found to be low. Then determine the right border in the third and fourth interspaces; liver dullness renders percussion in the fifth interspace of no value unless the diaphragm is low.

Normally the right atrium extends 1 to 2 cm. to the right of the sternal border in the third and fourth interspaces. Very light percussion is required to demonstrate this; often the change is indicated by impaired resonance rather than dullness. If dullness extends well out to the right of the sternum in this area it suggests enlargement of the atrium, pericardial effusion, displacement of the heart or the presence of pulmonary disease at that site.

On the left, the size and shape of the area of dullness depend upon the contour and position of the heart. An average measurement would be 9 or 10 cm. to the left of the midsternal line in the fifth interspace. In any case, dullness should be found as far laterally as the apical impulse (p. 178). The total transverse diameter of the area of cardiac dullness should be less than one-half the transverse diameter of the thorax.

Often the measurements obtained by percussion do not seem to correspond with those found by x-ray. The total transverse diameter may seem the same, but on the film the right border is seen farther to the right; the left border and apex are nearer to the sternum than found on percussion. One reason for this discrepancy is shown in Figure 130.

In addition to this area of dullness, one should be able to demonstrate a small area of flatness over the heart near the sternum if very light percussion is used. A thin wedge of lung lies between the left lateral border and the chest wall. Anteriorly there is an area not covered by lung; this is where flatness can be elicited. Since resonant lung partially encircles the heart, some authors prefer to speak of relative and absolute dullness when referring to these areas.

SUPRACARDIAC DULLNESS

The area of supracardiac dullness should then be outlined by percussing in the first and second interspaces, both to the right and to the left of the sternum. Normally, dullness does not extend any appreciable distance lateral to the sternal border in this region. A widened area of dullness can be due to such abnormalities as an enlarged substernal thyroid, engorgement of the superior vena cava, dilatation, tortuosity or aneurysm of the ascending limb of the aorta, or the presence of a thymoma or other superior mediastinal tumor.

XII

Auscultation of the Lungs

Auscultation is often the most informative procedure in examination of the lungs. It also provides information to supplement or confirm your previous observations.

PRODUCTION OF BREATH SOUNDS

For generations the accepted explanation for the production of breath sounds as heard by the ear or through a stethoscope held firmly against the chest wall was that they were due in part to vibrations produced by air flowing through the upper respiratory tract, larynx, trachea and bronchi, and in part to the separation and distention of the alveoli by the inrushing current of air. In recent years certain observations have been published which cast some doubt on this concept; apparently such factors as muscular contractions and the movements of the thorax must also be considered. At present, it seems safe to say that the exact details are still unknown. This, however, does not alter the fact that various types of breath sounds are known to be associated with certain pathologic changes in the tracheobronchial tree and in lung tissue.

TYPES OF BREATH SOUNDS

Vesicular Breath Sounds. These are the sounds you will hear over most portions of normal lung tissue; the exceptions will be discussed later. Vesicular breath sounds are soft and rustling in character and low in pitch, ranging down to 100 vibrations per second. They are audible all during inspiration and continue without any appreciable break through the first part of expiration. Then they fade out and become too faint to be heard, although they can still be recorded by instruments more sensitive than the human ear. The ratio of audible inspiration to expiration during quiet breathing is roughly 5:1 or 5:2, as opposed to the physiologic ratio of 5:6. The breath sounds are louder during inspiration than during expiration.

——Tracheal Breath Sounds.   These are the sounds you will hear if you place your stethoscope over the side of the neck in the region of the thyroid cartilage. They are harsh and high-pitched, with a distinct pause between inspiration and expiration; the latter is even longer, harsher and higher-pitched than the former.

——Bronchial Breath Sounds.   Bronchial or tubular breath sounds closely resemble—but are not identical with—the sounds heard over the trachea. They may be loud or they may be faint, but the typical characteristics are unchanged. Inspiration is harsh and even higher-pitched

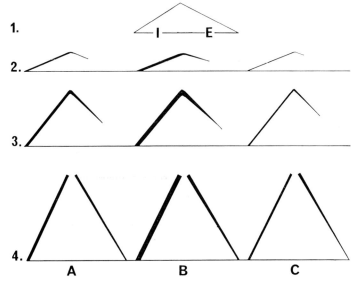

Fig. 131.   Breath sounds. In these drawings the relative pitch is indicated by the acuteness of the angle, and the intensity by thickness of the lines. The drawings also indicate average or normal (A), increased (B) and decreased (C) breath sounds of each type.

1. Physiologic ratio of inspiration to expiration; normally this is 5:6.

2. Vesicular breath sounds. Inspiration is soft and low-pitched; only the first part of expiration is heard.

3. Bronchovesicular breath sounds. The pitch is higher and much of expiration is audible. Decreased bronchovesicular breath sounds are often confused with increased vesicular breathing. The duration seems much the same but the distinguishing feature is the difference in pitch.

4. Bronchial breath sounds. Inspiration and expiration are harsh and high-pitched. There is a distinct pause between the two sounds. Expiration is longer and often higher pitched than inspiration.

than the tracheal inspiratory sound. There is a definite pause between inspiration and expiration, and the expiratory sound is louder, longer and of higher pitch than inspiration; it may even rise in pitch. Bronchial breathing is never heard over any normal lung tissue.

The higher pitch of expiration in bronchial breathing can be explained on an anatomic basis. During inspiration the negative pressure within the thorax tends to exert traction on the walls of the bronchi and bronchioles; they become slightly longer and larger in diameter. With expiration the reverse change occurs; the shorter, smaller tubes produce a higher-pitched note.

Bronchovesicular Breath Sounds.   This term is applied to breath sounds which fall between the two extremes—vesicular and bronchial. As the name implies, they seem to combine certain features of each. Obviously the spectrum is wide; the sounds may range from almost vesicular to almost bronchial in character. To recognize it, attention must be directed to expiration; this is longer and higher-pitched than in vesicular breathing, but does not meet the criteria listed for bronchial breath sounds. Physiologically, bronchovesicular breath sounds are heard normally in those areas in which fremitus is also increased—the right apex, the second right interspace anteriorly, and between the scapulae posteriorly. When heard in an adult at any other area, such sounds should be considered abnormal and usually are indicative of lung disease.

Since the explanation of the production of breath sounds is so uncertain, it would seem justifiable to further confound the issue by suggesting an analogy that has seemed to help students understand and interpret the sounds they hear. When excessive noise is present in a room, an acoustic engineer will cover walls, ceiling and other solid structures that reflect sound with some porous material that will absorb, scatter and diffuse the vibrations. The major component of the respiratory sound is produced by vibrations in the larger air passages, and we find that Nature has performed a similar sound-conditioning feat. By interposing a thick layer of porous lung tissue between the bronchi and the stethoscope, the vibrations are so scattered and diffused that they become merely a faint whisper (vesicular breath sounds). When the layer is not so thick, the bronchial element is more prominent and bronchovesicular sounds may be normal; this holds true in the areas mentioned above, where the bronchi lie close to the chest wall. If, however, the air is replaced by exudate as in pneumonia, by fibrosis or by a mass lesion, the damping effect of the air sacs is diminished or lost. Solids transmit the vibrations; bronchial or bronchovesicular breath sounds are heard, depending upon the relative proportion of solid tissue to air-containing lung.

In infants and very small children the normal breath sounds are very similar to those called bronchovesicular in an adult. Because the chest is so small, there is no area where a thick layer of lung tissue is interposed between the bronchi and your stethoscope. For similar reasons, the normal breath sounds in a person with a small, thin, flat chest will differ from those heard in one with a large deep thorax. Sounds that might be interpreted as bordering on bronchovesicular in the latter could be considered perfectly physiologic in a flat chest. Therefore it is advisable to establish a "normal" in each patient, just as a normal percussion note was determined (p. 188).

ALTERED BREATH SOUNDS

Absent Breath Sounds. Physiologically, breath sounds are never persistently absent over the entire thorax during life, but at times they may be so faint that they are difficult to hear, especially if respiration is very shallow. Pathologically, complete occlusion of a bronchus will result in absence of breath sounds over the area supplied by that bronchus, regardless of the status of the lung tissue distal to the obstruction. A massive pleural effusion may also block all transmission; so much of the sound is reflected at the lung-fluid and fluid-chest wall interfaces that nothing is heard. A large pneumothorax may also block breath sounds completely.

Decreased Breath Sounds. Physiologically these may be due to diminished sound production or to altered conduction. The former may be present in a healthy person at rest who is breathing slowly and shallowly, or in a person with generalized muscular weakness. Poor conduction may be due to massive muscles, adiposity, large breasts or edema of the chest wall. Pathologically the production of breath sounds will be decreased whenever respiration causes pain as with pleurisy or fractured ribs, with localized muscular weakness or paralysis due to nerve injury or disease, or with thoracic rigidity or restricted diaphragmatic movement due to intrathoracic or intra-abdominal disease. Transmission will be decreased somewhat if there is a pleural effusion of moderate size, partial pneumothorax or thickening of the pleura due to fibrosis or tumor. The characteristics of the breath sounds will depend upon the status of the underlying lung tissue.

Exaggerated Breath Sounds. This term denotes only an increase in the intensity of the breath sounds without change in their fundamental characteristics. Both inspiration and expiration become louder and more of the expiratory phase is audible. It is normal in children (puerile breathing) since the respiratory rate is rapid, or in adults after exercise. It should not be confused with bronchovesicular breathing.

ABNORMAL BREATH SOUNDS

Asthmatic Breath Sounds.   In asthma the diameter of the bronchi is decreased by spasm, edema and secretions. During inspiration the bronchi open as much as possible, but during expiration there may be exaggeration of the collapse normally seen. Therefore inspiration tends to be short and gasping, while expiration is markedly prolonged and usually high-pitched. In addition, wheezes and rhonchi are heard during expiration and often during inspiration.

Cavernous Breath Sounds.   These are low in pitch; expiration is longer and lower in pitch than is inspiration. Cavernous breath sounds may be heard over a large superficial thin-walled cavity or over an open pneumothorax. It is attributed to reinforcement of the low-pitched component of the breath sounds by the large air-containing space.

Amphoric Breath Sounds.   These are high in pitch and metallic in quality. They may be heard over a tense, thick-walled, superficial cavity or over an area of pneumothorax. Forceful breathing is often required to produce amphoric or cavernous breath sounds.

Metamorphosing Breathing.   Occasionally the breath sounds may be faint and indistinct at the start of inspiration, but suddenly become much more intense and often altered in quality. This is thought to be due to the sudden opening of a partially occluded bronchus as the lung expands; it is also known as the veiled puff of Skoda and as "trap-door" breathing.

Cog-wheel Respiration.   Instead of producing a soft, continuous sound, inspiration becomes a series of puffs or jerks and pauses. This results from irregular inflation of the pulmonary tissue. When due to parenchymal or pleural disease the interruptions occur at irregular intervals; this is usually heard over the upper lung fields. In the more common type the variations are synchronous with the heart beat; the adjacent lung expands rapidly during systole. This phenomenon is best heard over the lower portion of the left lung; it is of no clinical significance. It may be mistaken for a faint systolic murmur, but it disappears when the patient holds his breath.

Emphysematous Breath Sounds.   With pulmonary emphysema the breath sounds are always diminished; the markedly restricted movement of the thorax and diaphragm limits the amount of air moved with each breath. This produces few vibrations, and the transmission of these is poor. Inspiration may be very faint or inaudible; expiration may be more easily heard and is relatively low-pitched.

VOICE SOUNDS

The procedure for eliciting vocal resonance is the same as for testing tactile fremitus (p. 176), but auscultation is substituted for palpation. When a person speaks in a normal manner you will hear a confused indistinct sound as you listen over the chest wall; the words themselves cannot be recognized. This normal vocal resonance has the same origin as tactile fremitus and will be decreased or increased for the same physiologic reasons and by the same pathologic processes.

Bronchophony.   Literally, this means the sound heard over a large bronchus. It denotes vocal resonance which is loud and seems very close to the ear; the words are more distinct but still slightly distorted. Pathologically it occurs over an area of pulmonary consolidation of any etiology, with atelectasis or compression of lung tissue, with partial compression of a bronchus by an extrinsic mass, and sometimes over a thin-walled cavity. It is usually associated with increased tactile fremitus, percussion dullness and bronchovesicular or bronchial breath sounds. It will not be heard if the bronchus is completely occluded proximal to the point at which you are listening.

Pectoriloquy.   This is the transmission of syllabic speech to the chest wall. The most useful form is whispered pectoriloquy. Have the person whisper slowly words such as "one, one, one" or "ninety-nine, ninety-nine." Normally these sounds will be faint or inaudible over the thorax, and the words themselves will not be recognizable. With consolidation or other disease processes that produce bronchophony, the sounds will be heard without difficulty and the words will be clear and distinct. This change is often very helpful in picking up small areas of consolidation; the adjacent lung tissue may serve to mask or alter the other abnormal signs one might expect to find.

Egophony.   This is a modified form of bronchophony; the sounds are less resonant and higher in pitch. There is a nasal quality which to Laennec resembled the bleat of a goat (*aix*, goat; *phone*, voice). It also resembles what is incorrectly called "talking through the nose," when actually the nasal passages are occluded. It is heard most often just below the apparent level of a pleural effusion, especially when this overlies compressed or consolidated lung. It is of value because it helps to differentiate uncomplicated consolidation from consolidation with effusion; the former rarely, if ever, produces egophony.

↘ Don't Have egophony

ADVENTITIOUS SOUNDS

This is a term applied to sounds that are added; they are not merely alterations of sounds physiologically produced, such as breath sounds

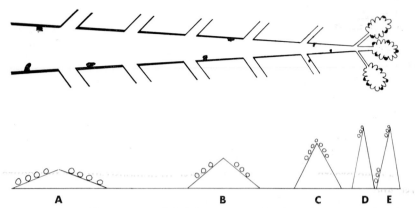

Fig. 132. Rales. *A,* Musical (sibilant; sonorous) rales. These are produced by vibrations of thick tenacious mucus and are usually most easily heard during expiration but may be heard almost continuously during both phases of respiration. *B,* Coarse (bubbling; gurgling) rales arise in the larger bronchi. These may be heard shortly after inspiration starts, and during most of expiration. *C,* Subcrepitant (medium; crackling) rales due to excess moisture in the smaller bronchi and bronchioles. These tend to occur during late inspiration and early expiration. *D,* Crepitant (fine; consonating) rales, indicative of exudate or transudate in the alveoli. These are most prominent at the end of inspiration, as air distends the alveoli. *E,* Post-tussive crepitant rales. These may be heard with the cough, at the start of inspiration or at the end of inspiration.

or vocal resonance. They are abnormal, and indicate the presence of intrathoracic disease.

Rales

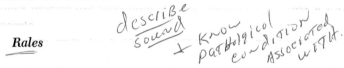

Rales of one type or another are the most commonly heard adventitious sounds. They were mentioned by Hippocrates; Laennec first attempted to classify them, but even today there is no unanimity concerning nomenclature.

Rales may be heard during one or both phases of respiration when there is excess fluid of any sort in the alveoli or in any portion of the tracheobronchial tree. Since they are produced by vibrations of fluid, regardless of its viscosity, terms such as "dry rales" or "moist rales" are not merely confusing; they are etiologically incorrect.

Crepitant (Fine; Consonating) Rales. These are very fine and high-pitched and are most commonly heard at or near the end of inspiration. They can be simulated by holding a lock of hair close to the ear and rubbing it between the thumb and fingers. Movement of the stethoscope on a hairy chest wall produces a similar sound and may lead to erroneous conclusions; wetting or greasing the hair may be necessary to diminish or abolish this extrapulmonary source of confusion.

Crepitant rales usually occur in showers and are thought to be produced by the separation of the moist walls of collapsed alveoli or alveolar ducts as air enters and distends them. When persistently present they are indicative of alveolar exudation, congestion or inflammation. They occur primarily with pulmonary infection of any type or with pulmonary congestion due to circulatory disturbances.

Crepitant rales may be accentuated by cough; occasionally they are heard only after cough. These are called latent or *post-tussive rales*. To elicit them, have the subject exhale as completely as possible, apply a final squeeze by giving a short cough *without* taking a breath, and then take a deep breath. You will probably have to demonstrate this procedure first, and then have him practice it; usually he tries to take a short breath before coughing. When he finally learns to do this properly, listen while he coughs and as he takes the deep breath. Crepitant rales may be heard with the cough, at the start of inspiration or occasionally only near the end of inspiration.

Marginal (Atelectatic) Rales. During normal respiration the lungs are never fully expanded. Small areas at the extreme periphery remain unaerated and secretions tend to accumulate, especially in the most dependent portions. With a deep breath, these areas are re-expanded. By listening carefully over the lower lung margin as the patient takes his first deep breath or two, crepitant-like rales may be heard. Unlike true crepitant rales, which persist, these marginal rales disappear after a few deep breaths. That is why they are seldom found during a routine examination of the chest; the patient has already been breathing deeply for other procedures. Marginal rales are of no pathologic significance.

Subcrepitant (Medium; Crackling) Rales. These are lower-pitched and coarser in quality than crepitant rales. They resemble the sound produced by the "fizz" of a carbonated beverage when the bottle is first opened, or the crackle of a dry cigar rolled between the fingers. They are thought to originate in the bronchioles and smaller bronchi, and occur in many of the conditions that produce crepitant rales also.

Coarse (Bubbling; Gurgling) Rales. These are low-pitched, coarse and relatively loud. They arise in the larger bronchi and trachea, or in cavities. They are often altered or abolished by a vigorous cough. In an extremely ill person with a depressed or absent cough reflex, the accumulation of secretions in all parts of the tracheobronchial tree gives rise to a vast number of bubbling rales—the so-called death rattle.

Musical Rales (Rhonchi). These are sounds which Laennec and many others since him have improperly called "dry rales." They are produced by vibrations of thick, tenacious, wet mucus in bronchi of various sizes. When originating in smaller bronchi the sounds are high-pitched and sometimes are called *sibilant;* those arising in larger bronchi are lower in pitch or *sonorous.*

These rales may be audible as a "wheeze" at some distance from the patient. They are most prominent during expiration, although they are usually heard in both phases of respiration, and may produce an almost continuous sound. They often vary in intensity with the phase of respiration and become higher-pitched in expiration as the bronchial lumen becomes smaller. If few in number they may be altered or even temporarily abolished by cough; the mucus is dislodged and no longer vibrates.

Often the history or other physical signs suggest the presence of asthma, emphysema or some other disease in which one would expect to find musical rales or rhonchi, but none are heard. In such instances it may be possible to elicit them by having the person exhale as completely as possible while you listen just below the clavicle.

Narrowing of the bronchial lumen may also result in the production of musical rales. This may be due to swelling of the mucosa from hyperemia or edema, to spasm, to extrinsic pressure on the bronchus or to an intrinsic endobronchial lesion such as a carcinoma or an adenoma. In such cases the rales are heard in a localized area only.

Friction Sounds

The parietal and visceral pleural surfaces are normally smooth and glistening and slide silently over one another during respiration. When one or both of these layers become roughened, a friction rub can result.

For a close approximation of this sound, rub your thumb and forefinger together close to your ear. A friction sound seems very superficial, as though it originated in the bell of the stethoscope; sometimes it may, if you carelessly allow the instrument to slip over dry skin. Firm pressure on the thorax with a hand or with the stethoscope will often increase the intensity of a friction sound, as will a deep breath. Usually a pleural friction rub will be audible in both phases of respiration; occasionally it may be heard only during inspiration, particularly near the end. Since the excursion of the lung is greatest at the base laterally and anterolaterally, friction rubs are more common there and the loudest ones are usually heard in that area. Only rarely will you hear friction at the apex, since motion is minimal at that point. When sufficiently intense, the vibrations may be palpable as well as audible.

It is often difficult to differentiate friction sounds from a localized patch of rales or from muscle sounds in a tense, nervous or shivering patient. In addition to the characteristics mentioned above, pain on inspiration suggests the presence of pleurisy, which could give rise to a friction rub. Cough may alter or abolish rales; it does not affect a friction rub, even when you can persuade the patient to cough. If both are present, as they frequently are, there may be a change in the sounds heard after the cough.

A friction rub is evidence of pleural changes, but is not diagnostic of any specific disease. Inflammation (pleurisy) is the most common cause; occasionally this is primary in the pleura but usually it results from underlying lung disease that has spread to involve the visceral layer. Trauma to the chest wall, infection of those tissues or a fractured rib can produce changes in the parietal layer. With uremia, the patient often has a harsh, dry friction rub; dehydration may be responsible for this.

Succussion Splash

Succussion splash was first described by Hippocrates, and is pathognomonic of the presence of both fluid and air, either in the pleural cavity or in some other large space. To elicit it, have the patient bend quickly from side to side, or grasp his shoulders and shake him gently; listen for the splashing sound. When heard over the thorax it indicates either hydropneumothorax or herniation through the diapragm of a large hollow viscus containing both air and fluid, such as the stomach or colon. Over the lower ribs of the left hemithorax anteriorly or over the upper abdomen a normal gastric succussion splash may be heard; this should not cause confusion.

Metallic Tinkle

Metallic tinkle is a clear, vibrant musical sound which has been likened to the distant tinkling of a silver bell. It may be heard with hydropneumothorax when there is a bronchopleural fistula below the level of the fluid; air from the lung bubbles through the pleural fluid.

Bell Tympany

Bell tympany is a clear bell-like sound elicited by the coin test. Hold one silver coin flat on the anterior chest wall as the pleximeter; strike this with the edge of another silver coin. Listen with a stethoscope over the posterior chest wall. Bell tympany is heard only when air is present in the pleural space, but it is not invariably demonstrable.

XIII

Diseases of the Lung

and Pleura

When one or more abnormal physical signs are found on examination of the lungs, the next step is to attempt to reach a tentative explanation. Differential diagnosis requires a broad knowledge of medicine not possessed by students early in their training. However, it should be possible to reach a conclusion as to the nature of the pathologic changes present, even though the etiology may not be determined.

In previous chapters the possible variations in physical signs were described and the cause or causes for these were discussed. In this chapter an attempt will be made to group various signs together to arrive at a pathologic diagnosis. For example, dullness on percussion over the right upper lobe area is not by itself diagnostic, but if limited expansion, increased fremitus, bronchial breath sounds and whispered pectoriloquy are also found, one is justified in concluding that consolidation is present.

This is a pathologic diagnosis. The next step is to establish an etiologic diagnosis, if possible. Here the history and other physical findings are often of great importance. If the illness came on suddenly with a chill, chest pain, cough and expectoration, and if there are high fever, tachycardia and prostration, the most probable diagnosis is acute pneumonia of some type. Tuberculosis or extensive primary or metastatic carcinoma might produce the same physical signs in the lung, but the history and the general appearance of the patient would be entirely different.

One must think first of the various changes in the lungs or pleura that can produce each abnormal sign, then decide which one of these could explain the entire group of signs that have been found. Finally, one must see whether additional information (the history and the examination of other parts of the body) will point to some specific disease process. Remember always that the abnormal findings do not depend upon the

202

disease itself, but upon the abnormal physiology and the alteration in the physics of sound produced by changes in the underlying or involved tissues. A few of the more common diseases will now be discussed, in an attempt to point out this correlation.

DISEASES OF THE BRONCHI

Acute Bronchitis

This is usually a complication of an acute respiratory infection, but occasionally it occurs in a systemic disease such as measles, or as a result of the inhalation of irritating fumes or dusts.

Pathologic Changes.   Initially there are edema and hyperemia of the bronchial mucosa. Increased production of mucus soon follows; later the secretions become mucopurulent or purulent. With recovery the inflammatory changes disappear.

Physical Signs.   The abnormal signs are the result of excess secretions in the bronchial tree, plus the general physiologic changes produced by infection. A slight or moderate elevation of temperature is often present. With fever the respiratory rate is somewhat increased; otherwise it is normal. If the secretions are abundant, rhonchal fremitus will be felt. The lung parenchyma is not ordinarily involved; therefore the percussion note will be physiologic and the breath sounds will not be altered. However, small areas of atelectasis (p. 214) may occasionally develop intermittently, due to temporary plugging of small bronchi by viscid secretions. Subcrepitant rales and rhonchi will be heard over much or all of the chest.

History.   With acute bronchitis there is dull discomfort, soreness or a "raw" sensation beneath the sternum and the adjacent areas of the chest anteriorly. If the temperature is moderately elevated, intermittent episodes of chilliness may be annoying; headache and malaise might also be present. Initially the cough is dry and rasping; it is the result of inflammatory changes in the bronchi. As the secretion of mucus increases the cough becomes more and more productive; bacterial infection produces the typical mucopurulent sputum. With recovery the secretions become scanty and tenacious; these plus the residual inflammatory changes continue to stimulate the cough reflex long after the infection has been eliminated and the physical signs have disappeared.

Chronic Bronchitis

This may occasionally be the end result of repeated attacks of acute bronchitis; it can also be produced by prolonged exposure to dusts or irritating fumes. Chronic sinusitis is frequently present; this may be the focus that leads to repeated reinfection of the bronchi. Asthma also seems to produce a fertile soil for implantation of infection, as does the pulmonary congestion present with certain types of chronic heart disease.

Pathologic Changes.   The mucosa will be swollen and hypertrophic in the earlier stages, with excess mucus or mucopus. After months or years the mucosa becomes thinned and atrophic and partially replaced by scar tissue. Weakening of the walls may lead to dilatation with the production of bronchiectasis (below). Microscopically, round cell infiltration of the entire bronchial wall may be seen.

Physical Signs.   As with acute bronchitis, rales and rhonchi are the principal findings; the characteristics of these depend upon the size of the bronchi in which they are being produced. They will be altered if cough temporarily moves or expels mucus, but they recur as soon as secretions reaccumulate. When chronic bronchitis is accompanied by asthma or emphysema, the signs of those conditions will be added to the findings due to the bronchitis itself.

History.   Chronic cough that slowly becomes more frequent, more severe and more productive is the principal symptom. In the earlier stages the cough may decrease or almost disappear during the summer, only to recur in the fall and persist throughout the winter. Eventually it is perennial, with seasonal or periodic exacerbations.

Bronchiectasis

In this disease bronchi and bronchioles are enlarged, leading to increased amounts of secretion and the pooling of the secretions in the bronchial tree. Infection is always present.

Pathologic Changes.   The bronchial dilatation may be fusiform, cylindrical or saccular; it may be limited to a portion of one lobe or it may involve several lobes. It occurs more frequently in the basal segments of the lungs than in the apices, and if unilateral it is more commonly found in the left lower lobe.

In addition to the dilatation, there is chronic infection of the bronchial wall and usually of the peribronchial tissues, as well as tenacious secretions that are not easily expectorated. Often the peribronchial infection flares up and patches of pneumonia develop, or an entire lobe may become consolidated and mimic the picture of lobar pneumonia. If the infection spreads to the pleura, considerable fibrosis and thickening may develop.

As the disease progresses, the bronchial dilatation tends to become more pronounced and the intervening lung tissue becomes fibrotic and shrunken. Purulent sputum may spill over into other areas, to initiate changes in previously healthy bronchi.

Physical Signs.   There is less aerated lung tissue, as well as an increased amount of solid tissue from fibrosis and exudate in the peribronchial areas, and excessive amounts of retained secretions. The latter may produce temporary occlusion of bronchi and bronchioles, with atelectasis distal to those points. Therefore, the physical signs will depend upon the extent and severity of the disease.

On inspection the patient may appear perfectly healthy or he may look sick. With severe bronchiectasis, clubbing of the fingers and even of the toes usually develops (p. 355). Expansion may be limited over the involved area. Palpation will confirm the decreased expansion; rhonchal fremitus may be felt. With extensive involvement of the lung parenchyma fremitus will be increased, but if the bronchi are temporarily filled with secretions fremitus will be decreased. It will also be decreased if the pleura is thickened. The percussion note is usually impaired or dull, depending upon the amount of disease present.

On auscultation the breath sounds and voice sounds may be normal if the diseased bronchi are relatively free of secretions at that time and if the lung tissue is not seriously involved. More commonly the breath sounds are bronchovesicular, and rales and bronchi will be heard; these will be altered but not entirely abolished by cough. If pneumonic consolidation is present, the breath sounds will become bronchial if the bronchi are patent.

History.   Chronic productive cough is the principal symptom. Usually this is paroxysmal and persists until some sputum is raised. It is most liable to start with change of position; secretions that have accumulated in one area shift to a new spot and initiate a cough reflex. With extensive bronchiectasis the daily volume of sputum may amount to several hundred milliliters. Characteristically it is composed of soft globules of mucopurulent material plus thin watery mucus; when allowed to stand in a suitable container, the former settle to the bottom. The odor is sweetish or slightly musty; it is entirely unlike the foul or putrid odor that is present with lung abscess.

Later in the disease, when parenchymal involvement occurs, there may be repeated attacks of "pneumonia" involving the same lobe each time.

With abnormal lung signs plus a typical history, bronchiectasis can be suspected. The usual chest roentgenograms are of little help; bronchoscopy may also be inconclusive. To establish the diagnosis the secretions must be removed as completely as possible and the appropriate segments of the bronchial tree outlined by the introduction of a suitable radiopaque contrast medium. Then the roentgenogram (bronchogram) will clearly show the degree and extent of bronchial dilatation and distortion.

Asthma

This is a manifestation of allergy, with hypersensitivity to one or more extrinsic or intrinsic allergens.

Pathologic Changes.   During inspiration, normal bronchioles are slightly dilated by the negative intrathoracic pressure and the pull of the lung tissue; with expiration they tend to constrict. Therefore expiration is slightly more difficult and more prolonged than inspiration. In asthma, regardless of the specific cause, the primary change is narrowing of the lumen of the bronchioles. There is edema of the mucosa, increased secretion of mucus and a variable amount of spasm of the bronchiolar muscles. All of these interfere somewhat with inspiration, but expiration becomes much more difficult; some air is trapped in the lungs. Early in the course of asthma these changes are temporary, but in the late stage one finds thickening and other irreversible alterations in the walls of the bronchioles and emphysema of the lung parenchyma.

Physical Signs.   During a severe acute attack the patient is obviously in distress. He prefers to sit leaning forward, often with his arms supported by some firm object such as a table or a chair. The accessory muscles of respiration in the neck are prominent. Cyanosis may be present. Wheezing is frequently audible even at a distance from the patient. There is unproductive cough of increasing severity; neither the edema of the mucosa nor the thick mucus that characterizes the early stage can be dislodged. Thoracic movement is slight, and in contrast to the short rapid inspiration, the expiratory phase is very prolonged as the air drifts out through the narrowed bronchioles.

Palpation will confirm the abnormal thoracic movements. Rhonchal fremitus is usually striking. Percussion may yield either normal resonance or hyperresonance, depending upon the degree of emphysema; this increases in chronic asthma.

On auscultation one may hear no normal breath sounds; they are inaudible because of the cacophony of "musical" rales, which resemble music about as much as do the sounds produced by the members of an orchestra when they are "tuning up." As the paroxysm subsides the cough becomes more productive, the sputum becomes increasingly more fluid, and the physical signs revert toward normal. Between attacks the lungs may seem perfectly healthy, but even in the asymptomatic phase, *forced* expiration may produce a few scattered rhonchi, especially in the subclavicular or apical regions.

History.   Asthma may be paroxysmal or it may be more or less continuous from the start. The initial episodes may be relatively mild and brief, but occasionally the first attack is very severe. Without appropriate treatment the attacks tend to become more severe and more prolonged, and may eventually lead to continuous mild asthma with intermittent severe paroxysms or to a very severe attack that lasts for days (*status asthmaticus*).

The patient becomes aware of slight shortness of breath, an unproductive annoying cough or a sense of tightness in the chest; he is conscious of the *need* to breathe. These symptoms increase in severity, then gradually abate. He may go to the window to "get fresh air" and stay there until the attack subsides. Subsequent attacks tend to be more severe and more prolonged.

Not infrequently the initial attack occurs during an acute respiratory infection, and the person blames all his symptoms on his cold. It is not until the attacks persist and become more frequent or troublesome that someone suggests that he might have asthma; then he sees his doctor.

Bronchogenic Carcinoma

Whatever the etiologic factor may be, this disease is occurring more frequently that it formerly did.

Pathologic Changes.   Initially there is a localized focus of irritation in the wall of the bronchus. As the tumor grows there is progressive decrease in the lumen of the bronchus; this may lead to complete stenosis. Invasion of the lung parenchyma is common; direct extension or lymphatic spread to the pleura often occurs. The mediastinal lymph nodes are involved early in the disease and may be considerably enlarged. Metastasis to distant sites such as the brain or skeleton can produce symptoms that tend to draw attention away from the chest.

Physical Signs.   These are extremely variable and usually mimic some other disease. Partial bronchial obstruction may lead to emphysema of the lung tissue distal to the tumor; complete obstruction will give rise to atelectasis. Secretions may intermittently convert partial obstruction into complete bronchial occlusion, giving rise to signs that change from day to day. Retention of secretions produces rhonchi and a variety of rales localized to the involved area. Infection often develops and pneumonia or lung abscess can follow. Consolidation may also be produced by direct extension of the tumor into the lung tissue. Pleural involvement can cause pleuritic pain; pleural effusion (usually hemorrhagic) may be the most striking abnormality.

Mediastinal involvement can destroy the ipsilateral phrenic nerve; the diaphragm on that side will be paralyzed and elevated. Partial or complete obstruction of the superior vena cava can follow compression or invasion of that vessel. Involvement of the cervical sympathetic chain will produce Horner's syndrome (p. 75); this is fairly commonly seen with tumors involving the apical segment, or with the so-called superior sulcus or Pancoast tumor, which also invades the brachial plexus.

History.   In a person over 50 years of age who develops a productive cough of increasing severity, carcinoma of the bronchus should be suspected. Blood-streaked or pink sputum should further heighten the suspicion; so should the presence of a "wheeze" or "rattle" in the chest that is localized to one area. A "virus infection" or "pneumonia" that does not resolve normally, or that recurs in the same area, is another clue. Appropriate studies at that time may be life-saving; if physical signs such as those mentioned above are already present it is usually too late for anything other than palliative measures.

DISEASES OF THE LUNGS

Bronchopneumonia

This may occur as a terminal complication of any chronic or wasting disease or with systemic infections such as measles, pertussis (whooping cough) or sepsis. More commonly it evolves from a milder respiratory infection. The course is extremely variable, depending upon such factors as the virulence of the causative organism and the general health of the person.

Pathologic Changes.   Infection spreads outward from the bronchi. Inflammatory changes develop in many of the terminal bronchioles and the surrounding lung tissue, giving rise to patches of consolidation of various sizes, together with compensatory emphysema of the surrounding uninvolved lung tissue. The areas may be few in number and small, or they may be so numerous and large that practically an entire lobe seems involved (*confluent bronchopneumonia*). The bronchi also contain abnormal secretions. With recovery the consolidated areas gradually become aerated and the lung tissue returns to normal.

Physical Signs.   There is increased solid tissue (consolidated lung) with a corresponding decrease in the amount of air present. There will be some respiratory distress and the rate will be moderately increased. The pulmonary signs will depend upon the amount of lung involved and the location of these areas of consolidation. Small, deeply situated patches may produce no demonstrable abnormalities. Over superficially situated areas there will be decreased resonance or dullness on percussion, bronchovesicular breath sounds and subcrepitant or crepitant rales; occasionally bronchial breath sounds or rhonchi will be heard. Over an adjacent uninvolved area the findings may be normal. A pleural friction rub may be heard if a pneumonic area is situated peripherally.

History.   The onset is usually insidious; occasionally it is very rapid. The person has had a cold or bronchitis that did not respond to home remedies or proprietary cold cures. Chilly sensations followed by warmth and sweating may recur repeatedly; a sharp chill is uncommon. The temperature rises gradually and tends to fluctuate. Headache and malaise develop; the person feels sick but is not prostrated. The cough increases in severity. The sputum becomes somewhat more profuse but is not bloody. Pain is not commonly present and is rarely severe.

Lobar Pneumonia

The introduction of antimicrobial drugs has made the classic picture of full-blown lobar pneumonia a rarity, especially in many hospitals. Prompt treatment in the early stages halts the infection before the typical lung changes develop. When therapy is ineffectual or is started late, complete consolidation may be present. In any case, the physical signs will vary according to the stage of the disease.

Pathologic Changes. Initially there is intense congestion, followed by pouring out of exudate into the alveoli and bronchioles (the inflammatory response). Gradually vast numbers of alveoli become completely filled with exudate; the lobe becomes larger than normal and relatively solid, but even at the height of the disease there are still some aerated alveoli and air is present in the bronchi. When the infection is overcome, naturally or by appropriate therapy, the exudate is gradually absorbed and the lung slowly returns to normal.

Very early in the disease the larger bronchi may be plugged temporarily by thick secretions; for a few hours the pulmonary signs resemble those of atelectasis (p. 214), but the typical signs of pneumonia soon develop.

Physical Signs. In the diseased area, solid material (exudate) has almost completely replaced the air normally present; this decreases oxygenation of the blood. The skin is flushed (fever); occasionally the face shows a greater flush on the side of the lesion. The expression is anxious; the nostrils flare with inspiration; herpes simplex may be present on the lips or face. Respiration is rapid and shallow; expiration may be accompanied by an audible grunt. Cyanosis may be apparent; the blood that circulates through the unaerated lobe is not oxygenated. The affected side may appear larger than the normal side, but the respiratory excursion of the thorax is decreased over the involved area and increased over the opposite hemithorax.

Palpation confirms this inequality of expansion. Since there is more solid material (exudate) and less air, fremitus is increased over the involved area. If secretions cause bronchial obstruction, fremitus may be decreased temporarily; if the patient can cough and expel this plug, exaggerated fremitus will again be found.

On percussion, dullness can be demonstrated over an area corresponding roughly to one or more of the lobes (Fig. 106); adjacent to this there may be skodaic resonance.

On auscultation, breath sounds may be bronchovesicular in the very early stage when there is little exudate in the alveoli, but they soon become bronchial in character. With resolution, the amount of exudate decreases and aeration increases; the bronchial element fades and eventually vesicular breath sounds return. Vocal fremitus waxes and wanes in a similar manner. Very early in the disease, when there is only a small amount of exudate in the alveoli, crepitant rales will be present (*crepitus indux*). Later, when most of the alveoli are filled, these largely disappear and subcrepitant rales can be heard. With resolution and absorption of the exudate, crepitant rales will again appear (*crepitus redux*); these also eventually disappear.

A pleural friction rub is often heard at some stage of the illness; if pain is severe the patient may refuse to breathe deeply enough to permit this sign to be elicited.

History.   The onset is usually rapid, often with a single sharp chill; high fever, malaise and prostration soon develop. Cough quickly follows; the sputum is thick and tenacious. It may contain bright red blood, but more commonly it is brown or "rusty" in appearance; later it becomes mucopurulent. Involvement of the parietal pleura results in pain with respiration or with cough. If the diaphragmatic pleura is involved as in lower lobe pneumonia, pain may be referred to the neck and shoulder, or sometimes to the abdomen, suggesting intra-abdominal disease.

Tuberculosis

This is a disease of such protean manifestations that it would be impossible to discuss here all of the changes that might be produced in the lungs.

Pathlogic Changes.   Exudation and fibrosis are the primary pathologic processes; loss of lung tissue (cavitation) may occur later in the disease. Although tuberculosis can develop in any part of the lung, it is more common in an upper lobe, especially in the subapical or apical area. Involvement of a lower lobe alone is uncommon, and it occurs in females more often than in males.

Physical Signs.   These may be entirely absent with a minimal lesion well below the pleural surface; only the roentgenologist or the pathologist can find such a process. A large area, or one that is near the chest wall, will produce definite signs.

If exudate predominates, one or more areas of consolidation will be present and the signs will simulate those of bronchopneumonia. The presence of crepitant or post-tussive rales is the most significant finding.

If fibrosis is present in an upper lobe there will be retraction of the overlying ribs and interspaces, and the trachea may be pulled toward that side. The muscles, skin and subcutaneous tissues will show some atrophy; this collar of degeneration corresponds to the distribution of the third, fourth and fifth cervical nerves. The apex will be retracted and Krönig's isthmus will be narrowed or obliterated (p. 188).

With fibrosis the aeration is decreased; therefore fremitus is increased. Breath sounds are transmitted more readily; they lose their vesicular quality and become bronchovesicular. Rales are mainly subcrepitant; they are produced by secretions retained in the distorted bronchioles and smaller bronchi.

If cavitation is present the percussion note, fremitus and breath sounds will be further altered as described in previous chapters.

History. Tuberculosis may be so mild that it produces no definite symptoms, or it may be rapidly progressive and misdiagnosed as pneumonia—the so-called "phthisis florida" or "galloping consumption." Symptoms such as cough, expectoration, fever and weight loss will be roughly proportional to the severity of the process.

Whenever a patient has chronic cough, it is wise to assume that he has tuberculosis until this possibility has been ruled out. This advice is given for your protection. Some of you will heed it; others will start to worry after they have seen the patient's chest films.

Emphysema

Literally, emphysema means a tissue puffed up with air. Although emphysema may occur in other tissues, the term when used alone is considered synonymous with pulmonary emphysema. This is often subdivided into various types such as compensatory, senile, obstructive and hypertrophic; the last is the most common. Physiologists and pathologists still disagree as to the exact mechanism by which hypertrophic emphysema is produced, and as to the relative significance of the various tissue alterations, but all seem to agree that chronic cough, loss of elastic tissue and partial obstruction of many small bronchi and bronchioles are three of the essential factors in the production of this disease.

Pathologic Changes. These will depend upon the duration and the severity of the disease; the findings in well-established hypertrophic emphysema have been selected for this discussion.

The lungs are overinflated and there is loss of the normal elasticity of the tissues. The alveoli are dilated and many of the septa are destroyed, giving rise to large sacs or bullae. The bronchi and bronchioles usually are the site of chronic inflammatory disease (chronic bronchitis) or have the characteristic changes of long-standing asthma.

With thinning and loss of alveolar walls the capillary bed is markedly decreased. Oxygenation of hemoglobin is incomplete and carbon dioxide tends to accumulate in the blood. An added burden is thrown on the right ventricle to force blood through the limited number of capillaries still present. Compensatory or secondary polycythemia develops; nature provides more erythrocytes in the vain hope of capturing more oxygen for the anoxic tissues. These added cells help to increase the viscosity of the blood; the rate of flow is decreased, more strain is thrown on the heart and right ventricular hypertrophy or *cor pulmonale* develops. Death may be due to right heart failure, to generalized tissue anoxia and wasting, or to an acute pulmonary infection that seems mild but is just enough to add the straw that breaks down the precarious balance of gaseous exchange.

Physical Signs.   The amount of lung tissue is decreased; the amount of air is markedly increased. The patient is dyspneic, but this may show little variation with change of position. Inspiration is short; expiration is prolonged because the elastic recoil is poor and the bronchioles are narrowed. Often the patient breathes through his mouth to eliminate the slight obstruction to air flow imposed by the nasal passages. A variable degree of cyanosis is present. Small dilated venules may be seen on the skin overlying the line of attachment of the diaphragm.

The contour of the chest provides another clue to the diagnosis; it looks as if the person had taken an extremely deep breath and then held it. The ribs may be almost horizontal, and the costal angle is wide. The sternum is pushed forward and the thoracic spine shows exaggerated bowing (*kyphosis*). The anteroposterior diameter may equal or exceed the transverse diameter, giving the classic barrel-shaped chest (Fig. 110). With inspiration the thoracic cage expands but slightly; instead, it is pulled up as a unit by the accessory muscles of respiration in the neck. The shoulders are elevated and held somewhat forward, making the neck appear short. The clavicles and supraclavicular fossae are unduly prominent. Occasionally there is retraction of the lower ribs on inspiration due to contraction of the already flattened diaphragm (Hoover's[1] sign). The cardiac impulse will be minimal or entirely absent over the chest, but there may be exaggerated pulsations visible in the epigastrium.

Palpation confirms the lack of expansion and the absence of the apex beat. Fremitus will be decreased by the excessive amount of air in the lung, but it is rarely abolished.

Percussion yields a hyperresonant or even a tympanitic note; this extends much lower than would be expected. Excursion of the diaphragm is limited or absent. There will be little change demonstrable

[1] Charles Franklin Hoover, American physician, 1865–1927.

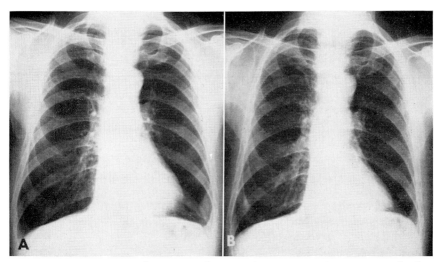

Fig. 133.   Severe pulmonary emphysema. *A*, Inspiration; *B*, expiration. The diaphragm is very low and practically horizontal; there is almost no movement with respiration. The lung fields show excessive aeration. (Courtesy of Dr. R. H. Chamberlain.)

between deep inspiration and forced expiration, but extreme dyspnea may limit the patient's ability to cooperate for this determination. The area of cardiac dullness is considerably diminished because of the interposition of overinflated lung tissue between the heart and the chest wall (Fig. 133).

On auscultation, breath sounds tend to be feeble and distant; little air is being exchanged and the large air-containing sacs interfere with the transmission of sound. Inspiration may be almost inaudible; expiration may be harsh, but unlike bronchial breathing, it is low in pitch. Coarse rales and rhonchi may be heard if chronic bronchitis or asthma is present; forced expiration may be needed to elicit these. The heart sounds are usually faint but the pulmonic second sound is generally accentuated.

History.   Interference with expiration is an important factor; a history of chronic asthma or of chronic bronchitis can be obtained in most instances. Chronic cough due to prolonged inhalation of irritating fumes or dusts is sometimes an important factor. Since emphysema develops slowly over a period of years, the onset is insidious. It is not until the disease is well advanced and a large amount of functioning lung tissue has been lost that the individual begins to notice increasing dyspnea on exertion, or reduced exercise tolerance. He attributes this to the fact that he doesn't exercise often enough, isn't "in condition," is getting older or has been smoking too much recently. The flight of stairs seems longer; the hill seems steeper. Finally he realizes that he has to slow down even when walking on the level; eventually he decides to see a doctor about this. In the far-advanced stage, the slightest exertion leaves him breathless; even talking becomes an effort.

When emphysema develops in an asthmatic patient the increasing dyspnea may be attributed to the asthma itself; to the patient, the asthma is just getting worse. When emphysema is due to chronic bronchitis, there may be repeated episodes of acute respiratory infection or a history of a "touch of pneumonia" at frequent intervals, especially during the winter. The "cold" seems to hang on longer than usual, but improves or even disappears when summer comes, only to recur the following winter.

Occasionally the time of onset seems to be more specific and related to a definite severe respiratory infection. The disease was actually fairly far-advanced before this, and the increased secretions and added endobronchial swelling merely aggravated and accelerated the process.

Compensatory Emphysema.   This term is applied to the overinflation that occurs when one lung or part of one lung expands to fill a space formerly occupied by aerated lung tissue. For example, if the right middle lobe is removed surgically, the right upper and lower lobes will become somewhat overinflated. If chronic fibroid tuberculosis reduces the right upper lobe to a fraction of its normal size, the remaining lung tissue will expand.

The physical signs will depend upon the primary disease process present and the amount of hyperaeration of the healthy lung tissue. The increased amount of air will produce the predictable changes, but these will be relatively less dramatic than those described above because the remaining lung tissue is essentially healthy but overinflated, not diseased.

Obstructive Emphysema.   This develops distal to some lesion that produces partial occlusion of a bronchus or acts as a check valve. Air enters the lung segment but some of it cannot be expelled. If a small bronchus is involved the signs may be minimal; the diagnosis will be made by fluoroscopy or by comparing films taken during inspiration and expiration; a localized area of hyperaeration will be seen. If a large bronchus is involved the signs will resemble those found in compensatory emphysema.

Senile Emphysema.   This is primarily a pathologic diagnosis. In this condition there is moderate atrophy of alveolar walls but little loss of elastic tissue; dyspnea is rarely a distressing symptom.

Atelectasis

This term denotes lack of expansion or lack of aeration of lung tissue. It may be neonatal (fetal atelectasis) or it may develop in previously aerated lung tissue. In a newborn infant the lung is completely unaerated (atelectatic). As soon as the baby starts to breathe the lung begins to expand, but not all areas participate equally; patches of atelectasis may persist for several days. Occasionally the infant's lung never becomes adequately aerated; death soon occurs. In children or adults several types of atelectasis are recognized.

Functional Atelectasis.   This is a term sometimes applied to small areas of unaerated lung resulting from shallow respiration; usually these develop at the margins of the lobe, especially at the base of the lung. The only significant finding is the presence of atelectatic rales when the person takes a few deep breaths and re-expands the unaerated segments.

Compression Atelectasis.   This may develop in a healthy aerated lung or portion of a lung as a result of pressure, as from pleural effusion or a huge heart. The primary disease often masks the pulmonary signs, but since the tissue is practically airless and the bronchus is not occluded increased fremitus, dullness to percussion, bronchovesicular or bronchial breath sounds and crepitant rales may occasionally be demonstrable.

Obstructive Atelectasis.   This is the most important form; it develops as a result of occlusion of a bronchus or bronchiole of any size. Small areas may occur with bronchitis or asthma; usually these give no definite physical signs. Obstruction of a lobar or main stem bronchus will

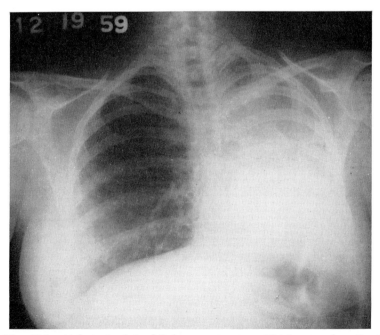

Fig. 134.   Atelectasis of the left lung, postpartum. The heart and mediastinum are drawn to the left; the entire left hemithorax has a hazy appearance. The left dome of the diaphragm is elevated. The right lung is overinflated (compensatory emphysema). A plug of tenacious mucus was removed bronchoscopically; the following day the chest x-ray appeared normal. (Courtesy of Dr. R. H. Chamberlain.)

produce the condition variously known as *massive atelectasis, massive collapse* or *drowned lung*. Most commonly the obstruction is caused by retained secretions or occurs postoperatively or in an acutely ill patient, when deep breathing and cough may be painful or impossible. Sometimes it is due to compression by an extrinsic mass such as a tumor or a rapidly enlarging lymph node, or to an endobronchial process such as a growth or an inhaled foreign body.

This clinical entity had been known for years as "postoperative pneumonia." The role of retained secretions in the production of this syndrome was not generally recognized until 1924, when Leopold[2] published his report entitled "Postoperative Massive Collapse and Drowned Lung." Bronchoscopy was a relatively new procedure but Leopold postulated: "If bronchoscopic examination during a collapse attack will demonstrate complete bronchial obstruction in the bronchus supplying the collapsed and 'drowned' lung, then this explanation would seem correct for those cases that occur postoperatively." Tucker[3] soon confirmed this hypothesis by bronchoscopic observations.

Pathologic Changes.   Absorption of air from the alveoli and bronchi, transudation of fluid into the normal air chambers and vascular engorgement all contribute to convert the involved area into a dense solid mass. In pneumonia, some air is present in the bronchi and in a few of the alveoli; with atelectasis the air is absorbed or replaced by fluid. These changes may develop within a few hours.

Physical Signs, Obstructive Atelectasis.   It should be emphasized that, although this process is sometimes called "massive collapse," the lobe or lung *does not* collapse away from the chest wall; it merely becomes much smaller. To adjust for this, the ribs over the involved area are pulled downward (as in expiration), the intercostal spaces are drawn inward, the diaphragm rises, and the heart and mediastinum shift toward the affected side. The uninvolved lung tissue becomes overinflated (compensatory emphysema).

With obstruction of a main stem bronchus, the patient looks anxious and prostrated. The respiratory rate is increased; cyanosis is often marked. The affected side of the thorax is smaller and barely moves with respiration; the ribs slope downward and the interspaces are sunken. The uninvolved side shows increased expansion and a more horizontal position of the ribs. The cardiac impulse is shifted toward the midline with right-sided atelectasis, and to the left and upward to the fourth interspace or higher if the left lung is involved.

Palpation confirms these findings; tracheal deviation toward the affected side is also demonstrable. Fremitus is markedly decreased or

[2] Simon S. Leopold, Philadelphia physician, 1892–1957.

[3] Gabriel Tucker, Philadelphia physician, 1880–1958.

absent over the atelectatic lung, since the primary bronchus to the area is obstructed.

Percussion yields a dull or flat note over the collapsed areas; hyperresonance is found over the aerated portions. If the right lung is involved, the heart may be shifted so far to the right that the area of cardiac dullness cannot be demonstrated. The left border will be near or under the sternum and the right border will blend with the solidified lung tissue.

On auscultation, breath sounds and vocal fremitus will usually be absent while the bronchus is occluded; rarely, faint bronchial breath sounds may be heard. If the mucus or other obstructing object is removed, the breath sounds promptly become bronchial in character. After bronchial patency has been restored the fluid is gradually reabsorbed and the lung re-expands and returns to its former condition.

When only one lobe is involved the general signs will be less dramatic but the changes over the collapsed area will be the same. Since the volume of that lobe is decreased, the abnormal findings will be less extensive than expected.

History. This will depend upon the cause of the atelectasis. When due to an endobronchial tumor the symptoms usually develop insidiously. With compression atelectasis the primary disease process may overshadow the lung changes. When atelectasis is due to obstruction by secretions or a foreign body, the onset is usually rapid. Dyspnea, cough and fever develop promptly; pain may be present at the outset or it may appear later.

PULMONARY EDEMA

This may be either acute or chronic. It is most commonly due to some type of chronic heart disease in which the left atrium or ventricle is abnormal or bears an excessive burden; some of these conditions will be discussed in Chapter XV. It may follow an acute insult to the left ventricle such as a myocardial infarction. It can occur with severe nephritis or uremia, with pulmonary infarction, in the moribund patient or after the injudicious removal of an excessive amount of fluid or air from the pleural cavity. Acute pulmonary edema is sometimes called "cardiac asthma," a confusing and altogether misleading term. Wheezes may be audible but the fundamental disease process is entirely different and the treatment is not the same.

Pathologic Changes. Blood enters the pulmonary vessels from the right ventricle more rapidly than the left ventricle can remove it.

This discrepancy in output need not be great. If the right ventricle expels only one drop per beat more than the left ventricle, blood can accumulate in the lungs at a rate of 4 ml. or more per minute.

As the volume of blood in the lungs increases, pressure in the pulmonary circulation rises; fluid tends to escape through the capillaries into the alveoli. Aeration is decreased; oxygenation of the blood is incomplete.

Physical Signs.   The amount of air in the lungs is markedly decreased and the relative amount of solid tissue (fluid) is increased because of the distention of the blood vessels and the presence of transudate in the tracheobronchial tree and the alveoli.

With acute pulmonary edema the patient appears apprehensive. Usually he will sit upright or lean forward somewhat, resting the arms on a support as does the asthmatic patient. The accessory muscles of respiration are active. Tachypnea and cyanosis are obvious. Inspiration is short; expiration is moderately prolonged. Cough appears and increases in severity; the sputum is watery, frothy or foamy, and is often blood-tinged. The skin may be cold and moist ("clammy"). Fremitus will be increased unless the patient is too dyspneic to phonate properly. The percussion note will be impaired; it may even be dull in dependent areas. On auscultation, bronchovesicular breath sounds may be heard, or even small areas of bronchial breathing, but usually the breath sounds are obscured by rales. Initially these will be crepitant as fluid appears in the alveoli; later, subcrepitant rales become more numerous as the bronchioles begin to fill. Eventually the entire bronchial tree contains excess fluid; this plus congestion and edema of the mucosa results in a medley of sounds difficult to differentiate from those present during an asthmatic attack.

The heart sounds may be completely obscured; if not, abnormalities may be audible. The blood pressure is often elevated if pre-existing hypertensive cardiovascular disease is the primary factor; in asthma the blood pressure is usually normal.

With chronic pulmonary edema the onset is gradual and much less dramatic; rales may be the most important clue.

History.   In acute pulmonary edema the onset is generally sudden; often the patient is awakened by dyspnea and cough. A history of hypertension, angina pectoris or other manifestations of cardiovascular disease may be elicited, or precordial pain from myocardial infarction may have preceded the development of pulmonary edema. Age is another helpful clue; a sudden attack of dyspnea in a middle-aged or elderly person is rarely due to the onset of asthma.

With chronic pulmonary edema the dyspnea develops more slowly; symptoms of the underlying disease process may predominate.

DISEASES OF THE PLEURA

Pleurisy

Except in those rare instances in which pleural damage results from direct trauma to the chest wall, pleurisy is secondary to some other disease. It can occur with lung disease that extends to the pleura or impinges upon it. It may also result from spread of infection from the mediastinum, the pericardium, the peritoneal cavity (by extension through the diaphragm) or by way of the blood stream. Rheumatic fever, gout and uremia may also be accompanied by pleural changes.

Pathologic Changes. The pleura is the site of inflammatory changes; the severity and extent of the lesions will depend upon the etiology of the primary disease process. Spasm of the intercostal muscles overlying this area is commonly present early in the course of acute pleurisy and is responsible for much of the pain on respiration. When pleurisy is due to an acute inflammatory process it may resolve completely, or there may be formation of adhesions between the parietal and visceral layers. Such adhesions are commonly found at autopsy in elderly persons, due probably to repeated respiratory infections with minimal amounts of pleurisy. In some cases pleural irritation produces a fairly rapid accumulation of fluid in the pleural cavity (pleural effusion).

Physical Signs. Since deep breathing or cough usually brings on or intensifies the pain, respiration is shallow and the rate is increased. There is restriction of motion on the affected side. The patient may prefer to lie on that side, thus limiting thoracic expansion, or he may assume some other position that achieves the same result. Palpation confirms the limited movement of the chest wall; firm pressure may decrease the pain by further limiting thoracic expansion. In rare instances a friction fremitus may be felt. The percussion note will not be influenced by the pleurisy itself, but it may be altered by the underlying pulmonary disease or by fluid in the pleural cavity.

The diagnosis is established by finding a friction rub. This may be heard over a wide area or it may be sharply localized. In most instances it is heard at or near the end of inspiration; occasionally it is present during expiration also. It is most frequently heard over the lower portion of the lung laterally or somewhat anteriorly. The characteristics of the breath sounds will depend upon the nature of the underlying lung disease that has produced the pleurisy.

History. Pain on breathing is the complaint that points to pleurisy; this may be slight or may be extremely severe. Other symptoms will depend upon the disease producing the pleural reaction. This pain is often relieved promptly by drugs that decrease muscular irritability or produce muscular relaxation, by nerve block or by frosting the skin over the involved area with an ethyl chloride spray. The patient can then inhale more deeply; the friction rub will become more easily audible.

Diaphragmatic Pleurisy

When the pleural surface of the diaphragm is affected the clinical picture is altered. The outer portion of the diaphragm is supplied by the six lower intercostal nerves; referred pain will therefore be felt in the anterior abdominal wall, which is the area supplied by the sensory fibers of these nerves. This may simulate an acute abdominal process such as appendicitis or gallbladder disease. The central portion of the diaphragm is supplied by the phrenic nerve, and referred pain will be felt in the neck or at the tip of the shoulder.

Firm pressure over the lower ribs will restrict thoracic expansion but tends to increase the excursion of the diaphragm, thus aggravating the pain. Abdominal pressure will limit the motion and decrease pain. Moreover, if there is referred abdominal pain, this is superficial. Light palpation may be as painful as firm pressure, which is not true if visceral disease is present.

Pleural Effusion

Depending upon the etiology of the primary disease, there may be slow or rapid accumulation of fluid in the pleural space; this may be serous, serosanguineous, sanguineous or frankly purulent (*empyema thoracis*). With the latter, adhesions may develop rapidly and sequester the fluid into separate pockets, producing isolated collections. Similar loculations may develop if there are pre-existing adhesions from a previous attack of pleurisy.

When fluid forms it tends to gravitate to the lowest point in the thorax; normally this is the costophrenic sulcus posteriorly. As the amount of fluid increases the lower portion of the lung begins to be compressed and the lung is pushed forward to some extent; however, it is still fixed to the mediastinum by the bronchus and blood vessels. With increasing amounts of fluid there is more and more pressure on the lung, which is now pushed upward and medially, but even with massive effusion the apical region remains aerated. The fluid does not form a layer at the bottom, with lung floating on top; it more closely resembles what you would see if, instead of the lung, you had a football attached at the hilar region. The fluid surrounds this and extends upward in an ever-thinner layer, giving rise to the apparent meniscus seen on roentgenograms.

Physical Signs. A layer of fluid separates the lung from the chest wall and interferes with the transmission of sounds. The lung itself contains relatively less air. The signs will vary, depending upon the quantity of fluid present and the amount of compression of the lung. They will also be altered if the underlying lung is consolidated or if the bronchus is obstructed. In this discussion it will be assumed that the bronchus is open, that the actual amount of lung disease is slight, and that the patient is sitting upright.

SMALL EFFUSION. An amount less than 300 ml. will produce no diagnostic physical signs but may be demonstrable radiologically. If there is a somewhat larger amount (500 ml.) signs can usually be elicited. There may be slight limitation of motion of the lower ribs on the involved side. Fremitus will be decreased at the base posteriorly but not elsewhere. As one percusses downward the note becomes impaired, then dull or flat as the thickness of the layer increases. Vocal fremitus will similarly decrease or be obliterated, as will the breath sounds, but they will remain vesicular in character.

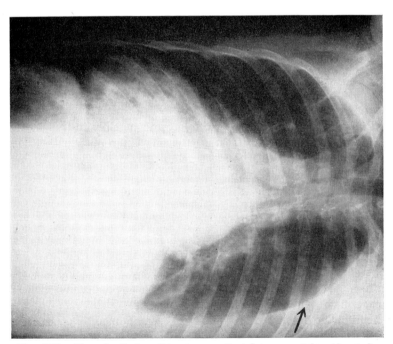

Fig. 135. Pleural effusion. PA view; patient lying on right side. A layer of fluid can be seen extending from the diaphragm to the apex; the lung floats above this. (Courtesy of Dr. R. H. Chamberlain.)

If the patient lies face downward for a few minutes, part or all of the fluid may gravitate to the lateral and anterior portions of the pleural cavity; the abnormal signs previously found posteriorly decrease or disappear (shifting dullness).

MODERATE EFFUSION.   If the amount of fluid is greater (1000 ml. or more) there will be compression atelectasis of the lower portion of the lung. Inspection will show that expansion is decreased on the affected side. The lower intercostal spaces may bulge slightly and do not retract with inspiration. Fremitus is decreased or absent at the base posteriorly and laterally. Flatness is present over the lower portion; dullness may extend to the level of the angle of the scapula or higher. It may seem to rise higher in the axilla and near the spine, giving rise to the so-called Garland[4] curve or S-line, of historic interest only. With right-sided effusion the position of the diaphragm cannot be determined; the flatness due to the effusion merges with liver flatness. With left-sided effusion there may be a sharp demarcation if the stomach or the splenic flexure of the colon contains gas. In either case the diaphragm is somewhat depressed and motion is restricted. On auscultation, distant bronchovesicular breathing may be heard near the upper limit of the effusion. This is transmitted through the thin layer of fluid from the partially collapsed and relatively unaerated portion of the lung. If there is a considerable amount of compression there may be an area where fremitus is increased and bronchial breath sounds are heard; egophony will also be present. Shifting dullness can usually be demonstrated and will tend to confirm the diagnosis of free fluid.

Unless the heart and mediastinal structures are anchored by adhesions, they will be pushed somewhat toward the uninvolved side. With a right-sided effusion the trachea is displaced to the left, the apical impulse will be farther to the left and possibly in the sixth interspace, and the area of cardiac dullness may seem enlarged. It may be difficult to decide whether there is actual cardiomegaly or whether the changes are all due to displacement. With a left-sided effusion the apical impulse is usually obliterated and cardiac dullness cannot be determined on the left, but it may be percussed several centimeters to the right of the midsternal line.

MASSIVE EFFUSION.   When the hemithorax contains 2 liters or more of fluid, most of the lung is compressed but the apical portion will still be aerated. The intercostal spaces on the involved side will show a definite bulge. Expansion will be almost absent and fremitus will not be felt except over the apex. The percussion note will be flat over most of the hemithorax; it may be resonant or even tympanitic at the extreme apex. Faint bronchovesicular or bronchial breath sounds may be heard

---

[4] George Minot Garland, American physician, 1848–1926.

over the uppermost portion of the effusion; lower down the breath sounds are absent. At the apex there may be amphoric breathing.

Occasionally one may hear loud bronchial breath sounds over a massive effusion, suggesting the diagnosis of pneumonia. This is apparently due to the fact that the intrathoracic pressure is very high, both with expiration and with inspiration. If this high positive pressure is relieved by the removal of a small amount of fluid the breath sounds become faint or disappear.

Mediastinal shift is usually very pronounced with a massive effusion; the diaphragm is also depressed and the liver or spleen may become palpable even though not enlarged.

Since the uninvolved lung must carry almost the entire load of respiration, there will be overinflation or compensatory emphysema on that side. Thoracic expansion will be increased, the diaphragm will be lower and its excursion will be augmented. The percussion note will often be hyperresonant and breath sounds will be loud but not pathologically altered.

Because the involved hemithorax is almost completely filled with fluid, there can be no appreciable shift of this fluid and there will be little or no change in signs with altered position of the patient.

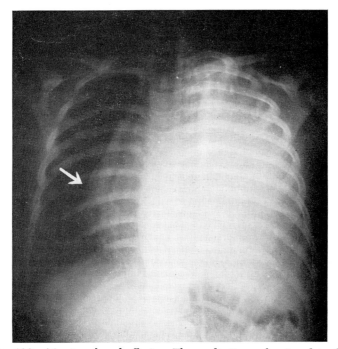

Fig. 136. Massive pleural effusion. The mediastinum, heart and trachea have been displaced to the right. (Courtesy of Dr. R. H. Chamberlain.)

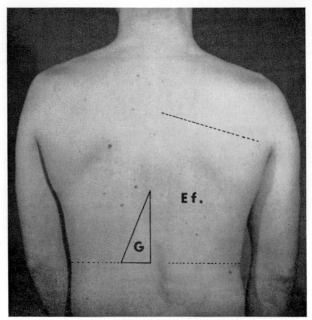

Fig. 137. Grocco's triangle. With a large pleural effusion, a paravertebral area of relative dullness will be present on the opposite side (G).

When a moderate or massive effusion is present there may be a paravertebral triangular area of dullness over the normal lung (Grocco's[5] triangle); the base extends outward 4 to 8 cm. from the midspinal line. The most plausible explanation for this is that the fluid deadens vibrations of the spine that normally contribute somewhat to the production of a resonant note. This damping effect is proportional to the pressure exerted by the fluid, which increases as one approaches the diaphragm; therefore the area of dullness extends farther outward from the midline there.

History.   The symptoms will be those of the underlying disease, plus a variable amount of dyspnea. If the fluid accumulates rapidly, dyspnea will soon become embarrassing. If it accumulates more slowly, a massive effusion may be present before the patient is handicapped. Respiratory difficulty is also somewhat proportional to the age of the patient; a young person will tolerate effusion much better than an elderly one whose lungs have lost their juvenile elasticity.

Hydrothorax

Fluid may accumulate in one or both pleural cavities in the absence

[5] Pietro Grocco, Italian physician, 1857–1916.

of any disease of the pleura or lungs. This is a transudate, not an exudate; the fluid has a low specific gravity (1.018 or less) and contains few cells. Hydrothorax may occur with cardiac failure, constrictive pericarditis, liver disease, renal disease, or various other conditions associated with altered circulation or abnormal fluid balance. When due to circulatory failure it almost invariably appears first in the right pleural cavity unless that has been obliterated by adhesions. If bilateral, the amount present on the right will be greater than the amount on the left.

The physical signs will be similar to those described for pleural effusion. The history will often point to the underlying disease responsible for the accumulation of the fluid.

Thickened Pleura

Thickening of the pleura results from acute or chronic infection of the pleural surfaces.

Pathologic Changes.   The parietal and visceral layers are fused by a dense layer of firm fibrous tissue. The thickness is variable, sometimes being as much as 2 or 3 cm. The underlying lung tissue may be the site of chronic infection, or it may show no residual damage following an acute infection.

Physical Signs.   A layer of solid tissue has been interposed between the lung and the chest wall; this is usually thickest at the base. The thickness of the pleura determines the amount of alteration in the physical signs.

Mechanically this fibrous tissue restricts movement of the overlying ribs and consequently of the lung tissue in that region. The diaphragm is often retracted upward; its motion is restricted. Fremitus will be decreased and the percussion note will be impaired or dull, depending upon the thickness of this layer. Breath sounds will be fainter but vesicular in character unless the underlying lung tissue is also involved.

The signs of thickened pleura are essentially the same as those produced by a small or moderate-sized effusion. It may be difficult to differentiate these two conditions by physical examination or by roentgenograms, especially if loculated effusion is present. Even thoracentesis may be misleading; a small amount of effusion may be missed and the physician attributes the "dry tap" to thickening of the pleura.

History.   The thickened pleura itself rarely produces any definite symptoms; one must search for the etiologic disease process. The history may suggest chronic lung disease such as bronchiectasis or tuberculosis, or there may have been an acute infection such as pneumonia, recently or in the distant past. Trauma causing hemothorax can also lead to pleural thickening.

Pneumothorax

This denotes the presence of air between the visceral and parietal layers of the pleura; it results from perforation of one of these.

Pathologic Changes. Pneumothorax is seen occasionally following injury of the parietal pleura, either accidental or surgical; however, in most instances the visceral pleura is breached. Although this may result from external force such as a broken rib or stab wound, it often occurs spontaneously and without obvious cause. In such cases a peripherally situated bronchiole apparently becomes partially constricted by acute or chronic inflammatory changes or by scar tissue formation. A localized area of emphysema develops distal to this and produces a subpleural bleb. This continues to enlarge and eventually ruptures, permitting air to escape into the pleural space.

The normal elasticity of the lung causes it to shrink in size; the negative intrapleural pressure produced by this elastic recoil continues to favor the escape of air into the pleural cavity. The rate at which the lung collapses depends upon several factors. If adhesions are present they will limit or prevent collapse of the adjacent lung tissue. If a small bronchiole is involved, collapse and compression of the lung tissue may close this bronchiole completely before much air has escaped. If the rupture communicates with a larger branch of the bronchial tree there may be complete collapse of the lung. Occasionally there is a valve-like action either in the bronchus or from the wall of the ruptured bleb. Air enters the pleural cavity with each inspiration but cannot escape during expiration. Gradually the intrapleural pressure increases and tension pneumothorax develops; this can be extremely serious if pressure is not relieved.

Physical Signs. A layer of air separates the lung from the chest wall; this conducts sound poorly. The lung itself is deflated; it contains less air. The signs will depend upon the amount of air in the pleural space or the amount of collapse of the lung.

SMALL OR PARTIAL PNEUMOTHORAX. If only a small or moderate amount of air escapes it tends to collect in the upper part of the thorax; with the patient erect the signs will be found in the apical region. On inspection there may be slight increase in the respiratory rate and deep inspiration may be uncomfortable or painful, suggesting pleurisy. Movement of the involved side will be normal or slightly restricted. Fremitus may be diminished over the upper portion on that side but normal over the lower interspaces. The percussion note will be hyperresonant and breath sounds will be diminished or absent over the upper thorax.

LARGE OR COMPLETE PNEUMOTHORAX. The lung has been markedly reduced in volume due to the elastic recoil of the pulmonary tissues. It is collapsed against the mediastinum; nowhere is it in contact with the chest wall. Dyspnea and tachypnea will be present unless the air has accumulated very slowly, allowing the person to become adjusted to the altered aeration. Expansion will be limited on the involved side. Fremitus will be markedly decreased or entirely absent. The percussion note will be hyperresonant or tympanitic. The area of cardiac dullness will be obliterated if the air is in the left pleural space. Breath sounds are usually absent; the coin test (p. 201) is positive. The uninvolved side will show increased respiratory excursions and signs of compensatory hyperventilation (compensatory emphysema).

TENSION PNEUMOTHORAX.   In this condition the lung is firmly compressed against the mediastinum, and since the air is under relatively high pressure the mediastinal structures will be shifted to the opposite side unless immobilized by adhesions. Dyspnea is obvious and the respiratory rate is increased. Movement of the affected side is markedly impaired; the interspaces may be obliterated or actually bulge slightly. Tactile fremitus will be absent, and the trachea will be shifted to the opposite side. The percussion note is usually tympanitic but with extremely high tension it may be impaired or almost dull. The diaphragm is depressed and motion is slight. Breath sounds are absent or amphoric in quality if heard at all. The coin test is positive. The area of cardiac dullness will be shifted away from the involved side, and may appear to be decreased in size.

History.   The onset is usually sudden, often with sharp pain resembling that of pleurisy. Dyspnea will be present if the rate of col-

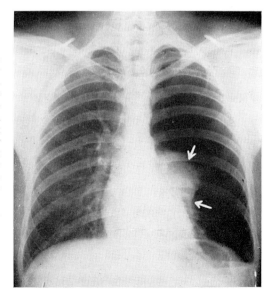

Fig. 138. Pneumothorax. The left lung has collapsed completely; the lung tissue forms a rounded mass to the left of the heart, as indicated by the arrows. No lung markings are seen in the left hemithorax. The heart and mediastinum are normally situated, indicating either that they are fixed by adhesions or that the intrathoracic pressure on the left is not excessively high, as was true in this case. (Courtesy of Dr. R. H. Chamberlain.)

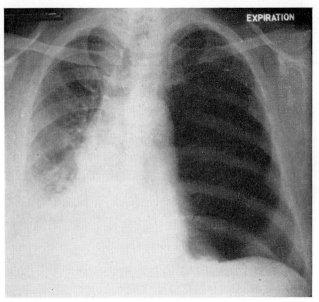

Fig. 139. Tension pneumothorax. This film, taken during expiration, shows a marked shift of the mediastinal structures to the right, indicative of high intrathoracic pressure on the left. The left dome of the diaphragm is also depressed. The patient was extremely dyspneic and cyanotic. A needle was promptly inserted through the thoracic wall to allow air to escape. Within 30 minutes the patient was much more comfortable. (Courtesy of Dr. R. H. Chamberlain.)

lapse is rapid; this may decrease or almost disappear after a few days as the necessary physiologic readjustments occur.

Pneumothorax may also result from accidental puncture of the lung during such procedures as nerve block, thoracentesis, pericardial paracentesis, liver biopsy, renal biopsy or splenic puncture. In such cases the needle usually enters or passes through normal lung tissue and a relatively small amount of air escapes before the opening is sealed. Occasionally air is deliberately introduced to permit better visualization of the pleural surfaces on roentgenography.

Benign spontaneous pneumothorax is primarily a disease of healthy young males; it is rare in females. When it occurs in an older person one should suspect emphysema, tuberculosis or other lung disease. Traumatic pneumothorax may develop at any age.

Hydropneumothorax

This denotes the presence in the pleural cavity of air plus fluid; the latter may be serous, purulent, hemorrhagic or pure blood (hemopneumothorax). The fluid may develop as a complication of pneumothorax, with spread of infection to the pleural space, by rupture of a blood vessel in the torn pleura or in a small adhesion that snaps, or possibly as a result of irritation of the pleural surface by the air. In other cases the air may be secondary to rupture of the pleura over a diseased area in the lung that has already produced the effusion. It may also follow thoracentesis for removal of fluid if the visceral pleura is inadvertently punctured.

Pathologic Changes.   These will depend upon the underlying disease process that produced the effusion and the pneumothorax.

Physical Signs.   Since there is fluid plus air, there will be a horizontal line at the junction of the two phases. This will remain parallel to the ground as the patient changes position; shifting dullness is easily demonstrable. In addition, a succussion splash is usually elicited. A metallic tinkle may be heard if there is an opening in the lung below the surface of the fluid.

Other signs will depend upon the amount of air and of fluid present. Over the lower (fluid) area the signs will be those of pleural effusion; over the upper portion the typical changes of pneumothorax will be found.

History.   This will depend upon the sequence of events. Occa-

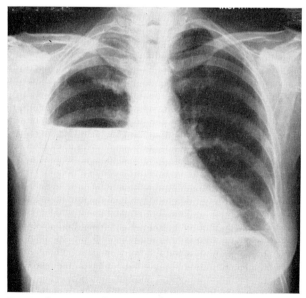

Fig. 140. Hydropneumothorax. On the right a small amount of air separates the lung tissue from the thoracic wall in the apical region. Below this there is uniform density due to fluid. The horizontal line indicates that both air and fluid are present. The mediastinal structures are not displaced in this film, which was taken after the removal of 1000 ml. of fluid and the introduction of a small amount of air. Prior to that they had been shifted somewhat to the left. (Courtesy of Dr. R. H. Chamberlain.)

sionally the patient is aware of the presence of fluid and feels it "splashing" as he changes position.

Mediastinal Emphysema

Although Laennec described this rare condition, it was Hamman[6] who revived interest in it.

Pathologic Changes.   With or without preceding trauma or strain, distended alveoli adjacent to a bronchus or a large blood vessel rupture. Air then dissects through the peribronchial or perivascular tissues and reaches the mediastinum. From there it may spread to the neck or to the subcutaneous tissues of the thorax. At times it ruptures the mediastinal parietal pleura and pneumothorax results, more commonly on the left. Compression of the venae cavae may lead to circulatory embarrassment or failure.

Physical Signs.   There may be some fullness in the tissues of the neck and the veins may be distended. Dyspnea and cyanosis are often present. On palpating the neck or thoracic wall a characteristic crackling or "sponge-like" consistency may be felt, due to air in the tissues. The area of cardiac dullness is difficult to delineate and may seem decreased in size. On auscultation a peculiar crunching, crackling or knocking sound is heard; this is synchronous with the heart beat and is usually systolic in time. It may be accentuated when the patient leans forward or to the left. If pneumothorax develops it will mask many of these signs.

History.   There may have been asthma, emphysema, infection or some other process that has been accompanied by severe cough. Pain is rather vague and dull initially but may become severe and related to respiration. Dyspnea of increasing severity is present; weakness or dizziness may result from circulatory disturbances.

---

[6] Louis Hamman, Baltimore physician, 1877–1946.

XIV

Auscultation of the Heart

★ Know 4 valves Areas +

This is the final procedure in the physical examination of the heart, and often the most important one. Before discussing the procedure and findings, certain facts learned in anatomy and physiology courses will be reviewed.

ANATOMIC CONSIDERATIONS

Position of the Heart. The heart lies obliquely behind the lower two-thirds of the sternum, and in a normally shaped chest it rests upon the upper surface of the diaphragm. When the heart is of normal size and in normal position, about two-thirds of it lies to the left of the midline.

With a normal-sized heart the base extends from the lower border of the second left costal cartilage to the upper border of the third right cartilage. The apex is in the fifth left intercostal space approximately 8 cm. to the left of the midsternal line. Most of the anterior surface is right atrium and ventricle; a small rim of left ventricle is visible along the left border and at the apex. The left atrium lies posteriorly.

The exact position of the heart varies with the configuration of the chest and the position of the diaphragm. One can visualize these changes by assuming that the heart is suspended from the aorta; therefore in a long thorax the heart tends to assume a vertical position, whereas in a short-chested person, or with elevation of the diaphragm, it may be almost horizontal. Forced inspiration and expiration will also produce definite changes in the position of the heart (Fig. 105, p. 157).

Heart Valves. The approximate anatomic position of the heart valves is indicated in Figure 144. However, the sounds produced by the various valves are best heard in other areas, as shown; these are known as the mitral area, aortic area, tricuspid area and pulmonic area.

231

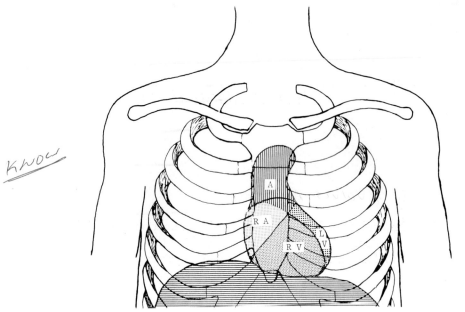

KNOW

Fig. 141.   Position of the heart. RA, right atrium; RV, right ventricle; LV, left ventricle; A, aorta. The left atrium lies posteriorly and is not visible if normal in size.

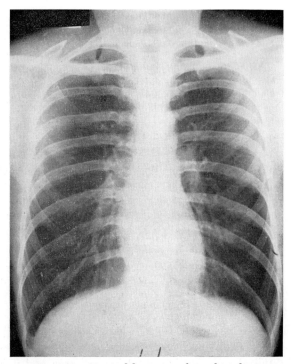

Fig. 142.   Vertical heart in a long thin chest.

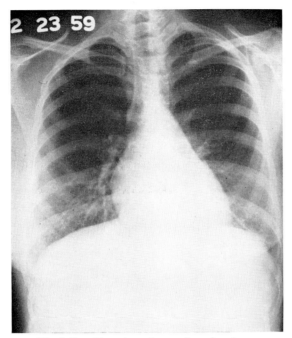

Fig. 143.   Heart in a shorter, broader chest.

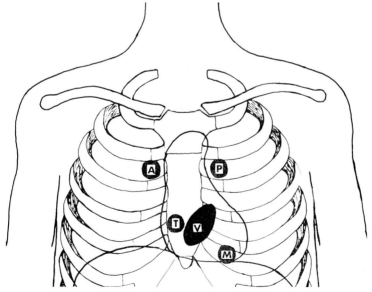

Fig. 144.   Valve areas. Anatomically, the valves are situated relatively close together (V). The sounds produced by each valve are most easily heard at the areas indicated: A, aortic valve area; P, pulmonic valve area; T, tricuspid valve area; M, mitral valve area.

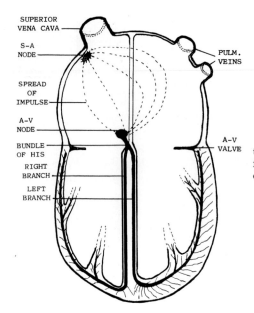

SUPERIOR
VENA CAVA

S-A
NODE

SPREAD
OF
IMPULSE

A-V
NODE

BUNDLE
OF HIS

RIGHT
BRANCH

LEFT
BRANCH

PULM.
VEINS

A-V
VALVE

Fig. 145. Electrical excitation of heart. Normal pathway of
impulses from S-A node to myocardium.

PHYSIOLOGIC CONSIDERATIONS

Electrical Excitation.   The electrical excitation of the myocardium
begins at the sinoatrial (S-A) node, spreads over the walls of both atria
and passes to the atrioventricular (A-V) node. It then passes down the
interventricular septum in the right and left branches of the bundle of
His;[1] the impulse is then carried to the ventricular muscle fibers from
the apex to the base by Purkinje[2] fibers.

Theoretically, any part of the conducting system or of the myocardium itself can initiate impulses, but since the rate of those arising
in the S-A node is normally the most rapid, this is usually the controlling
center or *pacemaker*. Ordinarily the contractions occur at regular intervals and at a rate of 70 to 80 times per minute in an adult at rest. If
for any reason there is a change in the rate or rhythm, the person may
be aware of it; such consciousness of cardiac action is called *palpitation.*
Often the person assumes that he has serious heart disease and that
his days are numbered; he may be right, but more often he is wrong.

Electrocardiography.   In the early days of the electrocardiograph
it was primarily an instrument for recording and studying irregularities
of cardiac rate and rhythm, which up to that time had been poorly
understood. Now that the mystery of these abnormalities has been

---

[1] Wilhelm His, Swiss anatomist and embryologist, 1831–1904.

[2] Johannes Evangelista Purkinje, Bohemian physiologist, 1787–1869. Lacking
laboratory facilities at the University, he made his early studies in his own house.
Later, a laboratory was built for him.

dispelled, the clinical diagnosis of them has become much easier; in the majority of cases this can be made at the bedside. The ECG is useful to confirm the diagnosis or to reassure the patient who considers a machine infallible. In an occasional case the physical examination leaves the physician completely baffled; in such instances the ECG is essential and may provide an answer.

However, the electrocardiogram has assumed new importance as a method of diagnosing abnormalities of other types, and especially those of the myocardium. For this reason it should be a part of the examination whenever there is reason to suspect heart disease. After the physician has completed his examination and formed his opinion, the tracing is helpful in confirming this. If he has erred, the physical examination should be repeated.

Origin of Heart Sounds. It has been known for generations that each complete cardiac cycle, or systole and diastole, results in the production of two principal sounds. One of these, the first heart sound, is heard at the beginning of *ventricular* systole; the second sound occurs at the end of systole.

Since the days of Harvey[3] and Laennec, dozens of theories have been advanced to explain the origin of the first sound. Despite all the newer techniques and instruments for measuring and recording heart sounds and their relationship to cardiac physiology, the argument continues. At present, it is generally stated that the major component, at least, is due to the abrupt closure of the mitral and tricuspid valves. However, there is a certain amount of newer evidence to indicate that those valves have already closed, and that it is the sudden tensing and contraction of the ventricular muscle fibers that plays the important role in the production of this sound.

The second heart sound is due to closure of the semilunar valves (aortic and pulmonic) at the end of the ejection phase of systole. In addition, other heart sounds may occasionally be heard in systole or in diastole; these will be discussed later.

PROCEDURE

For auscultation, the room must be quiet and warm and the patient must be comfortable; shivering or muscular movements may introduce extraneous sounds that might be confusing. Facilities should be avail-

---

* In timing heart sounds, *atrial* systole is ignored since it is usually inaudible; only ventricular systole and diastole are considered. A sound produced during the time of atrial contraction is classified as *presystolic* or *late diastolic*.

[3] William Harvey, English physician, 1578–1657. He first proved that the blood actually circulates in the arteries and veins.

able for examining the patient in the erect position and also lying supine or on either side. The examination must be carried out in a systematic manner, with certain definite questions in mind. The most important points to be determined are:

Identification. Which is the first heart sound? The second?

Intensity and character of the first heart sound. Is it decreased, normal or increased?

Intensity and character of the second heart sound, using the same criteria.

Interval between the first and second sounds (ventricular systole). This should be a period of silence; is there a murmur or other audible sound?

Interval between the second sound and the succeeding first sound (ventricular diastole). Is this silent, or are sounds heard?

Rhythm. Is it regular or irregular? Inspection of pulsations in the vessels of the neck and palpation of the radial pulse and of the precordium may have given clues; auscultation will supply additional evidence to confirm or change the original impressions.

Unfortunately the novice tends to overlook many of these points. He feels a glow of triumph if he hears a murmur; he ignores all else. As long as this attitude persists, he will remain a novice.

IDENTIFICATION OF HEART SOUNDS

When you place your stethoscope over the mitral or apical region of a normal heart, two different sounds will be heard. The first step is to determine which of these represents the first sound. One sound is low-pitched and rather dull; the other is shorter, sharper and somewhat higher in pitch. The former is the first heart sound; the latter is the second heart sound. Phonetically they are often represented as "lubb-DUP."

When the heart is beating slowly and the rhythm is regular, it is not difficult to differentiate between these two sounds. Also, diastole is definitely longer than systole; the interval between each *pair* of sounds is longer than the interval between the first and second sound. However, as the rate increases, diastole becomes relatively much shorter and the problem becomes more difficult. In such a case it may be possible to determine the timing by palpating the apical impulse; the first sound comes just before or with the thrust of the apex. The carotid artery can be used if the apex beat cannot be felt; the time relation is essentially the same. *Never* attempt to time the cardiac cycle by using the pulse at the wrist; the time lag renders this worthless.

In some instances it may be possible to slow the rate temporarily by having the patient hold a deep inspiration* or by exerting pressure over one carotid sinus area; diastole will then become relatively longer.

Another useful procedure is to listen first over the aortic valve area. Almost invariably the second sound will be louder than the first. Then slowly move the stethoscope downward over the precordium, concentrating on this second sound. Levine and Harvey[4] refer to this as "inching"; it is also useful for timing other sounds and their relation to the cardiac cycle.

Having properly identified these two sounds, the next problem is to determine whether they are normal or abnormal at each of the four valve areas. Physiologic variations must be borne in mind. Since the first sound is produced in the region of the mitral and tricuspid valves, it should be louder in those areas than in the aortic and pulmonic areas. Similarly, the second sound will be louder in the aortic and pulmonic areas than at the apex. In a normal person the first sound at the apex may be twice as intense as the second sound; at the aortic area the relationship is reversed (Fig. 147). However, both sounds should be audible at all four valve areas.

In describing heart sounds at various valve areas, certain abbreviations are commonly employed, even though they are open to criticism. For example, the first heart sound is produced by the mitral and tricuspid valves, yet one constantly sees phrases such as "the aortic first sound" instead of "the first sound at the aortic area." This in turn is abbreviated

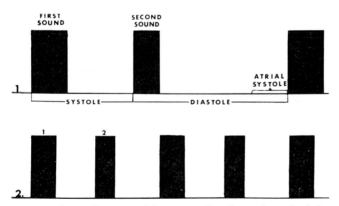

Fig. 146. Relative duration of heart sounds, of systole and of diastole when the rate is 70 (1) and when the rate is 140 (2). Diastole becomes relatively much shorter than systole.

* Remember—you should always do the same thing yourself.
[4] Samuel Albert Levine, Boston internist, 1891– ; W. Proctor Harvey, Washington internist, 1918– .

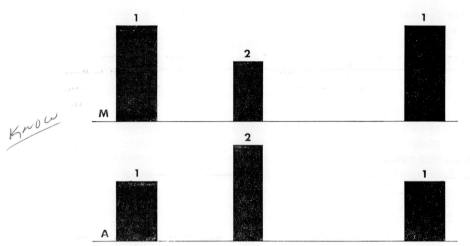

Know

Fig. 147. Relative intensity of first and second heart sounds at the mitral area (M) and at the aortic area (A).

and becomes "A₁." Bowing to common usage, the heart sounds will be designated by symbols such as A_1, A_2, M_1, M_2.

ALTERED INTENSITY OF HEART SOUNDS

Physiologic Alterations of Both Sounds. One must differentiate between altered intensity of both heart sounds as opposed to changes heard only in the first sound or in the second sound. Both sounds will be more intense (louder) in a person with a thin chest wall, or when the cardiac rate is increased by extracardiac factors such as exercise, nervousness or hyperthyroidism. The intensity will be decreased if anything is interposed between the stethoscope and the heart. Both sounds will be more difficult to hear if there is a thick muscular chest wall, a heavy layer of fat or a mass of mammary tissue interfering with the transmission of vibrations. An emphysematous lung may envelop much of the heart; sounds may be audible only over the sternum and the immediately adjacent areas or in the epigastrium. The same may be true with left-sided pneumothorax or massive pleural effusion.

increas **Increased Intensity of the First Sound.** This may be physiologic in a person with a very thin chest wall, or in anyone after exercise or with emotional tension. Pathologically it can occur in conditions such as mitral stenosis, hyperthyroidism, anemia or during an acute febrile illness. The time relationship between atrial and ventricular contraction is important. Normally, the atrial contraction starts 0.16 to 0.18 second before the ventricular contraction. If this time (P-R interval on the electrocardiogram) is shortened, a louder first sound can be expected. This has usually been attributed to the position of the mitral and tricuspid valve leaflets at the start of ventricular systole. A long P-R interval permits more complete filling of the ventricles; the leaflets float up on the blood and travel only a short distance as they close gently when systole begins. With a short P-R interval there is less blood in the ventricles and the leaflets must travel a greater distance; they snap or slam shut. However, there is some evidence to suggest that the valve leaflets are already closed by the time ventricular systole begins, and that the increased first sound is due to vibrations produced by the rapid shortening of muscle fibers in a ventricle that is only partially filled.

Decreased Intensity of the First Sound. Mitral insufficiency may be accompanied by a very faint first sound, especially when due to rheumatic involvement; thickening of the valve leaflets is believed to slow their movement. In cardiac failure the first sound may be almost inaudible. Prolongation of the P-R interval, as in certain types of heart block, will diminish the intensity of the first sound, as explained above. It should be emphasized that the intensity of the first heart sound is not diagnostic of the presence or absence of heart disease. A normal heart *usually* has a loud first sound at the mitral area; the failing or decompensating heart *rarely* does. However, this is merely one link in the chain of evidence that leads to the correct diagnosis.

Increased Intensity of the Second Sound. Normally the pulmonic second sound is louder than the aortic in children and often in young adults, and its intensity is greater when the subject is recumbent. Pathologically, it is louder when the blood pressure in the pulmonary circulation is increased. Therefore P_2 is accentuated when there are such conditions as pulmonary hypertension or arteriosclerosis, emphysema or pneumoconiosis. It will be accentuated with disease of the mitral valve that increases the amount of blood in the lungs, or with congenital anomalies giving left-to-right shunt, provided the right ventricle is able to maintain the increased blood pressure.

The aortic second sound is louder than P_2 in older persons and it is increased when the systemic blood pressure is elevated, provided the left ventricle remains competent. The elevated pressure may be physiologic (exercise; emotions) or pathologic, as in benign or malignant hypertension, glomerulonephritis or nephrosclerosis. The sound may also be increased when there are pathologic changes with loss of elasticity at the base of the aorta, as in old age or with syphilitic aortitis.

The amount of accentuation of the second sound is not an accurate index of the degree of hypertension present. Possibly it is not the actual pressure in the aorta or in the pulmonary artery, but the difference in pressure (pressure gradient) between the vessel and the ventricle that determines the speed of closure of the valve leaflets, and hence the intensity of the sound.

Decreased Intensity of the Second Sound.   Both second sounds (A$_2$, P$_2$) will be decreased in intensity when the blood pressure is very low as in syncope, in shock or in other states accompanied by hypotension and a lowered pressure gradient. Stenosis of either semilunar valve will result in a decreased second sound at that area. The same is true when there is any disease that destroys or seriously affects the mobility of the leaflets. Weakened contractions of either ventricle (myocardial failure) will result in decreased second sounds at the corresponding value area.

SPLITTING (REDUPLICATION) OF HEART SOUNDS

So far, we have assumed that there is a single first sound and a single second sound; this is not always true. Each of these sounds is produced by the closure of two separate valves—mitral and tricuspid; pulmonic and aortic. If both close practically simultaneously the two sounds blend or fuse into a single sound. If they do not, there will be splitting, or two distinct sounds. This is not rare; it may occur physiologically or it may be a sign of heart disease.

Splitting of the Second Heart Sound.   Since this is more common and is of greater clinical importance it will be considered first. During inspiration the negative intrathoracic pressure increases the return of blood to the right atrium and ventricle. The right ventricle requires more time to expel this extra amount of blood; closure of the pulmonic valve is slightly delayed. This negative pressure also tends to hold blood in the lung; the return flow to the left side is slightly decreased, so the aortic valve may close slightly sooner. Therefore, with inspiration the time interval between A$_2$ and P$_2$ increases; during expiration the interval becomes shorter or the two sounds merge completely. This appearance and disappearance or increase and decrease in splitting is physiologic. Since A$_2$ is normally louder than P$_2$, the splitting will be more easily audible at the pulmonic area; the fainter P$_2$ may be overshadowed or obliterated by A$_2$ at the aortic area. It should be remembered that with physiologic splitting, it is the pulmonic component of the second sound that shows the greater shift.

Obviously, any pathologic condition that delays emptying of the right ventricle will delay closure of the pulmonic valve. If the right branch of the bundle of His is injured or destroyed (right bundle branch block; R.B.B.B.) the activation of the right ventricle is delayed. There will be wide splitting of the second sound and this will increase during

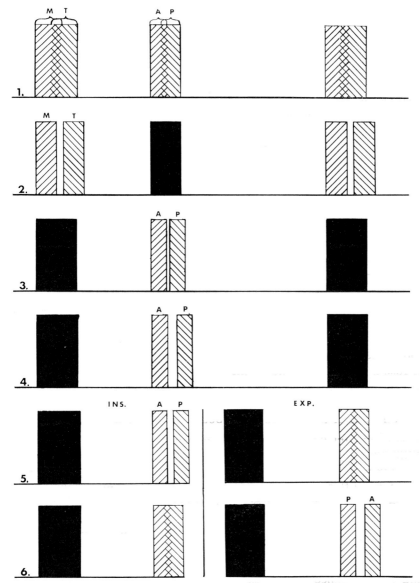

Fig. 148. Splitting of heart sounds: *1.* Normal sounds. The first sound is a combination of the mitral and tricuspid sounds (M, T); the second sound, of the aortic and pulmonic components (A, P). *2.* Split first sound. The mitral element occurs a few hundredths of a second before the tricuspid sound; two "first" sounds are heard. *3.* Slight splitting of the second sound; the aortic component precedes the pulmonic. This is usually heard best over the pulmonic area; at the aortic area, the louder A_2 tends to obscure the faint P_2. *4.* Wide splitting of second sound. This may be confused with the physiologic third sound (Fig. 151), an opening snap (Fig. 152) or a diastolic gallop (Fig. 153). The timing is important; it occurs earlier in diastole than those sounds. *5.* Physiologic variation with respiration. During inspiration P_2 tends to occur later; during expiration the two sounds merge. *6.* Paradoxical (reversed) splitting. During inspiration a single sound is heard; during expiration P_2 occurs at the normal time, but with slow emptying of the left ventricle A_2 is delayed.

241

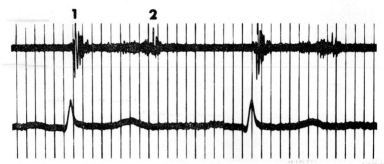

Fig. 149.   Simultaneous recording of heart sounds (upper tracing) and electrocardiogram. (Courtesy of Drs. C. C. Wolferth and C. F. Kay, Robinette Foundation,
Hospital of the University of Pennsylvania.)

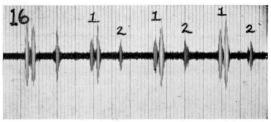

Fig. 150.   Phonocardiogram showing splitting of the first heart sound. The first
component may be mistaken for a presystolic murmur.

or atrial spetial defects

inspiration. Stenosis (narrowing) of the pulmonic valve will also produce
splitting because there is mechanical interference with emptying of the
right ventricle. However, this may be difficult to detect because the
blood pressure in the pulmonary artery is low and the pulmonic second
sound will be faint. The systolic murmur that precedes the second sound
tends to mask the aortic component and also makes P_2 less easily heard.
An atrial septal defect, with left-to-right shunt of blood, can overload the
right ventricle and produce increased splitting. In a majority of these
patients there is little variation with respiration because the right side
is constantly overfilled.

In some instances the split second sound is due to early closure of
the aortic valve. If the mitral valve does not close completely (mitral
insufficiency) a variable amount of blood leaks back into the atrium in
systole; therefore the left ventricle empties more rapidly and the aortic
valve closes earlier than normal, producing wide splitting of the second
sound.

Paradoxical (Reversed) Splitting.   In left bundle branch block
(L.B.B.B.) the excitation of the left ventricle is delayed; therefore the
pulmonic component will be heard first, then the aortic element. With
inspiration the pulmonic sound tends to show the normal variability and

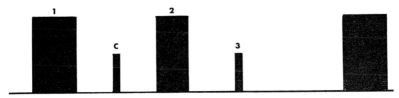

Fig. 151. Other physiologic heart sounds. Relative time in the cardiac cycle of midsystolic click (C) and of the physiologic third sound (3).

occurs later; therefore the two sounds become closer together or may merge. On expiration the splitting becomes wider. Also, the stenosis of the aortic valve A_2 may be delayed and paradoxical splitting can result.

Splitting of the First Heart Sound. This is frequently present in healthy subjects and is best heard at the apex or near the sternal border. It is not uncommon in older persons, and may be more prominent during expiration. It is sometimes misdiagnosed and called a presystolic murmur or an atrial gallop, even in the absence of other signs of heart disease. Occasionally it is due to bundle branch block; then it is significant.

OTHER PHYSIOLOGIC HEART SOUNDS

Midsystolic Click. Not infrequently a clicking sound, of maximum intensity near the apex, will be heard between the normal first and second sounds. The exact time relations may vary with respiration or with change of position. The cause is unknown, but it is usually heard in young people with no signs of heart disease.

Third Sound. A physiologic diastolic third sound may occasionally be present in a young person with no demonstrable cardiovascular disease, especially when the heart rate is slow. This comes early in diastole, usually about 0.15 second after the second heart sound. It is loudest when the person is supine or turned partially on his left side, and may wax and wane with expiration and inspiration. The exact cause is uncertain; it may be due to a sudden inflow of blood striking the wall of the ventricle early in the relaxation phase. No paTHological sign

ABNORMAL OR PATHOLOGIC HEART SOUNDS

Systolic Ejection Sound (Click). A short, high-pitched sound may be present at either the aortic or the pulmonic area; this is heard almost immediately after the first heart sound. An aortic ejection sound

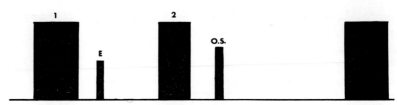

Fig. 152. Abnormal heart sounds. Relative time in cardiac cycle of systolic ejection sound (E) and opening snap of mitral stenosis (O.S.).

may occur with dilatation of the ascending aorta, stenosis of the aortic *Causes* valve, hypertension, coarctation of the aorta or other anomalies. A pulmonary ejection sound suggests stenosis of the valve, dilatation of the pulmonary artery or hypertension in the pulmonary circulation. These sounds are probably produced by vibrations in the respective vessels.

mitral stenos **Diastolic Opening Snap.** This sound is almost pathognomonic of mitral stenosis. It is a sharp snap or click heard shortly after the second heart sound. It is usually fairly sharply localized, and is most commonly present in the third or fourth intercostal space near the sternum. It occurs at the time when the ventricle begins to relax and a normal mitral valve would open. Sudden checking of the attempted opening of the stenotic valve leaflets is believed to produce the snap. It must be differentiated from splitting of the second sound and from a protodiastolic gallop (below). It can be heard in over half of the patients with mitral stenosis, and may be present when a murmur is difficult to elicit. Since the presence of the snap indicates that the edges of the valve leaflets are not excessively scarred or thickened, it is considered a favorable sign when surgical intervention is being contemplated.

Gallop Rhythm. This denotes the presence of three sounds, or possibly four, in each cardiac cycle. This gives rise to a triple rhythm resembling the sounds produced by a galloping horse. The extra sound may occur in systole or in diastole. It is usually faint, low-pitched and fairly well localized. It may appear and disappear repeatedly without obvious cause. It is rarely audible at the base, but is heard in the fourth or fifth intercostal space to the left of the sternum or near the apex. Some authors believe that sounds heard over the apex arise from the left ventricle, while those heard closer to the sternum arise in the right ventricle. In some instances the added sound may closely resemble the physiologic third heart sound or the midsystolic click. These occur in healthy persons; gallop is heard in various types of heart failure. It has been called "the cry of the failing heart." *AT Apex Rare at Base*

To determine the exact timing of a gallop sound, it is helpful to listen first at the base, where only two sounds are ordinarily heard, or occasionally at some other area. After identifying the first and second sounds and fixing their characteristics firmly in mind, move the stethoscope gradually downward and outward toward the apex until the third sound becomes audible. It is then fairly easy to determine the timing of this extra sound.

SYSTOLIC GALLOP.   An added sound is heard at the mitral area or apex, about midway between the first and second sounds; occasionally it can be heard at the aortic area also. The origin of this sound is unknown. It must not be confused with a split first sound, a midsystolic click or a systolic murmur.

DIASTOLIC GALLOP.   Here a third sound occurs after the second sound and before the next first heart sound. Three types have been described. With protodiastolic gallop the third sound occurs early in diastole, from 0.12 to 0.20 second after the second heart sound. It has been attributed to the sudden rise in ventricular pressure that occurs after the mitral and tricuspid valves open. It closely resembles the normal third heart sound but is accompanied by other obvious signs of cardiovascular disease.

PRESYSTOLIC GALLOP.   This is characterized by a third sound occurring late in diastole. Since this actually occurs during atrial systole, a better name might be atrial systolic gallop. It must be differentiated from splitting of the first heart sound and from a presystolic murmur. It is probably due to the sudden rise in the intraventricular pressure resulting from blood forced in by the contracting atria.

MESODIASTOLIC GALLOP.   The third sound is heard in middiastole. This is heard when diastole is short, as with tachycardia or A-V block. It is thought to represent the merging of a protodiastolic and a presystolic sound, and is often called a summation gallop. This is considered to be the most common and most significant type of gallop rhythm.

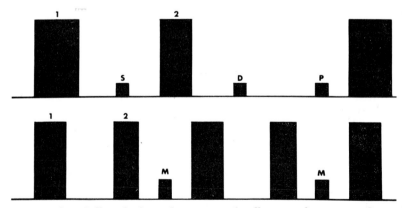

Fig. 153. Gallop rhythm. Three types of gallop may be present: S, systolic gallop; D, early diastolic gallop; P, late diastolic or presystolic gallop. With tachycardia, the diastolic and presystolic elements tend to merge, giving a mesodiastolic (middiastolic) or summation gallop (M).

Embryocardia.   With cardiac failure and tachycardia the first heart sound may be faint and the diastolic interval short. The first and second sounds at the mitral area or apex are much the same, and they occur at fairly evenly spaced intervals, like the ticking of a watch. Since fetal heart sounds are similar, this is known as embryocardia, fetal rhythm or tick-tock rhythm.

ALTERATIONS OF CARDIAC RATE

In an adult, a normal heart beats 60 to 80 times per minute. In young children the rate is more rapid; 130 to 140 may not be abnormal. Some of the physiologic variations have been mentioned in previous chapters; pathologic alterations will now be considered. In many instances the diagnosis cannot be proved conclusively without an electrocardiogram, but often the history and the physical examination will enable the examiner to arrive at a tentative diagnosis that is later confirmed by the tracing.

Sinus Tachycardia.   In this condition the rate is abnormally rapid, but the impulse arises in the normal pacemaker and spreads in a normal manner. When the rate is very rapid it may be difficult to determine which is the first heart sound and which is the second; measures that may help to solve this problem have already been discussed (p. 236). It should be pointed out that procedures that tend to slow the rate in sinus tachycardia do so in a gradual, regular manner; this is not true in other types of tachycardia.

Sinus Bradycardia.   Here again the impulse arises and travels in a normal manner. The rhythm is essentially regular, although there may be minor changes associated with respiration (sinus arrhythmia). This benign condition must not be confused with the potentially serious bradycardia of heart block, to be discussed later in this section.

Paroxysmal Atrial Tachycardia.   In this condition there is a sudden rise in the heart rate to 150, 200 or even 250 beats per minute; later this suddenly reverts to normal. The attack may be very brief, lasting only a minute or two, or it may persist for hours or days.

The diagnosis cannot be established unless the patient is actually examined during an attack. The rhythm will be regular and the sounds will not change from beat to beat except for the minor variations associated with respiration. Stimulation of the vagus, as by carotid pressure or having the patient hold a deep breath, will frequently end an attack abruptly; slow, normal contractions are resumed. In sinus tachycardia, vagal stimulation may produce gradual temporary slowing, but the rate promptly speeds up again when the stimulus is removed. In paroxysmal atrial tachycardia the rate is either entirely unaltered by this, or it drops promptly to normal.

A person with paroxysmal atrial tachycardia usually seems healthy, but is nervous and tense. Suddenly he realizes that his heart is racing, and just as suddenly the racing stops. The other symptoms depend largely upon the duration of the attack. It may last for only a few minutes and produce no apparent side effects. If it persists for hours or days there may be anginal pain due to myocardial ischemia, or signs of circulatory failure. Syncope is not uncommon during the attack; transient muscular weakness, paralysis or paresthesias are occasionally seen. If

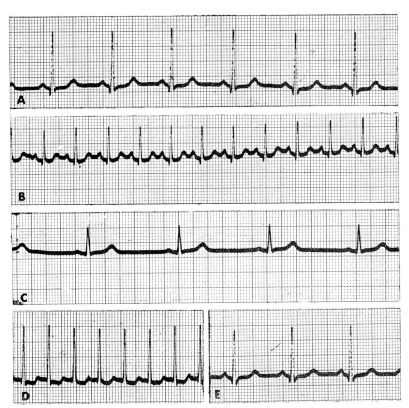

Fig. 154. Variations in cardiac rate. A, Normal adult, 70 beats per minute; B, sinus tachycardia (150) in a very nervous woman; C, sinus bradycardia (50) in an athlete at rest; D, paroxysmal atrial tachycardia (176); E, following unilateral carotid sinus pressure, the rate fell to normal (75) and the palpitation disappeared.

In these and subsequent tracings the standardization is such that one millivolt produces a vertical deflection of 10 mm. (10 small squares). The heavy vertical lines appear at intervals of 0.2 second; the faint vertical lines represent 0.04 second. Since there are 1500 vertical lines per minute, one method of estimating the cardiac rate is to count the number of lines appearing between any two comparable points in the cycle and divide this into 1500.

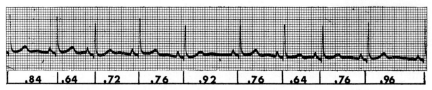

Fig. 155. Sinus arrhythmia. The interval between beats is indicated in seconds. The rate increases (short interval) during the early part of inspiration; it slows (longer interval) during expiration.

organic heart disease is already present, the results may be even more dramatic. Needless to say, the episode of tachycardia, whether brief or prolonged, does nothing to reassure the nervous, tense patient.

Paroxysmal Ventricular Tachycardia. In some respects this resembles atrial tachycardia. The onset is sudden; the rate ranges from 150 to 250 beats per minute; the cessation is usually abrupt. Unlike atrial tachycardia, this occurs most frequently in persons with severe myocardial disease such as coronary sclerosis, coronary thrombosis or severe valvular disease; only occasionally is it found in the absence of any demonstrable abnormality.

On auscultation, the rhythm seems regular but the consecutive beats are not *exactly* alike. The atria are contracting independently and more slowly than the ventricles; therefore the degree of ventricular filling and the position of the A-V valves will vary from one cycle to the next, and consequently the intensity of the heart sounds constantly changes. Moreover, vagal stimulation has no effect upon the ventricular rate. This abnormally rapid rate may revert to normal, or it may be followed by ventricular fibrillation.

ALTERATIONS OF CARDIAC RHYTHM

In this section no attempt will be made to describe all of the abnormalities of rhythm that may occur; only the more common ones that the student should learn to recognize at the bedside will be considered.

Sinus Arrhythmia. During the early part of inspiration the cardiac rate is increased; at the end of inspiration and during expiration it slows. This is attributed to varying degrees of vagal stimulation; if the breath is held the arrhythmia usually disappears. It is common in infants and children and is often called juvenile or respiratory arrhythmia. In adults it is much less noticeable and is of no significance unless accompanied by definite evidence of cardiac disease.

Sinus Pause. This is a rare condition in which there is sudden complete arrest of cardiac activity. It may be momentary; one or two beats may be lost. It may be more prolonged and lead to vertigo, syncope, convulsions or death. It is usually due to abnormal sensitivity of the carotid sinus, especially in elderly persons, or to a mass pressing on the sinus or involving the vagus nerve. Treatment in such cases is surgical.

Premature Contractions. In this arrhythmia an abnormal focus in the atrium, in the ventricle or in the A-V node sends out impulses that result in contractions at unexpected times. These are often referred to as "extra systoles"; actually they are not *extra* systoles, but *premature* ones. The term *extra systole* should be reserved for those rare instances in which there is an extra interpolated beat. Clinically, premature contractions are the most common cause of cardiac arrhythmia; bedside diagnosis is often possible.

VENTRICULAR PREMATURE CONTRACTIONS. These are much more common than either of the other two; therefore they will be considered first. An irritable focus somewhere in the ventricle (usually the left ventricle) sends out an impulse that then spreads to the rest of the myocardium and results in a contraction. This discharge occurs during diastole and frequently in early diastole. The auscultatory findings will depend upon the time at which the contraction begins. If it comes very early in diastole there will be little blood in the ventricles. The A-V

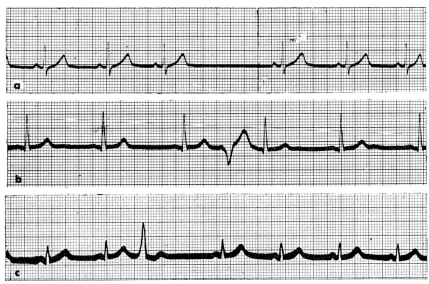

Fig. 156. Alterations of cardiac rhythm. *a,* Sinus pause; one beat is completely missing ("dropped beat"). *b,* An impulse arising in a ventricular ectopic focus produces a genuine "extra" systole, interposed between beats occurring at a relatively slow rate. *c,* Ventricular premature contraction. The complex is unlike the normal ones. The expected normal complex is absent; the next one appears after twice the normal time interval (compensatory pause).

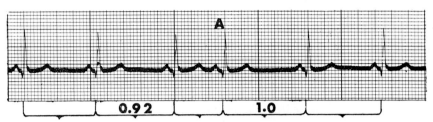

Fig. 157. Atrial premature contraction. In this patient the normal interval between beats was 0.92 second. An atrial premature contraction (A) occurred 0.48 second after a normal beat; the following normal contraction occurred at almost the expected time (1.0 second) after the premature contraction.

valves will be forced shut but there will not be enough pressure to open the semilunar valves. Therefore there will be only a single sound (first heart sound) occurring shortly after the normal second sound, and no pulsation occurs in the aorta or other arteries. If the contraction occurs a little later in diastole there may be enough blood to open the semilunar valves momentarily. A first and second sound will be heard, almost blending into one, and a faint pulse may be palpable in the carotid artery. If the impulse comes still later, the first and second sounds are more widely separated and a definite pulsation is produced in the carotids; this may or may not be palpable at the wrist.

The typical feature, which is frequently helpful in diagnosis, is that the next regular ventricular systole fails to appear at the expected time; it is completely ablated. Presumably the normal impulse from the atrium is blocked at the A-V node by the retrograde impulse from the ventricles, or if that impulse does reach the ventricles, they are in the refractory phase and cannot contract. The next contraction occurs when the second impulse spreads down from the atrium. The long pause between the premature contraction and the subsequent normal systole is known as the *compensatory pause*. The fundamental basic rhythm of the heart and of the pulse remains unaltered; at intervals one normal beat is missing when you palpate the radial artery, and an abnormal sound is heard on auscultation. Inspection of the jugular veins will show a regular rhythm, with an auricular wave at the expected time despite the missing ventricular contraction.

ATRIAL PREMATURE CONTRACTION.   These often present a different picture. The abnormal impulse arises too early in the cardiac cycle from an ectopic focus in the atrium, spreads through the tissues and arrives at the A-V node. From that point the conduction is normal, as is the ventricular response. The first heart sound may be slightly accentuated, because of incomplete filling of the ventricles; systole may be shortened and the second sound may be decreased in intensity. Again the exact findings will depend on the interval between the normal atrial systole and the abnormal excitation wave. The distinguishing feature is that the next normal beat frequently occurs at approximately the expected (normal) interval after the premature beat. The compensatory pause is missing; the rhythm changes.

To illustrate this in another way, let us assume that the rate is 60 beats per minute; each cycle takes one second. If a ventricular premature contraction occurs 0.4 second after a normal beat, the next contraction will occur 1.6 seconds later, or 2 seconds after the preceding normal beat. If an atrial premature contraction occurs 0.4 second after a normal impulse, the next contraction can occur approximately 1 second later, or 1.4 seconds after the preceding normal beat. With ventricular premature beats the rhythm remains regular; with atrial premature contractions the rhythm may be constantly changing; you can't dance to it.

NODAL PREMATURE CONTRACTIONS. These are rare and usually are diagnosed only by electrocardiography. The physical signs resemble those produced by atrial premature contractions.

MULTIPLE PREMATURE CONTRACTIONS. So far we have considered a single premature contraction following a normal beat. This is the most common situation; such ectopic systoles may recur at rare or at frequent intervals. However, one occasionally finds that each normal systole is followed by a ventricular premature contraction; this is known as coupling (Fig. 158). Because of the compensatory pause, the rhythm heard on auscultation becomes "strong beat, weak beat—long pause; strong beat, weak beat—long pause." This is one type of *bigeminal* rhythm. Depending upon the time and force of the premature beat, it may or may not produce a faint pulse palpable at the wrist. Therefore the radial pulse may exhibit the same rhythm as the heart, or it may be regular but slow when only the normal beats are producing a palpable impulse. If a premature systole follows every two normal beats, and does not produce a palpable pulse, the rhythm seems to be "beat, beat—long pause; beat, beat—long pause"; this is another form of bigeminal rhythm.

Two or more premature systoles may follow a normal beat; in such cases the rhythm may become very irregular and confusing, and an ECG may be required to differentiate this from atrial fibrillation. However,

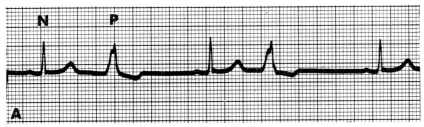

Fig. 158. Coupling. Each normal beat (N) is followed by a ventricular premature contraction (P).

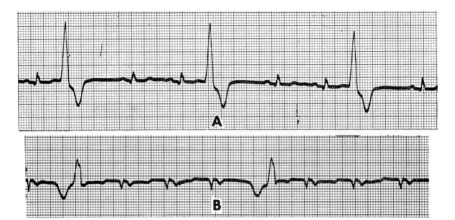

Fig. 159. Ventricular premature contractions following two normal complexes (A) and three normal beats (B).

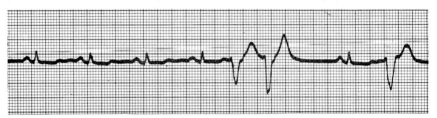

Fig. 160. Two ventricular premature contractions, a normal complex and a third PVC.

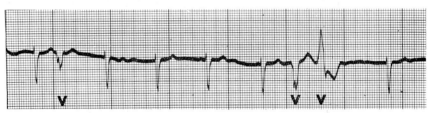

Fig. 161. Premature ventricular contractions (V) arising from different foci, as shown by the variations in the electrocardiographic pattern.

the diagnosis can often be suspected clinically if one remembers that only two types of beats will be heard—the normal and the premature contractions. The sounds produced by the normal contractions are essentially the same from beat to beat; those produced by the premature beats are different from those of the normal contractions, but they also all sound much the same.

SYMPTOMS.   The symptoms resulting from premature contractions are variable. In most patients, atrial premature contractions produce few subjective symptoms; ventricular premature beats are often annoying. Some persons are aware of the long pause: "My heart skips a beat" or "My heart seems to stop." Others are more annoyed by the forceful contraction that results from overfilling of the ventricle during the compensatory pause: "My heart thumps every once in a while"; "My heart seems to flop over"; "I feel a beating in my neck."

These ectopic beats are more liable to occur when the heart rate is slow and are often abolished by exercise. The person may have few or none while active during the day, but in the evening when he is quiet, or particularly after he has gone to bed, they become apparent. Just as he is falling asleep his heart starts to "act up." He gets up, wanders around, smokes a cigarette or two or watches TV. His heart is perfectly regular. He goes back to bed, the heart rate slows and the symptoms recur. The history alone may be almost diagnostic in such cases.

Why some apparently healthy persons develop premature contractions is still unknown. Emotional stress, nicotine, caffeine, alcohol and physical exhaustion are among the agents that have been accused but not always proved guilty. In other individuals none of these seem to play a part. It seems important to emphasize that in the absence of any other signs of heart disease, occasional episodes of premature contractions may be annoying but are not a danger sign. However, when heart disease is present, they may precede and portend more serious arrhythmias. Overdigitalization may also produce these.

Atrial Fibrillation. This is the most important of the common cardiac arrhythmias. In fibrillation, there is no orderly contraction of the atria. Instead, one finds distended and dilated atria with muscle fibers and groups of fibers contracting and relaxing in a totally disorganized manner and at an unpredictable rate. Each of these contractions results in an electrical impulse, many of which reach the atrioventricular node; there may be 400 or more per minute. Some of these are blocked at the node; others reach the ventricles. There the muscle may be in the refractory state, or it may respond. Consequently the ventricles contract at irregular intervals and at a rapid rate. Since the degree of ventricular filling varies from beat to beat, the heart sounds will also vary. With minimal filling the contraction may be too weak to open the semilunar valves; only a first heart sound will result, and no pulse wave is pro-

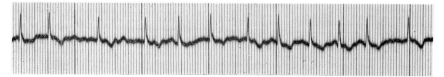

Fig. 162. Atrial fibrillation. The ventricular complexes occur at irregular intervals. No P waves can be identified; the fluctuations in the base line indicate erratic electrical activity of the atrium.

duced. At other times a very slight ejection occurs; this may be imperceptible at the wrist. As a result there will be a *pulse deficit;* the rate counted at the wrist will be less than the cardiac rate as determined by auscultation. Also, since the amount of blood ejected varies from cycle to cycle, the systolic blood pressure varies from beat to beat (p. 55).

Long before the stethoscope was introduced or the physiologic disturbance responsible for this arrhythmia was recognized, the pulse was described as *pulsus irregularis totalis et perpetuus.* Later, the auscultatory findings were aptly and vividly called *delirium cordis;* that description still has merit. For several seconds, sounds may assail the ear in a rush, tripping and tumbling over each other. Then there will be a lull with two or three fairly regularly spaced beats, but the peaceful interlude is brief; the tumult starts again.

DIFFERENTIAL DIAGNOSIS. To differentiate fibrillation from other arrhythmias is not always easy. Multiple premature ventricular contractions may produce a seemingly total arrhythmia, but certain differences will be heard if you listen carefully. Attention should be focused first on diastole. With premature contractions, two or more beats will occur in close succession, followed by a longer pause before the next beat. With atrial fibrillation the longer diastole may occur without the preceding rapid beats. Exercise tends to decrease the frequency of premature contractions, or to abolish them; the rate becomes more rapid but the arrhythmia decreases or disappears. With fibrillation the rate may increase slightly but the rhythm is unchanged by exercise. Also, variations in intensity of the first heart sound may occur that are roughly comparable to the duration of diastole. For practical purposes, if the cardiac rhythm is totally irregular, if the apical rate is 110 or more, if the pulse deficit is at least 10 beats per minute and if the force of the beats (blood pressure) is variable, one may assume that atrial fibrillation is present.

ETIOLOGY. The most common underlying etiologic factor is rheumatic heart disease with stenosis of the mitral valve. Fibrillation may also occur with other rheumatic processes, with hypertensive heart disease or as a result of coronary artery disease. It can also develop in hyperthyroidism, during an acute infection, during or after a surgical procedure or even in an apparently healthy person without obvious reason. It may be paroxysmal and last for only a short time; this is more common when there is no cardiovascular disease. If fibrillation continues for several days, it usually persists unless treated.

SYMPTOMS. Since the onset of fibrillation is sudden, it often produces an alarming deterioration in the condition of the patient. The heart that was damaged but was still able to maintain adequate circulation (compensated) now begins to fail (decompensate). Dyspnea, pulmonary edema and other signs of congestion appear and become progressively more marked unless the patient receives proper therapy. Digitalis and its derivatives will decrease or inhibit the transmission of impulses through the A-V node; the dosage can be adjusted so that 70 to 80 per minute reach the ventricle. At this relatively normal rate the circulatory dynamics are improved and symptoms decrease or disappear. At the same time the rhythm may show so little irregularity that it seems to be normal. However, it must not be assumed that the fibrillation itself has been controlled. Only the ventricles have benefited; the atria continue their delirious dance.

Atrial Flutter.   In this condition an ectopic focus in the atrium initiates *rhythmic* impulses at a rate of 250 to 350 per minute. The ventricles are unable to respond to each impulse but frequently they contract at half that rate (2:1 block), resulting in a pulse rate of 125 to 175. Occasionally a higher degree of block occurs (3:1; 4:1); in such cases the ventricular rate is correspondingly slower and may be within the normal range (Fig. 163). The bedside diagnosis is difficult; an ECG is usually needed. Flutter may be suspected if vagal stimulation produces a sudden marked drop in the pulse rate, as the 2:1 block becomes 3:1 or even 4:1; there may also be slowing with the appearance of ventricular irregularity due to 3:1 block mingled with 4:1. At times it is possible to see a-waves in the jugular vein occurring at the rapid atrial rate.

Ventricular Fibrillation.   This diagnosis is rarely made clinically. As in atrial fibrillation, individual muscle fibers and bundles of fibers contract irregularly; the ventricles cease to contract as a unit. No normal heart sounds will be heard since no blood is being ejected; occasionally

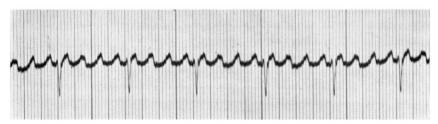

Fig. 163.   Atrial flutter. The atrial rate is 300 per minute. The ventricle is responding to every fourth atrial impulse (4:1 block); the rate is 75.

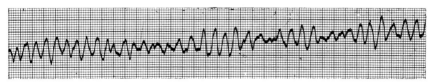

Fig. 164.   Ventricular fibrillation; ECG obtained a few moments before the patient died. In such a heart there is total disorganization of ventricular activity, resembling that seen in the atrium with atrial fibrillation. No heart sounds could be heard; no pulse or blood pressure could be obtained. Electrical defibrillation was attempted but was unsuccessful.

faint sounds due to atrial contractions will be audible. The diagnosis can be established only be the ECG or by direct inspection at the operating table. Ventricular fibrillation may persist for some time but irreversible brain damage develops quickly, since all peripheral circulation has stopped.

In many instances ventricular fibrillation is the terminal event in coronary artery disease or in other forms of heart failure. Occasionally it develops in a relatively healthy person as a complication of a minor episode of myocardial infarction, in the course of surgery with general anesthesia or after an electric shock. In such cases it may be possible to restore normal rhythm by using the electrical defibrillator, if adequate circulation and oxygenation can be maintained by open or closed (external) cardiac massage and mouth-to-mouth breathing until the necessary equipment can be secured.

Heart Block. If the A-V node or bundle of His fails to function normally the excitation wave will be delayed or completely interrupted. The resulting changes are classified as first, second or third degree heart block. Any of these may be produced by functional alterations in the conducting pathways, by organic disease of this tissue or by the action of certain drugs.

FIRST DEGREE HEART BLOCK. Conduction is slightly delayed but the rate and rhythm are normal. Since the interval between atrial systole and ventricular systole is increased, the first heart sound will often be faint but the second sound will be normal. In rare instances the faint sound of atrial contraction will precede the soft first sound, giving rise to a presystolic type of gallop. These findings will suggest block, but the diagnosis cannot be established without an electrocardiogram that shows a P-R interval of more than 0.2 second. Thereafter auscultation can be useful in determining progression or regression of the block.

First degree block may occur with active rheumatic infection, with diphtheria and occasionally with other acute infections. It can also appear in chronic heart disease, and frequently is the result of digitalis therapy.

SECOND DEGREE HEART BLOCK (PARTIAL BLOCK). If a slightly greater impairment of conduction is present, some atrial impulses fail to reach the ventricles (Fig. 165). The relation of atrial to ventricular contractions is expressed as a numerical ratio such as 10:9, 5:4, 2:1 or other appropriate figures. In some patients the block is due to acute or chronic disease of the conducting mechanism, as in first degree heart block, or to excessive amounts of digitalis. In others it may be due to fatigue of the tissues or inability of the ventricles to respond rapidly enough; for example, with atrial flutter the ventricular rate is usually one-half the rate of the atrium (2:1 block).

The auscultatory findings depend upon the degree of block present and the time elapsing between atrial and ventricular systole. With high degrees of block (2:1, 3:1) the rhythm will be regular and the sounds will be essentially identical from cycle to cycle. The first sound is often faint; the second sound is normal or increased. With lesser degrees, there will be a *regular irregularity*. For example, every sixth ventricular beat will be dropped in 6:5 block. Inspection of the jugular vein will show the typical a-wave at the proper time even though no heart sounds are heard.

In rare instances there is progressive lengthening of the P-R interval; eventually one atrial impulse produces no ventricular contraction. This is essentially an electrocardiographic diagnosis and is known as the Wenckebach[6] phenomenon.

THIRD DEGREE HEART BLOCK (COMPLETE BLOCK).   In this condition none of the atrial impulses reach the ventricles. However, the A-V node or the bundle of His appears capable of initiating slow rhythmic impulses that result in ventricular contractions; this is known as *idioventricular rhythm* (Fig. 166). The ventricular rate is usually from 30 to 40 beats per minute, but occasionally it is slower or faster than this. There is complete dissociation of atrial and ventricular contractions; the atria continue to respond to the S-A pacemaker and contract at a more rapid rate.

The diagnosis can often be made clinically. The pulse is slow and regular and does not increase appreciably with exercise, deep breathing

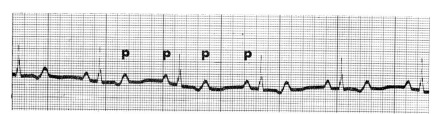

Fig. 165.   Second degree heart block, with 2:1 ventricular response. The atrial contractions (P) occur at regular intervals and at a rate of approximately 80 per minute; the ventricular rate is one-half as rapid (40 beats per minute).

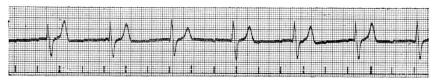

Fig. 166.   Complete heart block. The atria are contracting rapidly (about 144 beats per minute); the ventricular rate is slow (52). There is complete dissociation between the atrial and the ventricular contractions. Some of the atrial impulses are buried in the ventricular complexes (dotted lines).

[6] Karel Frederek Wenckebach, Dutch internist who later decided to live in Vienna, 1864–1940.

or other stimuli that would normally accelerate the rate. Inspection of
the jugular veins may show waves that are more rapid than the arterial
pulse. On auscultation faint sounds may be heard synchronous with the
jugular waves; occasionally a murmur will be heard. The most striking
finding is that, although the rhythm is regular, the intensity and quality
of the first sound usually change from beat to beat; this bears no relation
to the phases of respiration. If this is not obvious, it may be helpful to
have the patient breathe deeply or exercise a little; this will increase the
atrial rate but not the ventricular rate. With 2:1 heart block, which may
be confused with complete heart block, both the atrial and the ventricular rate will increase, but the first sounds will be unaltered. With complete block, the atrial rate might happen to be 80 while the ventricular
rate was 40; again the first sounds would seem similar. After exercise,
the atrial rate increases and the variations in ventricular filling make the
changes in the first heart sound obvious. The only exception to this would
be the presence of atrial fibrillation plus complete heart block. In this
situation, since the atria are not actually contracting, there would be no
change in the first heart sounds with or without exercise.

Etiology. In rare instances complete heart block is congenital;
usually it results from any one of a variety of diseases. It is often due to
coronary artery sclerosis, even without other signs of heart disease. It
also occurs with mitral stenosis or aortic stenosis, with hypertension, as
a complication of an acute infection such as rheumatic fever, diphtheria
or syphilis, or from scar tissue formation as a late sequel of such infections.

Symptoms. In some instances, when complete heart block develops it is permanent; this is not incompatible with life if the myocardium is relatively normal. In other cases partial block may suddenly
become complete, then revert to partial block or some other arrhythmia.
This sudden change from partial to complete block may be associated
with ventricular asystole that persists until the new center begins to
initiate impulses. Depending upon the duration of the cerebral ischemia
that occurs at such times, the patient may experience vertigo, syncope or
epileptiform seizures; such episodes constitute one form of the Adams-
Stokes syndrome. Similar symptoms may occur with other sudden
changes in rhythm, with asystole occurring during complete block, or
when the ventricular rate is extremely slow (12 to 15 beats per minute),
especially if the patient stands, walks or engages in other forms of activity. Implantation of a suitable electrical pacemaker may enable the
patient to resume a fairly normal life; it will supply the impulses to
initiate ventricular contractions at a predetermined rate.

Bundle Branch Block. In this conduction disturbance the impulse is delayed or blocked in either the right or the left branch of the
bundle of His. The impulse travels through the unaffected branch and

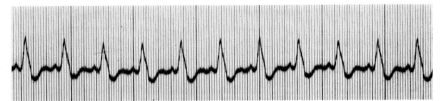

Fig. 167. Left bundle branch block. The impulse reaches the right ventricle in a normal manner but travels in a circuitous path to the left ventricle; the resulting QRS complex is wide and abnormal in appearance.

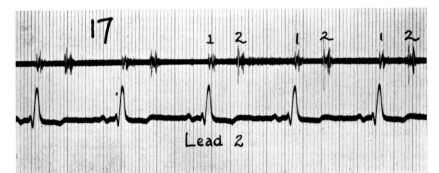

Fig. 168. Right bundle branch block. Both the first and second sounds are split, owing to asynchronous closure of the valves.

reaches the muscles of that ventricle in a normal manner; to reach the other ventricle it must travel a circuitous path and consequently it arrives later. Therefore the two ventricles do not contract simultaneously, and there will be splitting of the first heart sound, of the second sound, or of both sounds (Fig. 168). The variations in the degree of splitting produced by respiration have already been mentioned; although such findings are suggestive, the diagnosis cannot be established without an electrocardiogram.

Bundle branch block may develop as a result of any type of heart disease, but is most commonly found in patients with coronary atherosclerosis. Although it is usually an ominous sign under those conditions, it may occasionally be found—and persist for years—in persons who have no other demonstrable heart disease; more commonly these individuals have right bundle branch block.

MURMURS

A murmur is an abnormal or adventitious sound heard over the heart or a large artery. The more or less rhythmic vibrations are attributed to

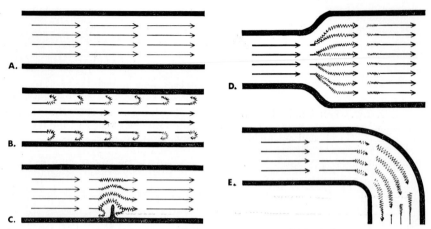

Fig. 169. Common causes of murmurs. *A,* Normal blood flow; no turbulence. No murmur heard on stethoscopic auscultation. *B,* Increased velocity of blood flow. Turbulence develops along the wall of the chamber. Tachycardia is often responsible for this; exercise may make a latent murmur audible, or increase the intensity of one already present. *C,* Obstruction. Most commonly this is a stenotic valve. It may also be due to a plaque or nodule in the heart or in the vessel wall, or to indentation produced by extrinsic pressure of any type. *D,* Sudden change in caliber, as with an aneurysm of the aorta or other large artery. Similarly, a murmur will be present if blood is flowing in the opposite direction—from a large vessel into a markedly smaller one. *E,* Sudden change in direction of blood flow. This is thought to be responsible for many of the murmurs so commonly heard in the pulmonic area, where blood entering the right pulmonary artery must change direction sharply.

turbulence or vortex in the blood stream, produced by some abnormality that disrupts the normal streamline flow. The most common mechanical factors are diagrammed in Figure 169. Various congenital or acquired diseases will produce changes in the heart or arteries that correspond to these sketches.

Valve leaflets that cannot open adequately constrict the blood stream at that point; this gives rise to turbulence and produces the murmur of *stenosis*. Leaflets that cannot close completely allow blood to escape through the opening in an abnormal direction; this produces the murmur of *regurgitation or insufficiency*. Obviously it is entirely possible to have a valve so damaged that it can neither open adequately nor close completely; two murmurs will then be produced at that site.

In addition, a murmur may result when there is tachycardia with increased velocity of blood flow, as with emotional stress, after exercise, with fever or with thyrotoxicosis. Decreased viscosity of the blood in severe anemia may also facilitate the production of turbulence, giving rise to the so-called *hemic* murmur, which disappears when the anemia is corrected. However, an increased rate of flow is also present with anemia; both factors probably play a part in the production of the murmur.

Position of Valve Leaflets.   At this point it seems appropriate to review the normal position of the valve leaflets in systole and in diastole and to mention the murmurs that may be produced by valvular abnormalities; other causes of cardiac murmurs will be considered later.

During ventricular systole the mitral and tricuspid valves should be completely closed. If either valve is damaged or cannot close completely for any other reason, valvular insufficiency is present. Blood will be forced back from the ventricle into the atrium, producing the systolic murmur of mitral (or tricuspid) insufficiency or regurgitation. At the same time, the aortic and pulmonic valves should be open. If they cannot open adequately a murmur will be produced; this is the murmur of aortic (or pulmonic) stenosis. These are all systolic in time.

During ventricular diastole the mitral and tricuspid valves should be open. If they are only partially open, turbulence results and a murmur indicative of mitral (or tricuspid) stenosis is produced. Also, the aortic and pulmonic valves should be closed; if not, a murmur of aortic (or pulmonic) insufficiency or regurgitation occurs. These are all diastolic in time.

During atrial systole the mitral and tricuspid valves should be open. If they cannot open adequately a presystolic murmur will be produced, provided the atria are contracting normally. This murmur is heard late in ventricular diastole, or just before the first heart sound.

Auscultation of Murmurs.   Whenever a murmur is heard you must determine and record certain important points including: (1) time in the cardiac cycle: systolic, diastolic or presystolic; (2) duration of the sound; (3) location of maximum intensity; (4) intensity, pitch and quality; (5) radiation and transmission; (6) effect of change of posture, respiration and exercise on the murmur.

TIMING OF MURMURS.   In rare instances there is a so-called continuous murmur heard throughout both systole and diastole, but in most cases a murmur occurs either during systole or during diastole. Therefore it is important to determine the relationship of the murmur to the first and second heart sounds. Many systolic murmurs are of little significance; a diastolic murmur almost invariably indicates severe organic heart disease.

A systolic murmur may start immediately after the first heart sound; it may accompany the first sound or it may begin with the first sound and entirely obscure it. Occasionally it will be heard in mid-systole only. Similarly, a diastolic murmur may follow, accompany or replace the second sound. It may be heard early in diastole, in mid-diastole only or it may not be heard until late in diastole. The latter is the presystolic murmur characteristic of mitral stenosis, which is not heard if the atria are not contracting normally.

DURATION.   The time of occurrence having been determined, the

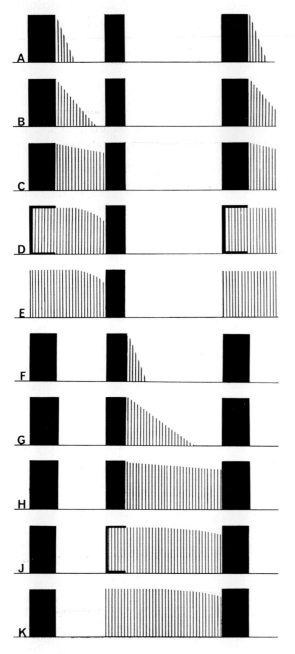

Fig. 170. Time and duration of murmurs. Systolic murmurs: *A,* Short systolic murmur following first heart sound; it is often of low intensity and difficult to hear. *B,* Systolic murmur following first sound and gradually fading before the second sound. *C,* Systolic murmur following the first sound and heard throughout systole. *D,* Systolic murmur beginning at the same time as the faintly audible first sound. *E,* Systolic murmur completely replacing the first sound and extending throughout systole.

Diastolic murmurs: *F,* Short diastolic murmur following second sound. Depending upon the location of the murmur, it may be the first auscultatory evidence of mitral stenosis or of aortic insufficiency. *G,* Diastolic murmur following the second sound which gradually fades before the next first heart sound. *H,* Diastolic murmur following the second sound and heard throughout diastole. *J,* Diastolic murmur beginning at the same time as the faintly audible second sound. *K,* Diastolic murmur completely replacing the second heart sound.

duration should be noted. A systolic murmur may end shortly after the first sound or it may persist throughout systole. The same is true of diastolic murmurs.

LOCATION.   The probable site of production of the murmur should then be determined. Most heart murmurs are due to valvular abnormalities; any such murmur is usually loudest over one valve area. If the murmur is relatively faint it may be heard only at that point; if more intense, it may be audible at some distance from the valve. A very loud murmur may be heard over the entire thorax and even over adjacent areas. Even in most of these cases it is usually possible to determine which valve is responsible; the murmur will be loudest at one of the four valve areas.

INTENSITY.   The intensity of a murmur depends upon the amplitude of the vibrations produced, but loudness is a subjective phenomenon and depends upon the observer's interpretation of the vibrations that reach his ears. Although these two terms are often used interchangeably, the physical principles should be remembered. Anything interposed between the site of production of a murmur and the tympanic membrane will alter the loudness; so will the auditory acuity and the subjective interpretation of the examiner. A fairly intense murmur may be heard only faintly after the vibrations have been damped by a heavy layer of fat or muscle. An experienced examiner will correctly interpret that faint sound which the beginner has missed completely.

A murmur may be so faint that it is barely audible; it may be so intense that a stethoscope is not needed. Quantitative measurements of the vibrations can be carried out experimentally but are not applicable in clinical practice. However, it is necessary to have some method whereby the examiner can record the relative intensity of the murmur, and at present many physicians use the "Grade" system. A Grade I murmur is one that is barely audible under ideal conditions for auscultation; it will usually be missed on a ward, in a noisy examining room or by the novice; a Grade II murmur is usually the faintest that is heard under such conditions. Grade III and IV murmurs are progressively louder, and Grade V is very intense. A Grade VI murmur is one that is still audible even when the stethoscope is lifted a short distance from the chest wall. In some cases, murmurs of Grade I and II may be unimportant; those of Grade III intensity or more are seldom heard in the absence of heart disease. With experience the examiner will find that this system is very helpful and relatively accurate.

PITCH.   The pitch of a murmur depends upon the frequency of vibrations. The human ear can perceive vibrations ranging from 16 or 32 cycles per second (c.p.s.) to about 16,000 c.p.s. A murmur is considered of low pitch if the vibrations range from about 30 to 80 c.p.s., of medium pitch in the range of 80 to 120 c.p.s. and high-pitched if the vibrations range upward to 700 or 800 c.p.s. or higher.

The absolute pitch of a murmur is of some diagnostic significance, but a more important point is that this fundamental pitch does not change as the stethoscope is moved from one area to another. The murmur may "sound" somewhat different because of changes in the relative intensity of the fundamental note and the various overtones, but the pitch cannot change. This is especially important in deciding whether you hear one murmur or two. For example, you hear a systolic murmur at the mitral area. As you move your stethoscope upward over the precordium the murmur becomes fainter, but then seems to increase in intensity over the aortic area. Is there one murmur, or two? Listen briefly at one area, concentrating only on the pitch of the murmur; then move the stethoscope quickly to the other area. Repeat this several times if necessary. If the pitch is not the same at the two areas, it cannot be one murmur; there must be two murmurs. If the pitch remains constant it almost certainly is the same murmur; the possibility of there being two murmurs of exactly the same pitch is very remote.

Apparent contradictions to this statement are the crescendo and decrescendo murmurs. In the former, the murmur initially is of low intensity and low pitch, but both of these increase rapidly; the typical example is the presystolic murmur, which may occur with mitral stenosis. A decrescendo murmur is just the opposite; it is heard most commonly early in diastole in a patient with mitral stenosis or slight aortic regurgitation. The variation in intensity is easily explained. With the crescendo murmur, the velocity of blood flow increases as the atrium contracts, and greater turbulence results. The decrescendo murmur starts when the pressure differential is high; this rapidly decreases as the pressure in the atrium or the aorta falls. The variation in pitch is more difficult to explain; it is probably related to changes in size of the resonating chamber (atrium or ventricle) associated with contraction or relaxation.

QUALITY.   The quality of a murmur depends upon the fundamental note plus overtones and other vibrations. The description of the resulting sound seems to depend upon the background or the imagination of the examiner. A partial listing would include such terms as blowing, harsh, musical, piping, rasping, roaring, rumbling, sawing, screeching, squeaking, whistling or "like the cry of a sea gull"; take your choice.

RADIATION AND TRANSMISSION.   When a murmur is produced at any given point the vibrations tend to radiate in all directions from that point. They should also decrease in intensity inversely as the square of the distance increases. A Grade II mitral murmur will be heard easily over the mitral area, but will be faint or inaudible at the aortic area.

However, certain murmurs do not seem to follow these principles of physics. An aortic systolic murmur will often be heard distinctly over the carotid artery at a point 10 cm. or more from the aortic valve site, yet it may be entirely inaudible in the second right intercostal space an equal distance away. It has long been taught that the murmur was "transmitted" by the blood, and in the direction of blood flow—to the carotid arteries in the example given. That failed to explain one well-established observation. In mitral insufficiency blood is flowing from the ventricle back into the atrium—from left to right—yet the murmur is "transmitted" in the opposite direction to the apex or axillary region. Recent studies suggest that the sounds are transmitted to a considerable degree by bone and other solid tissues, as well as by the blood stream.

CHANGE OF POSITION.   Cardiac murmurs frequently change in character and especially in intensity when the person changes position. A Grade II murmur heard when he is sitting or standing may disappear if he lies down; the reverse is also true. The faint diastolic murmur of aortic regurgitation may be heard only when the patient leans far forward. The presystolic murmur of mitral stenosis may be inaudible unless the patient exercises or lies on his left side, or does both.

CHANGES WITH RESPIRATION.   In full inspiration the inflated lung may partially cover the heart and decrease or abolish a murmur that is faintly heard in expiration. Changes may also be due to the relative position of the heart as it swings upward and outward when the left dome of the diaphragm rises with expiration. A pulmonic systolic mur-

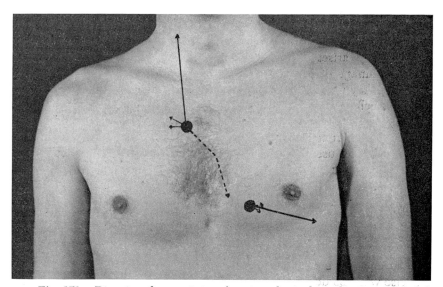

Fig. 171.   Direction of transmission of aortic and mitral systolic murmurs (solid lines) and diastolic murmurs (dotted lines).

mur often shows marked variation with respiration; this may depend
to some extent upon the changes in shape of the easily compressed
pulmonary artery. The alterations in cardiac filling must also be considered.

VALSALVA[7] MANEUVER.   This is sometimes helpful in determining
whether a murmur is produced in the right side of the heart or the left,
especially when it is heard at the base of the heart. Have the patient
take a deep breath, close his glottis and then attempt to exhale (strain).
This increases the intrathoracic pressure, interferes with the return of
blood to the right side of the heart and decreases the amount of blood in
the lungs. After several seconds have him resume breathing. If the
murmur is arising in the right side it will reappear or be increased after
one or two beats. Since the blood must refill and then pass through the
pulmonary vascular bed before reaching the left side, a murmur arising
at the mitral or aortic area will not be altered until several cardiac
cycles have occurred.

Exercise will accelerate the heart rate and increase the velocity of
blood flow in most instances; a murmur may become audible or definitely louder after physical exertion. With myocardial failure, the opposite effect may be observed; exercise may lesson the intensity of the
murmur.

INTERPRETATION OF MURMURS

The characteristics of a murmur having been ascertained, the next
question that arises is the significance of the findings. Does this imply
organic damage of the valve? Is it due to other changes in the heart?
If so, are they temporary or permanent? Or is it due to some physiologic
disturbance? Various classifications have been proposed, but none seems
entirely satisfactory. Some authors prefer such terms as "organic,"
"relative" and "functional"; others have proposed that "physiologic" and
"pathologic" be used instead. Some use "insufficiency" to indicate murmurs due to actual damage of the valve leaflets; "incompetence" is used
for other changes such as dilatation of the valve ring without structural
changes in the leaflets.

If a diastolic murmur is heard, organic heart disease is almost certainly present. Proper interpretation of a systolic murmur is much more
difficult. As mentioned before, various diseases that increase the cardiac
rate or accelerate the flow of blood may produce murmurs. Strenuous
exercise will also do this in a healthy person; the increased stroke volume
undoubtedly plays a part here. In children a murmur along the left

[7] Antonio Maria Valsalva, Italian anatomist, 1666–1723.

sternal border or in the pulmonic valve area is a fairly common finding; it may be due to turbulence as the blood stream suddenly changes its course, especially that going to the right lung. Systolic murmurs also appear during pregnancy and disappear after delivery. As a rule, these so-called "functional" murmurs are relatively short; they do not extend throughout systole. They are usually of Grade I or Grade II intensity, and tend to become fainter with inspiration. Occasionally, however, the murmur is heard only during inspiration; this is called a cardiorespiratory murmur. Sometimes a sound misinterpreted as a murmur appears to be due to the rate of movement of air in lung tissue as it is alternately compressed and expanded by changes in the cardiac volume (cog-wheel breathing, p. 196).

The most important point is that the significance of many murmurs cannot be determined without taking into consideration the history and the entire physical examination; very often a prolonged period of observation is also needed before a final decision can be made. For example, a faint mitral systolic murmur is heard (Grade II). This may be functional, but many organic causes must also be considered. A partial list would include such conditions as a minor congenital lesion, the presence of Aschoff[8] nodules on the valve leaflets, scarring due to healed rheumatic involvement, vegetations of bacterial endocarditis, dilatation of the mitral ring from long-standing hypertension with increased intraventricular pressure, and dilatation of the left ventricle, which would pull the chordae and valve edges downward, thus preventing complete closure. If the patient is a child with fever and swollen, painful joints, acute rheumatic endocarditis is probably producing the murmur. If such a murmur is found in an adult who has had fever without any obvious cause, if the murmur changes over a period of days, and if petechial hemorrhages are present, bacterial endocarditis is the most probable explanation. If the patient is elderly, hypertensive, dyspneic and edematous, dilatation of the ventricle or of the mitral ring might be the most appropriate diagnosis.

PERICARDIAL FRICTION RUB

A pericardial friction rub often resembles a pleural friction, but typically it is heard both in systole and in diastole, and is not influenced by respiration. Usually the sound does not extend entirely through either phase of the cardiac cycle, and occasionally it is audible in one phase only. Changes of posture often alter the intensity; generally the rub seems louder when the patient sits up. Increased pressure with the chest

[8] Ludwig Aschoff, German pathologist, 1866–1942.

piece of the stethoscope may also increase the intensity of the sounds. Although the rub may be audible over a very wide area, it is more common to find it localized to one small spot; the sounds are poorly transmitted to other areas.

When both the pleura and the pericardium are involved it may be more difficult to differentiate the two friction rubs. Having the patient hold his breath for a few seconds will eliminate the pleural rub; the pericardial friction sound will not be altered.

TO HERE

XV

Diseases of the

Cardiovascular System

Final

In recording the diagnosis of cardiovascular disease, the etiology is the first item; actually this represents the final conclusion based upon a careful history and complete examination. Even then the exact etiology may be in doubt. The most common causes are congenital anomalies, rheumatic fever, syphilis, hypertension and arteriosclerosis or atherosclerosis. Other less common causes include acute or chronic infection, thyroid dysfunction, trauma, toxins of various types, neoplasms and certain rare diseases. Some of the more common conditions will now be considered.

CIRCULATORY FAILURE

It is important to remember the pathologic changes produced by various diseases and the altered function that results from these. The symptoms will depend upon the specific lesions present and the amount of myocardial reserve. When the heart can no longer meet the strain and maintain adequate circulation, cardiac decompensation or failure results; this may develop slowly or rapidly.

Left-sided Failure. This is due to weakness of the left ventricle. It can follow trauma or infection; it may also result from myocardial ischemia due to narrowing of one or more of the coronary arteries. Very commonly it is the end result of the prolonged strain and extra work load imposed by conditions such as hypertension or valvular heart disease. Initially there is myocardial hypertrophy, which enables the heart to maintain adequate circulation, but eventually the heart begins to dilate. The person has dyspnea or other symptoms with less and less

269

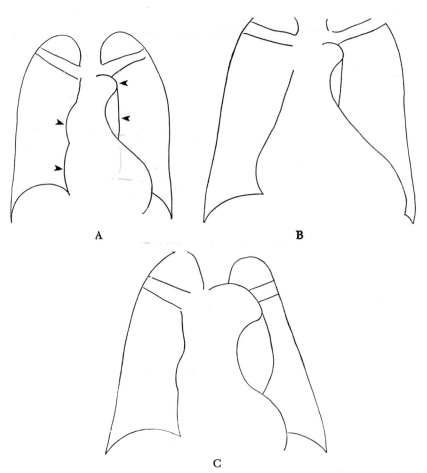

Fig. 172. *A,* Hypertension, anteroposterior view, without great increase in the total diameter of the heart. The left ventricle is concentrically hypertrophied; this is indicated by the long, prominent and somewhat bulging left ventricular salient. The ascending aorta is convex outward and extends as far to the right as the right atrial shadow. The knob is prominent and highly placed, indicating elongation of the aorta. The descending aorta is well visualized, indicating increased density.

B, Hypertension with dilatation, anteroposterior view. The left ventricular salient is long, but is not bulging. The right atrial shadow also extends to the right farther than normal. At the time this diagram was made the right ventricle had failed, as well as the left ventricle. The lungs were greatly congested.

C, Hypertension with dynamic distortion of the aorta, anteroposterior view. The aortic shadow is much exaggerated. At necropsy the aorta was not widened. The only gross change was moderate elongation. (Courtesy of Dr. T. M. McMillan.)

exertion; finally he is uncomfortable even at rest. Occasionally the onset is more sudden; this may follow physical strain of some sort.

Pulmonary congestion, severe dyspnea, tachypnea, pulmonary edema and pleural effusion are the most alarming symptoms. Cyanosis is commonly present. If pulmonary edema develops rapidly the patient may have rales, rhonchi and wheezing; the auscultatory findings are somewhat

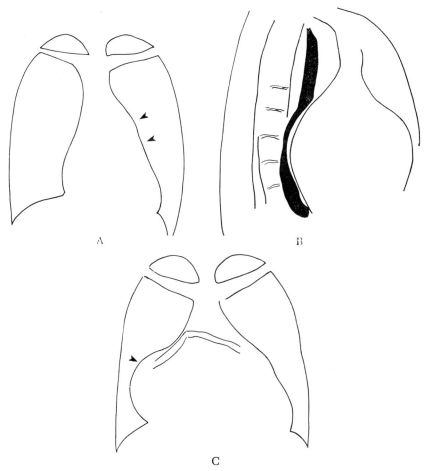

A   B

C

Fig. 173.   *A*, Mitral stenosis, anteroposterior view. There is unusual prominence in the conus region and the pulmonary artery salient. This has caused a disappearance of the waist with straightening of the left border. Note that the left ventricular salient is not abnormally prominent.

B, Mitral stenosis, right anterior oblique view, to show backward displacement of the barium-filled esophagus by the enlarged left atrium.

C, Mitral stenosis with left atrial aneurysm, anteroposterior view. There is great prominence along the left border in the region of the conus and pulmonary artery. The right side extends almost to the ribs. This great enlargement was the result of an enormous left atrium, which extended beyond the right atrium. Observe the upward displacement of the left main stem bronchus. (Courtesy of Dr. T. M. McMillan.)

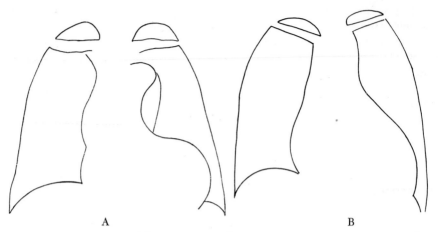

Fig. 174. *A,* Syphilitic aortic insufficiency, anteroposterior view. The left ventricular salient extends outward from the waist almost horizontally; this produces the characteristic "boot-shaped" appearance. The aorta shows some widening. (Courtesy of Dr. T. M. McMillan.)

B, Rheumatic aortic insufficiency, anteroposterior view. The left ventricle is enlarged, but the silhouette is not boot-shaped. The waist is fairly well preserved. The aorta does not appear to be diseased as in the syphilitic variety. (Courtesy of Dr. T. M. McMillan.)

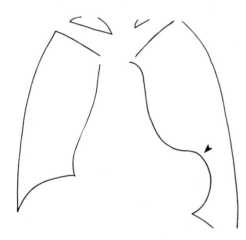

Fig. 175. Left ventricular aneurysm, anteroposterior view. There is a striking and bizarre bulge in the left ventricular wall. Fluoroscopically, no pulsations could be seen over this area. The patient showed electrocardiographic findings and had a history characteristic of an acute coronary occlusion several years before this diagram was made. (Courtesy of Dr. T. M. McMillan.)

like those of asthma (p. 206). The term "cardiac asthma" is sometimes incorrectly applied; this should be called acute pulmonary edema. Since these attacks frequently occur at night or while the patient is asleep, they are also referred to as paroxysmal nocturnal dyspnea.

Right-sided Failure. This may be secondary and due to the strain imposed by the elevated pressure in the pulmonary circulation that occurs with left-sided heart failure. It may also be primary, due to abnormalities of the pulmonary vascular bed such as those that develop with primary pulmonary hypertension, with pulmonary arteriosclerosis or with chronic lung disease such as emphysema. In the secondary type there are changes in both ventricles. In the primary type it is the right ventricle that hypertrophies, dilates and fails; this type is often called *cor pulmonale*.

With right heart failure the congestive phenomena are peripheral. The veins are distended; the liver is enlarged; fluid collects in the peritoneal cavity (ascites) and the tissues become edematous, especially in the dependent areas.

VALVULAR HEART DISEASE

The signs that accompany organic disease of the individual valves will now be described. It should be remembered that more than one type of deformity may be present, or that more than one valve may be involved. This in turn will produce additional or opposing changes and alter the physical signs.

Mitral Insufficiency (Mitral Regurgitation). If the mitral leaflets are unable to occlude the valve orifice completely during ventricular systole, blood will be forced back (regurgitate) through this incompetent valve into the atrium; a systolic murmur will be produced. Many conditions can give rise to a slight degree of valvular incompetence, with a Grade I or II systolic murmur, but when a murmur classified as Grade III or louder is present, it will usually be found that the valve has been damaged by rheumatic fever. At autopsy, the margins of such leaflets are distorted by scar tissue, making accurate apposition impossible. The chordae may be shortened, deflecting the valve margins downward.

To maintain adequate circulation despite the leak, the left ventricle must increase in size, contract more frequently, or do both. Depending upon the amount of regurgitation and the duration of the disease, the left ventricle will show a variable amount of hypertrophy. The apical impulse is seen to be displaced outward, and sometimes downward into the sixth intercostal space. On palpation the impulse usually seems more forceful than normal, although with decompensation it may be feeble. The area of cardiac dullness is increased. A systolic murmur is present, heard best near the mitral valve area or at the apex, and transmitted downward and outward toward the axillary region. If very loud, the murmur may be heard over the entire precordial area or over other parts of the thorax, anteriorly or posteriorly. If the amount of regurgitated blood is sufficient to produce congestion in the pulmonary vessels,

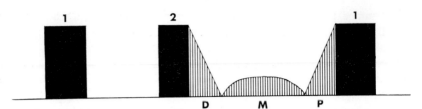

Fig. 176.   Murmurs that may be present with mitral stenosis: D, early diastolic; M, mid-diastolic; P, presystolic.

this may give rise to accentuation of the pulmonic second sound or variations in the splitting of the second sound.

Mitral Stenosis.   Almost invariably this is a late complication of rheumatic fever. The valve leaflets are fused together near the mitral ring; therefore only the central portion can open during diastole. This obstruction gives rise to turbulence and a murmur results. Since the left atrium cannot empty completely, it gradually enlarges and the pressure within it rises. This in turn leads to elevation of pressure in the pulmonary vascular bed.

On inspection, one may see flushing of the malar regions. Mitral stenosis is more common in women than in men, but this malar flush persists even after all cosmetics have been removed. On palpation, the apical impulse will not be displaced with mitral stenosis alone, but other valvular lesions are often present and can produce alterations in the size and shape of the heart. A presystolic sound ending with a sharp thrust or shock, usually localized and felt near the apex, is sometimes palpable; this is sufficient to establish the diagnosis. Changes in the cardiac contour are not easily demonstrable by percussion, but are often conspicuous on x-ray films. The pulmonary outflow tract is enlarged; the left border of the heart becomes straight or bulges outward. On auscultation three alterations of sounds may be heard. Since the left ventricle is incompletely filled, the mitral first sound will be accentuated. Elevated pressure in the pulmonary vascular bed will give rise to an accentuated pulmonic second sound. A diastolic murmur is usually heard over the mitral area. In the early stages of stenosis, this may be a low-pitched decrescendo murmur audible only in early diastole, when the overfilled atrium begins to empty. As the diastolic pressure differential decreases, the murmur fades and disappears. In other patients there may be a low-pitched rumbling mid-diastolic sound only. With more advanced disease, with a higher degree of stenosis or with greater atrial enlargement, the murmur is more prolonged and may extend through much or all of diastole. The classic murmur, which is considered diagnostic of mitral stenosis, is rumbling in character, crescendo in intensity and pitch, and presystolic in time. It is synchronous with, and usually attributed to, contraction of the atrium forcing blood through the stenotic valve orifice. This murmur may be inaudible when the patient is erect; having him exercise and then lie on his left side will often bring it out. If atrial fibrillation develops, there are no rhythmic contractions of the atria and this murmur disappears, but the early diastolic or mid-diastolic murmur will persist. Another auscultatory finding considered diagnostic of mitral stenosis is the opening snap (p. 244).

In addition to the low-pitched rumble, another higher-pitched diastolic murmur is occasionally heard near the left border of the sternum. This is known as the Graham Steell[1] murmur; it is believed to be due to incompetence of the pulmonic valve resulting from the high pressure in the pulmonary circulation. It must be differentiated from a diastolic murmur due to disease of the aortic valve.

Occasionally the left atrium becomes so large that it extends upward far enough to press upon the left recurrent laryngeal nerve; hoarseness due to paralysis of the left vocal cord will develop.

Mitral Stenosis and Insufficiency. Very often a mitral valve that has been damaged by rheumatic fever will become both stenotic and incompetent; it can neither open nor close completely. In such cases

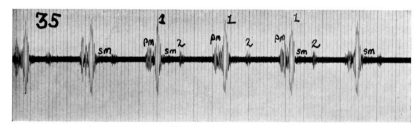

Fig. 177. Mitral stenosis with slight regurgitation. Presystolic murmur (*pm*), faint systolic murmur (*sm*) and accentuated first sound (1).

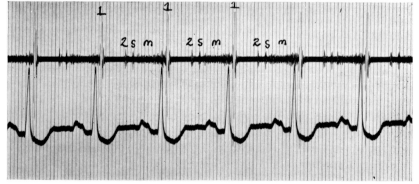

Fig. 178. Mitral stenosis. Opening snap (*s*) following second heart sound (2); diastolic murmur (*m*) with presystolic crescendo accentuation. Note loud first sound (1). No systolic murmur present.

[1] Graham Steell, English physician, 1851–1942.

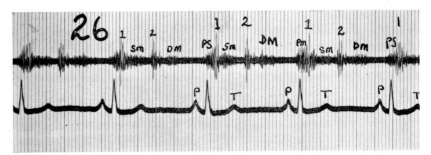

Fig. 179. Mitral stenosis and regurgitation. Presystolic (*ps*), systolic (*sm*) and diastolic (*dm*) murmurs.

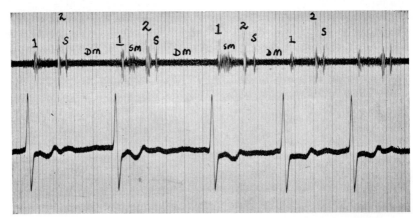

Fig. 180. Mitral stenosis and insufficiency; atrial fibrillation. Systolic murmur (*sm*); opening snap (*s*) shortly after the second sound (2); faint diastolic murmur (*dm*) without presystolic accentuation (atria fibrillating).

there will be a combination of the signs described above. In fact, it is uncommon to find a heart that has "pure" mitral stenosis or "pure" insufficiency, but often one of these lesions is much more severe than the other. The left atrium, a relatively weak muscle, has to bear the burden in stenosis; it is primarily the left ventricle that is affected by insufficiency. Determination of the relative severity of these two processes is often important if surgical intervention is contemplated. When valvulotomy is performed it decreases stenosis but increases the amount of regurgitation, thus shifting some of the strain from the atrium to the ventricle. If a marked degree of ventricular strain and insufficiency is already present, the end result of the operation would be poor.

Aortic Insufficiency (Aortic Regurgitation). The aortic valve leaflets are unable to occlude the orifice completely during diastole and blood regurgitates into the left ventricle, producing a diastolic murmur. The most common causes are rheumatic fever, syphilis and hypertensive heart disease with or without arteriosclerosis. With rheumatic valvulitis the leaflets are scarred and distorted; stenosis may also be present. With syphilis there is dilatation of the ring and separation of the commissures; the leaflets themselves show little abnormality. Hypertension presumably produces dilatation of the aortic ring; the murmur may become much fainter if the blood pressure is reduced.

Aortic insufficiency due to rheumatic fever usually develops in childhood or adolescence; it is often accompanied by other valvular lesions, especially of the mitral valve. When insufficiency is due to syphilis it tends to become apparent long after the primary infection, usually after the age of 40. Other valves are not involved and stenosis practically never occurs.

The physical signs will depend largely upon the degree of insufficiency and the amount of blood that regurgitates during diastole. In the early stage only a very faint diastolic murmur may be heard. As the disease progresses other signs appear; eventually the diagnosis becomes relatively easy. The findings that might be expected with a moderately severe lesion will be considered.

Blood pressure determination (p. 57) and palpation of the pulse (p. 49) have already supplied clues. The systolic pressure is elevated and the diastolic pressure is low; in some instances the sounds persist after all pressure in the cuff has been released. This wide pulse pressure is strongly suggestive of aortic regurgitation, although it may be found with other diseases.

Inspection can be extremely helpful. The face appears pale even when there is no anemia; this is in contrast to the malar flush of mitral stenosis. The peripheral arteries exhibit strong pulsations; the throbbing carotids may cause the head to jerk with each heartbeat (de Musset's[2] sign). Even the bed may vibrate if the patient is recumbent; this was the inspiration for Starr's[3] original ballistocardiograph. A capillary pulse (Quincke's[4] pulse) may be present; this is elicited by grasping the end of the finger (or toe) and depressing the nail slightly. Alternate filling and emptying of the arterioles and capillaries will cause the nail bed to flush in systole and blanch in diastole. A pocket flashlight held under the fingertip often accentuates this. The pulsation can also be demonstrated at the mucocutaneous junction of the everted lip by pressing a glass slide against it, or on the forehead by rubbing vigorously to produce a narrow band of hyperemia, which then flushes and blanches with systole and diastole.

Since the heart is enlarged, particularly the left ventricle, the apex beat is displaced downward and to the left. Forceful or heaving pulsa-

[2] Louis Charles Alfred de Musset, French poet, 1810–57. He died of heart disease, presumably luetic aortic insufficiency. He was aware of this "jerk" which was accurately described in a biography written by his brother Paul, who was not a physician.

[3] Isaac Starr, Philadelphia physician, 1895– .

[4] Heinrich Irenaeus Quincke, German neurologist, 1842–1922.

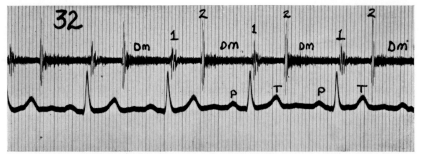

Fig. 181. Aortic insufficiency. The second sound (2) is followed by a long decrescendo diastolic murmur (*dm*).

tions may be seen as low as the seventh intercostal space; *cor bovinum* (ox heart) is a term frequently applied to such a huge heart. The precordium may bulge outward if the disease began in childhood, while the ribs were still relatively pliable.

Palpation verifies the site and character of the cardiac impulse. At times a diastolic thrill may be felt over the aortic area or in the third or fourth left intercostal space. One of the most dramatic signs of aortic insufficiency is the collapsing, water-hammer or Corrigan pulse; this has already been described (p. 49).

Percussion confirms the cardiac enlargement; there may also be some widening of the area of supracardiac dullness to the right of the sternum produced by dynamic dilatation of the aorta.

Auscultation adds the final bit of evidence. A diastolic murmur will be heard, either over the aortic valve area or in the third or fourth left intercostal space near the sternum; occasionally it is best heard to the right of the sternum. With minimal involvement of the valve the murmur may be soft, blowing and short, and heard only when the patient leans far forward. As the disease progresses it increases in intensity and duration. The first heart sound is usually decreased in intensity because of overfilling of the ventricle. The second sound may be audible; generally it is replaced or obliterated by the murmur.

A mitral systolic murmur will develop if there is significant enlargement of the left ventricle with stretching of the mitral ring or displacement of the papillary muscles and chordae downward, thus producing relative mitral insufficiency. An Austin Flint[5] murmur is sometimes heard at the apex. This is a late diastolic or presystolic murmur that is liable to be misinterpreted as the presystolic murmur of mitral stenosis. In his original description Flint stressed the fact that this murmur was heard in patients who subsequently died and showed no changes in the mitral valve. There are various explanations for this murmur. One that is widely accepted at the present time is that it is due largely to regurgi-

[5] Austin Flint, American physician, 1812–86.

tating blood striking the anterior leaflet of the mitral valve and displacing it, thus partially closing the valve and producing a relative obstruction to the flow from the left atrium into the ventricle.

Auscultatory findings are sometimes present over the peripheral vessels of a patient with aortic regurgitation or with a high pulse pressure from other causes. Sudden distention of a large artery such as a femoral produces a sharp snap known as Traube's[6] pistol shot sound. Firm pressure with the stethoscope at this point may produce a double murmur (systolic and diastolic) known as Duroziez's[7] murmur.

Aortic Stenosis. If the aortic valve leaflet cannot open completely, or if the aortic ring is narrowed, a systolic murmur will be produced. When stenosis of the aortic valve develops in a young person, almost without exception it is due to rheumatic fever. In elderly persons calcific deposits in the ring and at the base of the leaflets may be present; this led to the belief that arteriosclerosis was the etiologic factor. It now seems generally agreed that in the majority of these cases rheumatic valvulitis was the primary disease and that this led to deposition of calcium; arteriosclerosis is probably much less commonly the cause.

Inspection may show displacement of the cardiac impulse, but often no impulse at all can be seen. The carotid artery pulsations are also inconspicuous, in contrast to the bounding vessels seen with aortic regurgitation.

Palpation can practically establish the diagnosis if a systolic thrill is felt and is of maximum intensity over the aortic valve area; this may be faintly palpable over a wide area. Absence of a thrill does not invalidate the diagnosis, since the turbulence in the blood stream may not be of sufficient magnitude to produce palpable vibrations in the tissues of the thorax even though a murmur is present.

Percussion may show a heart of normal size; occasionally there is some enlargement of the left ventricle.

Auscultation is the most rewarding procedure. A rough systolic murmur is heard, usually of maximum intensity over the aortic valve area but occasionally loudest at the apex. Generally the murmur tends to become fainter as the stethoscope is moved toward the apex or xiphoid process, but it is often easily heard in a carotid, subclavian or even a brachial artery.

This murmur is often called "diamond-shaped." It begins shortly after the first sound, increases in intensity during the first half (or more) of systole, then rapidly fades away, as shown in Figure 182. This characteristic may be helpful in differentiating it from the systolic murmur of mitral regurgitation, especially when either one is heard best at some area other than the expected one.

[6] Ludwig Traube, German physician, 1818–76.
[7] Paul Louis Duroziez, French physician, 1826–97.

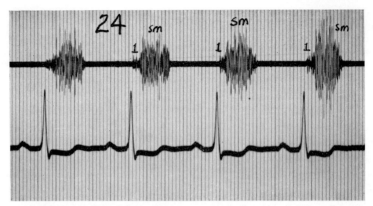

Fig. 182.   Aortic stenosis (calcareous). Faint first sound (1) and loud, coarse systolic murmur with characteristic so-called "diamond" configuration (sm). The second sound is obscured by the murmur.

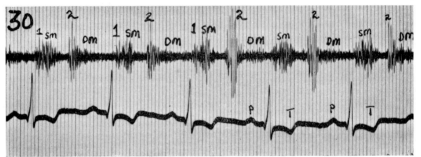

Fig. 183.   Aortic stenosis and regurgitation. Loud systolic murmur (sm) and decrescendo diastolic murmur (dm).

The second heart sound at the aortic area is usually decreased or inaudible; a normal pulmonic second sound is present.

Tricuspid Insufficiency (Tricuspid Regurgitation).   Organic disease producing insufficiency of the tricuspid leaflets is relatively rare; rheumatic fever and bacterial endocarditis are the two most common causes. Relative or functional insufficiency develops when there is dilatation of the right ventricle; although the leaflets are not altered, they are unable to occlude the valve orifice completely. This is found most frequently in patients with severe mitral stenosis or other diseases that produce elevation of the blood pressure in the pulmonary circulation; this leads to right ventricular strain and eventually to right-sided failure. Blood then regurgitates into the right atrium and obstructs the normal emptying of the venae cavae. Venous stasis produces engorgement of the peripheral veins, especially those of the head and neck, edema of the extremities and effusion into serous cavities, especially the peritoneal cavity (ascites). The liver becomes large and tender, and may expand

and contract synchronously with the heart beat; this late systolic pulsation must be differentiated from a nonexpansile pulsation transmitted from the underlying abdominal aorta.

On inspection, cyanosis is usually obvious. The venous distention is easily seen; pulsations may be observed in the jugular veins if they are not too tensely distended. Enlargement or even pulsation in the hepatic region may be visible.

On palpation, a systolic thrill is occasionally felt in the tricuspid valve area. A slight amount of pressure applied to the distended liver may be followed by a definite pulsation in the jugular veins (*hepatojugular reflux*). However, it may be difficult to differentiate this from the pulsations already present, and brute force can produce a reflux even in the absence of tricuspid valve disease.

On percussion, enlargement of the heart can be demonstrated, both to the left and especially to the right of the sternum.

A systolic murmur of maximum intensity over the lower part of the sternum is present. This may be transmitted to the apex, and is easily misinterpreted as a mitral systolic murmur. The pulmonic second sound is not accentuated.

The diagnosis of tricuspid insufficiency often depends more upon the collateral signs of right-sided failure than upon auscultation.

Tricuspid Stenosis. This exceedingly rare lesion is usually accompanied by mitral stenosis. Signs of right-sided failure are apparent but are not diagnostic. A presystolic impulse may be seen or felt in the distended jugular veins; it can be timed by simultaneous palpation of the aortic or carotid pulsation. A presystolic thrill may be felt over the sternum or in the right third or fourth intercostal space. There is enlargement of the right side of the heart, especially of the right atrium. The first sound is accentuated at the tricuspid area. A diastolic murmur is present and a presystolic murmur may be heard if fibrillation has not developed. These murmurs resemble those heard with mitral stenosis, but they are heard best over the lower part of the sternum and to the right of the midline.

Pulmonary Insufficiency (Pulmonary Regurgitation). Insufficiency due to organic disease of the valve is rare. Relative insufficiency may develop as a result of prolonged elevation of pressure in the pulmonary artery produced by mitral stenosis or by some chronic lung disease such as emphysema. The presence of a diastolic murmur heard over the valve area is suggestive of the diagnosis; when associated with mitral stenosis it is called a Graham Steell murmur.

Pulmonary Stenosis. Although a systolic murmur at the pulmonic area is a very common finding, in most cases this is a functional murmur. Pulmonary stenosis is a rare lesion, and almost invariably it is congenital. The pulmonic second sound will be faint or inaudible.

CONGENITAL HEART DISEASE

Although congenital anomalies of the cardiovascular system are not common, a number of types can be cured and others can be benefited by appropriate surgical procedures. The exact diagnosis often requires angiography, cardiac catheterization and other special studies, but certain physical signs may be very suggestive in some types. A few of these abnormalities will be discussed.

Septal Defects

Atrial Septal Defect. In this anomaly the blood is shunted from the left atrium to the right; therefore cyanosis is absent early in the disease. The added volume of blood leads to enlargement of the right atrium and ventricle and of the pulmonary artery and its branches. This excessive load may eventually lead to reversal of blood flow and a variable degree of cyanosis. The left atrium and ventricle are unaffected until late in the disease.

On auscultation, a moderately loud systolic murmur is heard, usually maximum over the pulmonic area; this rarely extends through systole. A short diastolic murmur may be present if dynamic insufficiency of the pulmonary valve has developed. Wide splitting of the second sound results from slower emptying of the overfilled right ventricle.

Variations are not uncommon. If the defect is low in the septum (*ostium primum* type) the atrioventricular valves may also be deformed, leading to additional auscultatory signs and circulatory disturbances. Pulmonary hypertension or pulmonary stenosis may also be associated with atrial septal defects. These will alter the heart sounds or produce additional murmurs.

Patent Foramen Ovale. In the fetus, there is a valve-like communication that permits blood to flow from the right atrium to the left, thus bypassing the unaerated lungs; at birth this closes. However, excessive pressure in the right atrium may reopen this communication and permit blood to be shunted from the right atrium into the left. It can also allow an embolus originating in a peripheral vein or in the right atrium to pass directly into the systemic circulation (*paradoxical embolism*). Occasionally both atria become enlarged; the septum will be stretched and the foramen may be reopened. The findings will then resemble those in other types of atrial septal defects.

Lutembacher's[8] Syndrome. This eponym means that there is an atrial septal defect plus congenital or acquired mitral stenosis; this combination is exceedingly rare, and many question its existence.

[8] René Lutembacher, French physician, 1884– .

Ventricular Septal Defect (Roger's[9] Disease).   The usual site for this communication is in the upper membranous portion of the interventricular septum. Since the shunt is from left to right, cyanosis is absent in uncomplicated cases, but this may change if other abnormalities are present.

The significant auscultatory finding is a loud systolic murmur of maximum intensity along the left sternal border. It extends throughout systole and may be accompanied by a thrill and by splitting of the second sound. If found in a very young child, such a murmur should suggest the possibility of septal defect. This murmur is easily confused with the systolic murmur of mitral insufficiency or of aortic stenosis. A history of rheumatic fever, followed by the development of a murmur, would be more suggestive of valvular disease.

Tetralogy of Fallot.[10]   In children and adults, this is the commonest congenital lesion accompanied by cyanosis. As the name implies, four defects are present: pulmonary stenosis; enlargement of the right ventricle; a ventricular septal defect; overriding or dextroposition of the aorta. Abnormal development of the septum and malrotation of the embryonal vessels are the primary defects producing this condition.

The pulmonary stenosis limits the amount of blood that can pass through the lungs to be oxygenated; the rest of the blood is shunted through the septal defect to the left ventricle, or escapes into the overriding aorta (right-to-left shunt). This mixture of oxygenated and unoxygenated blood accounts for the variable degree of cyanosis that is a characteristic feature of this disease.

Tissue anoxia leads to secondary polycythemia; clubbing of the

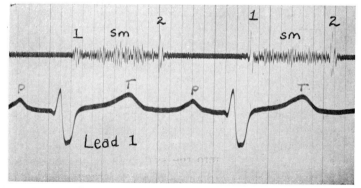

Fig. 184.   Loud, coarse murmur through systole, with systolic thrill. Microphone in third left interspace. Child, 8 years of age, with cyanosis, clubbing, right ventricular hypertrophy and diminished pulmonary vascularity. Tentative diagnosis: tetralogy of Fallot.

[9] Henri Louis Roger, French physician, 1809–91.
[10] Étienne-Louis Arthur Fallot, French physician, 1850–1911.

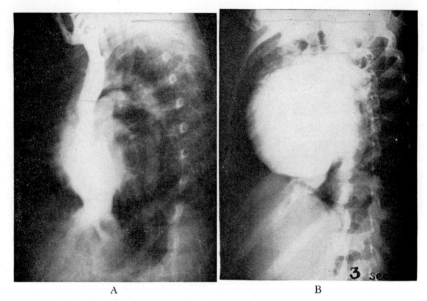

A   B

Fig. 185. Angiocardiogram, interatrial septal defect. The opaque material is injected rapidly and at high pressure into an antecubital vein.

A, The opaque has filled the right heart, refluxed into the hepatic veins and crossed the interatrial septum, opacifying the left atrium before filling the pulmonary artery or lung vessels. Shunting of the blood from the right side of the heart to the left side occurs only when the pressure in the right side exceeds that of the left. This is an abnormal pressure relationship, but may be present if the pulmonary artery is stenotic, as was the case in this patient. Cyanosis would be expected in such a condition and was present to a marked degree.

B, On this film, made 1 second later, the dilated pulmonary artery is filled. The dilatation is post-stenotic. In the interval between the two exposures the hepatic veins have emptied. The artificially increased pressure due to the injection itself is sometimes sufficient to cause the contrast medium to flow from the right side of the heart directly to the left through a septal defect. (Roentgen interpretation by Dr. Paul Eyler.)

fingers and even of the toes is common. Physical development is often retarded. A systolic thrill may be palpable to the left of the sternum, and one or two systolic murmurs will be heard. The septal defect and the pulmonary stenosis should each produce a murmur, but the latter may be intense enough to prevent recognition of the septal murmur. Roentgen examination shows right-sided cardiac enlargement, but the pulmonary vasculature is less prominent than normal, since some of the blood is not passing through the lungs.

Dyspnea is a common complaint, and syncopal attacks may occur; aching in the legs may also be present. These symptoms are decreased if the child squats; such a history should immediately suggest the presence of the tetralogy. Anastomosis of a large systemic artery to the pulmonary artery beyond the constricted area will increase the amount of oxygenated blood and ameliorate the symptoms, but this does not

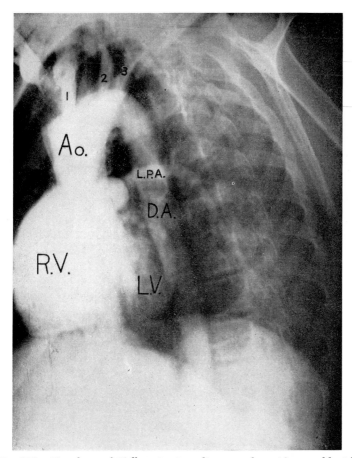

Fig. 186. Tetralogy of Fallot. Angiocardiogram of an 18-year-old girl taken 2 seconds after injection of the contrast medium into an antecubital vein. The aorta (Ao.) is opacified simultaneously with the enlarged right ventricle (R.V.), and before opacification of the left ventricle (L.V.). This indicates that the aorta overrides the right ventricle and receives unoxygenated blood from it. The small left branch of the pulmonary artery (L.P.A.) is seen crossing the descending aorta (D.A.). Note the absence of any significant pulmonary vasculature. The small artery and inadequate pulmonary vasculature result from the pulmonic stenosis that is a part of the tetralogy of Fallot. The numbers mark the vessels arising off the aortic arch. (From Zinsser and Kendrick: Pennsylvania M.J., 52:1665–1670, 1949.)

cure the disease. Direct approach by open-heart surgery with correction of the defects is now being performed.

Eisenmenger's[11] **Complex.** The important features are a large ventricular septal defect, pulmonary hypertension and enlargement of the right ventricle; overriding of the aorta may also be present. The pulmonary artery is normal in size or dilated. A moderate amount of blood passes from the right ventricle to the left, or directly into the aorta. The

[11] Victor Eisenmenger, German physician, fl. 1897.

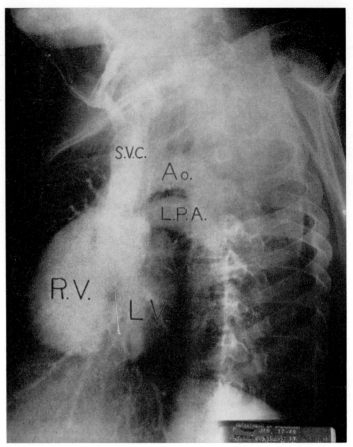

Fig. 187. The Eisenmenger complex. Angiocardiogram of a male patient aged 17 taken 2 seconds after injection of the contrast material into an antecubital vein. The aorta (Ao.) is opacified simultaneously with the enlarged right ventricle (R.V.). The left ventricle (L.V.) is not opacified, although contrast material is seen in pulmonary vessels running through this region. This indicates that the aorta overrides the right ventricle and can receive blood from it. However, in contrast to Figure 186 the pulmonary vasculature is prominent and the left pulmonary artery (L.P.A.) is large, approaching the aorta in size. This difference occurs because there is no pulmonic stenosis as there is in the tetralogy of Fallot. The superior vena cava (S.V.C.) is also opacified. (From Zinsser and Kendrick: Pennsylvania M.J., 52:1665–1670, 1949.)

resulting unsaturation of the arterial blood produces a variable degree of cyanosis, and clubbing of the fingers and toes may develop. A systolic impulse due to the thrust of the right ventricle may be felt near the left sternal border, and a systolic thrill may be present near the base. In the second or third left intercostal space near the sternum a loud systolic murmur can be heard; this rarely extends throughout systole. The pulmonic second sound is accentuated. Later in the disease the pulmonic ring may be dilated by the prolonged hypertension; a pulmonic diastolic murmur will then be heard.

VASCULAR MALFORMATIONS

Patent Ductus Arteriosus.   During fetal life the ductus arteriosus shunts blood from the pulmonary artery to the aorta, bypassing the nonfunctioning lungs. It should close shortly after birth and disappear completely within the first few weeks of life. A persistent ductus permits blood to flow from the aorta into the pulmonary artery. In such cases, the systolic blood pressure may be higher than expected, and the diastolic pressure low; a Corrigan type pulse may be present. A thrill is sometimes palpable in the pulmonic valve area. The most striking finding is a continuous harsh murmur ("machinery murmur") heard best over the pulmonic area. This may vary in intensity as the pressure in the aorta fluctuates with systole and diastole.

Early recognition of this lesion is important. It can be corrected surgically, but the operative mortality rises with increasing age. Also, subacute bacterial endarteritis ("endocarditis") is prone to develop in these patients, adding to the morbidity and mortality.

Coarctation of the Aorta.   In this condition there is a constriction of varying length at a point distal to the origin of the left subclavian artery. As a result, the blood pressure above that point is markedly increased; below the constriction it is decreased. To establish collateral circulation there is enlargement of other arteries, noticeably of the intercostal vessels. Coarctation should be suspected whenever a child or young person is found to have hypertension in the brachial artery.

Inspection or palpation may elicit the pulsating intercostal arteries. The pulses in the femoral arteries will be poor and there will be an appreciable lag or delay in filling when compared with the radial pulse. If the blood pressure in the thigh is measured, the systolic pressure will be low. A systolic murmur may be heard over the base of the heart, but with coarctation the murmur should be of maximum intensity over the

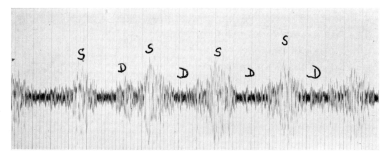

Fig. 188.   Patent ductus arteriosus. "Machinery murmur" with marked systolic accentuation (S) and less diastolic accentuation (D).

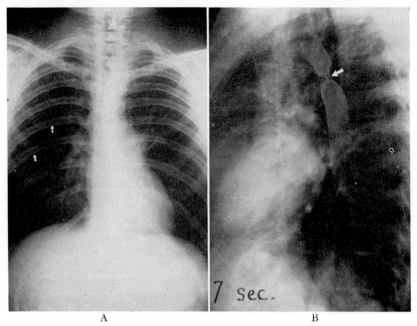

A   B

Fig. 189. Coarctation of the aorta. *A*, The plain chest film shows notching of the ribs, which is particularly well seen at the points marked by the arrows. Also to be noted is the lack of a definite prominence of the aortic knob, which is ordinarily present on the upper left border. *B*, Angiocardiogram taken 7 seconds after injection of the contrast medium into an antecubital vein. The aorta is opacified, and the site of the coarctation is seen at the point marked by the arrow. The photograph has been slightly retouched for clarity in reproduction. (Roentgen interpretation by Dr. Harry Zinsser.)

back, along the vertebral column and in the interscapular area. A roentgenogram may show scalloping or notching of the lower margins of the ribs caused by pressure from the enlarged pulsating arteries. The aortic knob may also be absent. The intra-arterial injection of a suitable contrast medium will delineate the exact site and size of the constriction.

Surgical correction is usually possible, but best results are obtained if this is done during childhood or adolescence. If the condition is unrecognized or uncorrected, cardiac or cerebrovascular complications may result from the long-standing hypertension.

AORTIC ANEURYSM

Weakening or destruction of the media of an artery will lead to gradual enlargement of the lumen and development of an aneurysm.

Syphilis, untreated or inadequately treated, and Marfan's[12] syndrome are the diseases usually responsible for aortic aneurysms developing before the age of fifty; degenerative changes account for most of those appearing later in life.

An aneurysm of the ascending aorta produces various physical signs. An expansile pulsating mass may be visible and palpable in the right second or third intercostal space; a systolic thrill and a diastolic shock may also be felt in that area. Palpation may elicit a tracheal tug (Oliver's sign, p. 120). Dullness or flatness will be present to the right of the sternum in the supracardiac area. A systolic murmur is usually present; with syphilis there will probably be an associated aortic insufficiency giving rise to a diastolic murmur also. There may be an appreciable difference between the radial pulses and the blood pressure in the two arms if the orifice of the subclavian or innominate artery is involved.

An aneurysm of the transverse portion of the arch or of the descending aorta produces few signs but may produce symptoms by pressure on the trachea, esophagus, thoracic duct, left main bronchus or left recurrent laryngeal nerve. Erosion of vertebrae or ribs can occur; occasionally a mass will protrude posteriorly to the left of the vertebral column.

An aneurysm of the abdominal aorta presents as a definitely expansile pulsating mass between the xiphoid and the umbilicus. It must be remembered that pulsations are normally visible and palpable in very thin persons; the diagnosis of aneurysm should not be made unless the aorta is definitely enlarged. These aneurysms are almost invariably due to degenerative changes and occur in elderly people. The prognosis is poor; life expectancy is short unless a suitable graft can be implanted.

Dissecting Aneurysm.   This is due to a tear in the intima, usually in the first portion of the thoracic aorta; hypertension may have preceded this. Blood is forced into the subintimal tissues, stripping the intima from the media. The onset tends to be sudden, with severe pain which mimics an acute myocardial infarction or some other catastrophic process. As the dissection proceeds, partial or complete occlusion or tearing of various branch arteries develops, leading to random and scattered signs of arterial insufficiency. Retrograde dissection may extend to the base of the aorta; the aortic ring may be partially avulsed and the action of the valve will be compromised. A systolic or diastolic murmur may appear suddenly and change rapidly. Rupture into the pericardial sac causes cardiac tamponade and death. Prompt surgical intervention when the dissection is first diagnosed may be life-saving.

[12] Bernard-Jean Antonin Marfan, French pediatrician, 1858–1942.

PERICARDITIS

Infection is the most common cause of pericarditis. Acute rheumatic fever and viral infections must always be considered, as well as extension of tuberculosis, pneumonia or other infections from the lung, the mediastinum or more distant sites. Pericarditis can also follow direct trauma or may develop as a result of myocardial infarction. In uremia, the pericardial surface may be roughened by extensive deposits of fibrinoid material with little inflammatory reaction; this also occurs when metastatic lesions are present.

Acute Fibrinous Pericarditis.　　The symptoms are variable. Usually the patient has substernal or precordial pain; sometimes this develops rapidly and is so severe that it mimics the pain of acute myocardial infarction. When pericarditis is due to infection the patient has fever; this finding is of limited diagnostic value if the underlying infectious process is active. Inspection will usually be unrewarding except that the patient appears ill. Palpation may occasionally be helpful; rough vibrations may be felt synchronous with the heart beat. The heart size is unaltered at this stage, but usually the previous size is unknown. On auscultation a to-and-fro friction rub will be heard; this may be very faint or it may loud and harsh. Increasing the pressure on the chest piece of the stethoscope may increase the intensity of the sounds. Very often the rub will disappear and reappear within minutes or hours. If the infection subsides or is cured at this stage there may be no demonstrable residual damage.

Pericarditis with Effusion.　　If the pericarditis persists fluid accumulates in the pericardial sac. This may appear insidiously or rapidly; in some instances the circulatory handicap imposed by a massive effusion overshadows the underlying disease. The stretched pericardium and the fluid itself interfere with venous return and with diastole; signs of cardiac decompensation appear.

The patient often appears apprehensive and cyanotic; dyspnea is common. At times he assumes some special position in which he seems most comfortable (Fig. 190). The neck veins are distended; other superficial veins may be unduly prominent. The cardiac impulse may not be visible, but this is significant only if it had been present previously. In children the precordial area may bulge outward. Compression of the lower part of the left lung may occur; expansion of the thorax over that area will be decreased and the costal margin will not flare outward with inspiration.

The pulse is rapid and feeble; a paradoxical pulse may be present. With a moderate amount of effusion a cardiac impulse may still be palpable; with massive effusion this disappears. The area of cardiac dullness is increased, both to the right and to the left of the sternum. It may be greater when the patient is erect than when he lies down; when he is recumbent the dullness at the base of the heart may increase in width. Compression of the adjacent left lung may result in dullness over the involved area (Ewart's[13] sign). On auscultation a friction rub may be heard if the amount of fluid is small, but this disappears if fluid completely surrounds the heart. The heart sounds become distant and faint as the effusion increases, and may show considerable change in intensity as the patient leans forward, sits erect and lies down. The pulmonic second sound may be accentuated if the pressure in the pulmonary vascular bed is increased. Bronchial breath sounds are usually heard over the compressed segment of the left lung.

Physical signs may be inconclusive even when a large effusion is present, and fluoroscopy or films may not help. Injection of a suitable contrast medium intravenously may demonstrate heart chambers that are much smaller than anticipated from the apparent size of the cardiac silhouette. Pericardial paracentesis and withdrawal of fluid establishes the presence of effusion and may yield an etiologic diagnosis.

Chronic Adhesive Pericarditis. This often develops after acute infectious pericarditis is cured. No characteristic signs are present; the diagnosis is usually made only during the course of cardiac surgery or at autopsy. Adhesions are present between the visceral and parietal pericardial surfaces, partially or completely obliterating the pericardial space.

Chronic Constrictive Pericarditis. In this type the adhesions are thick and firm, and calcification may be present. Of greater importance

[13] William Ewart, English physician, 1848–1929.

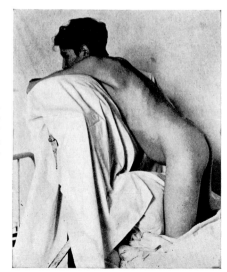

Fig. 190. A boy with rheumatic heart disease and pericardial effusion maintained this position almost continuously for weeks during an acute exacerbation. The effusion was not large.

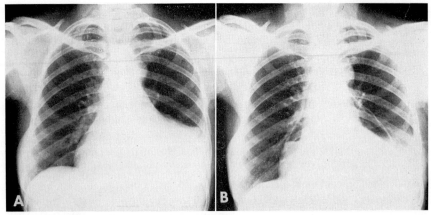

Fig. 191. *A*, Massive pericardial effusion. *B*, The suspected diagnosis was confirmed by pericardial paracentesis with removal of fluid and partial replacement with air (hydropneumopericardium). A moderate amount of pleural effusion is also present on the left. (Courtesy of Dr. R. H. Chamberlain.)

are adhesions that develop and bind the pericardium to the mediastinum, the diaphragm or the chest wall. The heart must perform extra work with every beat, and the dense sac in which it is encased hinders or prevents hypertrophy. Cardiac failure that develops without hypertension or signs of valvular disease should suggest the possibility of this condition, regardless of the size of the heart, but especially if the heart is normal in size. The physical signs are variable and depend upon the amount of constriction and the extent of the external adhesions.

On inspection there may be deformity of the precordial area. The apical impulse may be invisible or it may be very forceful; a systolic retraction is sometimes seen. The apex beat does not change its position when the patient turns from side to side. Palpation confirms these observations. The area of cardiac dullness may be normal, or it may be greatly increased if hypertension, valvular lesions or other disease preexisted; there is little or no change in this area of dullness with inspiration and expiration. On auscultation there are no characteristic findings of the disease itself.

During systole there may be retraction of the left eleventh and twelfth ribs and interspaces posteriorly; this has been attributed to adhesions between the heart and diaphragm, with tugging on the latter every time the heart contracts. This is known as Broadbent's[14] sign; it is commonly seen on examination papers.

---

[14] Sir William H. Broadbent, English neurologist, 1835–1907.

XVI

The Abdomen

Physical examination of the abdomen often fails to yield definitely diagnostic signs; radiologic and laboratory studies may be needed to establish the nature of the abnormalities present. However, that does not justify hurrying through this part of the survey; performed carefully, the basic procedures can yield a surprising amount of valuable information. One handicap is that the abdominal wall, often several centimeters thick, is interposed between the examining hand and the viscera. Another problem is that complaints in abdominal diseases are often vague and ill-defined, and that pain or discomfort is rarely sharply localized; it may be referred to some area of the abdomen distant from the actual disease. However, a careful examination will usually warrant conclusions that are subsequently verified by other studies.

TOPOGRAPHY

It is customary to divide the abdomen into four quadrants; the two imaginary lines run from the xiphoid to the symphysis pubis and transversely through the umbilicus. Less commonly, nine areas are designated. In addition, certain landmarks are used as points of reference, such as Poupart's[1] ligament.

The *linea alba*, formed by the midline fusion of the fascial sheaths of the rectus muscles, is usually visible and palpable from the xiphoid to a point just below the umbilicus; then it becomes very narrow and practically invisible. *Linea nigra* is the term applied to the pigmented line extending from the umbilicus to the symphysis pubis; it is often especially prominent in women who have borne many children. The *linea semilunaris* marks the lateral border of the sheath of the rectus muscle and extends from the ninth costal cartilage to the pubic spine. The

---

[1] François Poupart, French anatomist, 1616–1708.

293

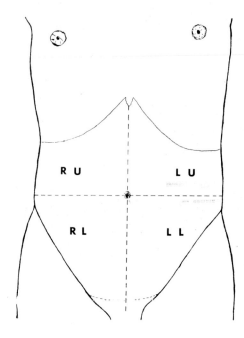

Fig. 192. The four quadrants of the abdomen: RU, right upper; LU, left upper; RL, right lower; LL, left lower.

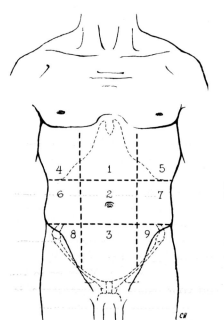

Fig. 193. The nine regions of the abdomen; (1) epigastric, (2) umbilical, (3) pubic, (4 and 5) right and left hypochondriac, (6 and 7) right and left lumbar, (8 and 9) right and left iliac regions. (After Walker, H.: Physical Diagnosis. St. Louis, C. V. Mosby Company, 1952.)

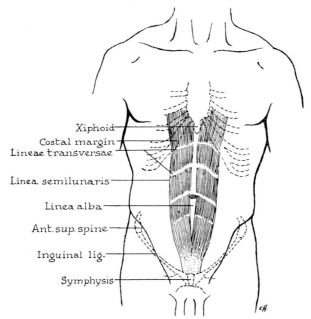

Fig. 194. Surface markings of abdomen. (After Walker, H.: Physical Diagnosis. St. Louis, C. V. Mosby Company, 1952.)

lineae transversae may be visible in a well-muscled person with little subcutaneous fat; these cross the rectus muscles transversely.

PROCEDURE

For proper examination of the abdomen, the patient must be lying supine on an examining table or on a fairly firm bed. Don't ask an ambulatory patient to lie down *on his back;* if you do, he will usually lie on his abdomen. Just say, "Now I want you to lie down, please," and he usually does what you want. Then he puts his hands above his head, or under it; that increases muscular tension and makes the examination more difficult or unsatisfactory. Have him place his arms at his side, or preferably clasp his hands across his thorax; this provides relaxation and keeps his arms out of your way (Fig. 195). The head should be raised by a small pillow to provide further relaxation. Needless to say, the room must be warm and so should your hands and stethoscope; icy fingers will produce muscular spasm and possibly other reactions. The abdomen must be completely bared from the lower ribs to the pubis.

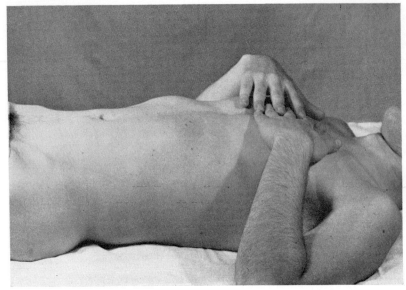

Fig. 195. Proper position of patient for examination. Abdomen completely bared; knees slightly flexed; hands resting on thorax.

Adequate illumination is essential so that minor abnormalities will not be overlooked.

INSPECTION

Inspection should be performed both from the side and from the foot of the bed; abnormality of contour or inequality of the two sides is often more noticeable from the latter position. Sit or kneel in such a position that your eyes are only a few inches above the abdomen.

Contour.   The general shape of the abdomen is apparent at once. It may be scaphoid or flat, or may show slight to tremendous protuberance. A scaphoid abdomen is often physiologic in a young asthenic person; in others it is usually indicative of malnutrition or of chronic illness that has resulted in significant weight loss. In severe emphysema, a normal abdomen may have much the same appearance because of the tremendous increase in the A-P diameter of the thorax. Protuberance may be due entirely to fat, especially in the abdominal wall and omentum. It may also be caused by physiologic or pathologic enlargement of one or more of the intra-abdominal organs such as a gravid uterus or a large ovarian cyst. Intestinal obstruction will result in gaseous distention. Ascites will also produce protuberance; often there will be excessive bulging of the flanks.

A localized area of prominence may be due to a benign or malignant tumor of the abdominal wall, to a hernia or to pathologic enlargement of one or more organs. Some of the more common processes are passive congestion, primary or metastatic carcinoma of the liver; polycystic kidneys, hydronephrosis or renal carcinoma; splenomegaly associated with blood dyscrasias; large benign tumors (fibroids) of the uterus; distention of the urinary bladder; ovarian, pancreatic or mesenteric cysts.

Retraction of the abdominal wall, especially noticeable in the epigastrium, occurs during inspiration if there is interference with respiration or severe dyspnea. A localized area of retraction is usually the result of postoperative adhesions or scarring.

In thin persons, and especially if the abdomen is scaphoid, pulsations in the abdominal aorta may be visible anywhere between the xiphoid and the umbilicus. With emphysema, the cardiac impulse may also be prominent below the sternum or in the left subcostal region.

Peristalsis. This is rarely visible in a healthy person, but when gastrointestinal disease is present one or several localized areas of bulging may slither slowly or fairly rapidly across the abdomen. The waves of gastric peristalsis cross the epigastrium from left to right; if they are visible, pyloric obstruction should be suspected. Peristalsis in the small intestine is most commonly seen around the umbilicus (Fig. 196). In the large bowel, waves may be present anywhere along the course of the colon but often they are most noticeable in the right lower quadrant.

Diastasis. Before completing this first phase of inspection, have

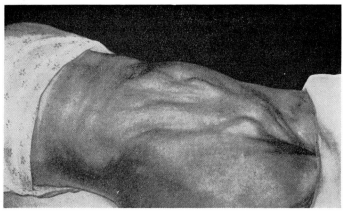

Fig. 196. Visible peristalsis, showing the characteristic ladder pattern in a case of strangulated right femoral hernia, which can also be seen. (Bailey, H.: Physical Signs in Clinical Surgery. 12th ed. Bristol, John Wright & Sons, Ltd., 1954.)

the patient raise his head and shoulders slightly, to tense the abdominal muscles. Weakness or separation of the fasciae along the linea alba (*diastasis recti*) is not rare; abdominal viscera will bulge forward. Other areas of protrusion or retraction may also become apparent.

The Skin. Normally this should have the same characteristics as the skin elsewhere. Marked weight loss will result in wrinkled, flabby skin. Enlargement of the abdomen will stretch the skin, which then becomes smooth and glistening. Overstretched skin will show sinuous vertical *striae*, which are silvery and feather-like in appearance; they result from tearing of the cutis and atrophy of the connective tissue layers. They frequently develop during pregnancy, but may occur in other conditions that stretch the skin rapidly. Purple or reddish striae may develop in Cushing's syndrome. The amount, character and distribution of suprapubic and abdominal hair should also be noted. Abnormal pigmentation or dermatologic lesions may be seen; they should be described.

Scars. These deserve particular attention; their location and appearance often give clues to the operative procedure and the postoperative course. A radiating area of puckered skin follows drainage; a very broad scar may indicate superficial infection, opening of the incision (*wound dehiscence*) or other complications during healing. Multiple scars over various areas suggest that the patient has chronic recurrent abdominal disease, abnormality of many organs, porphyria or a personality pattern that has misled the surgeon into a variety of operative procedures in an attempt to alleviate nonexistent organic disease.

Veins. Dilatation of superficial veins may develop if there is obstruction of the inferior vena cava, of the superior vena cava or of the portal vein (Fig. 197). The direction of flow should be determined. Normally, veins over the lower half of the abdominal wall carry blood downward and empty into the saphenous veins; those in the upper half drain upward into the thoracic veins. With obstruction of the inferior vena cava, some blood will be shunted to the superior vena cava through the superficial abdominal veins. In this case the normal direction of blood flow over the lower half of the abdomen is reversed; it flows upward. Obstruction of the superior vena cava occasionally produces enlargement of the superficial veins; blood drains downward over the upper abdomen and enters the inferior vena cava. With portal obstruction some of the blood reaches the superficial circulation around the umbilicus; the direction of blood flow from this point onward is normal. In rare instances these periumbilical veins become markedly enlarged and tortuous; some day you may be lucky enough to see such a *caput medusae*.[2]

---

[2] Medusa, mythical Greek Gorgon, renowned for her undulating serpentine tresses; probably this is the first recorded permanent wave.

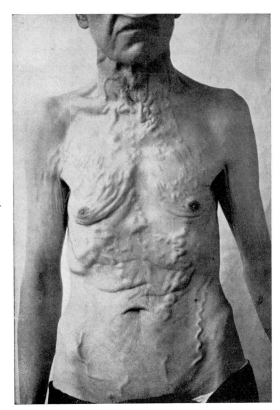

Fig. 197. Venous obstruction. (Phillips.)

The Umbilicus. Normally this is depressed below the level of the adjacent abdominal wall. Protrusion may be due to obesity, pregnancy, ascites, an umbilical hernia or some other condition that raises intra-abdominal pressure. Carcinoma of an abdominal organ occasionally metastasizes and gives rise to periumbilical nodules; ulceration may occur in these.

With intraperitoneal hemorrhage a bluish discoloration may be present (Cullen's[3] sign). Infection occasionally is present (*omphalitis*), especially when personal hygiene is poor; an area of cellulitis surrounds the umbilicus. A patent urachus may give rise to intermittent discharge of a few drops of urine.

PALPATION

Palpation is usually the most informative and rewarding part of the

[3] Thomas S. Cullen, Baltimore surgeon, 1868–1953.

examination but it is worthless unless the musculature is as relaxed as possible. It is advisable to have the patient flex the thighs and legs somewhat, or to place a pillow under the knees to improve relaxation. Abdominal respiration increases the relaxation, especially during expiration; breathing through the mouth often encourages this. If the patient is ticklish this should be ignored; continued light pressure will usually be rewarded by relaxation of the muscles. It is also helpful to distract the patient's attention by asking additional questions about his illness or preferably by discussing some totally irrelevant subject in which he is interested.

Initially, palpation should be very light; the hand barely rests on the abdomen. With slight flexion movements of all four fingers the general characteristics of the abdominal wall are determined. It is best to slide the hand an inch or two at a time as you move from one area to another; lifting it up and reapplying it results in some slight momentary muscle resistance. If the patient has complained of an area of abdominal tenderness, *never* palpate that area first; start at some distant point and gradually approach the painful area.   *& masses*

Muscular Rigidity.   This is best determined by light palpation; it may be localized or generalized. When rigidity is localized it usually denotes underlying intraperitoneal inflammatory disease—acute appendicitis or acute cholecystitis, for example. When generalized rigidity is slight it may be mistaken for poor relaxation. In the most pronounced form the abdominal wall becomes boardlike and resists all ordinary pressure; this is indicative of widespread peritoneal irritation or infection. If it develops rapidly, rupture of a hollow viscus has probably occurred.

Tenderness.   Tenderness on palpation may be slight or very severe; it may occur alone or be accompanied by any degree of rigidity. It may be fairly sharply localized, or diffuse and vague. In the initial stage of acute appendicitis, for example, slight pain may be present in the epigastrium or periumbilical region and tenderness will be minimal. *Visceral Dispeors* Later, the complaints shift to the right lower quadrant. As the inflammation increases the tenderness becomes more severe and more localized, and increasing rigidity of the overlying abdominal wall develops.

If pressure over a painful area is maintained, tenderness due to intra-abdominal infection will usually remain constant or increase in severity; when due to distention or spasm of a hollow viscus it often decreases. Then ask the patient to tense his abdominal muscles while you continue to press. Tenderness due to a visceral lesion will be decreased or abolished; that due to an abnormality of the abdominal wall will be unaltered or increased. The sensory nerve supply of much of the anterior abdominal wall is from the lower dorsal nerves; intrathoracic disease can give rise to referred pain and superficial tenderness. Disease of the abdominal muscles or other tissues in the wall may also be the cause of such pain.

Rebound Tenderness. This is a sign of peritoneal irritation, usually from infection. To elicit this sign, make firm pressure over any part of the abdomen for several seconds, then release it suddenly. The patient will experience a momentary stab of pain at the involved area. If the disease is minimal it may be necessary to press directly over the suspected spot. Watch the patient's face; often his expression will supply the answer before he can tell you that he has such pain.

PERCUSSION

Percussion is helpful to confirm the size of various organs and to demonstrate the presence of excessive amounts of fluid or gas; light percussion gives best results. Since a small amount of air is normally present in the gastrointestinal tract, chiefly in the stomach and colon, a tympanitic note will be elicited over scattered areas of the abdomen. This will be of variable pitch, depending upon the size of the underlying "tube"; it will be high-pitched over loops of small intestine, relatively low-pitched over the stomach, and of intermediate pitch over the colon. Obstruction at any point will result in abnormal distention of the loops of bowel proximal to that point and will alter the percussion note.

Procedure. A definite routine is advisable. Start over the left thorax laterally and percuss downward. At the ninth interspace the resonant note may suddenly become tympanitic, due to gas in the splenic flexure. Dullness or flatness in this area suggests enlargement of the spleen or of the left kidney. In a similar manner, percuss the right side. The upper limit of hepatic dullness laterally should be obvious at the level of the seventh interspace. Continue downward until tympany is elicited; this should mark the lower border of the liver. The apparent size of the liver in this region should then be confirmed by repeating the procedure during forced inspiration and forced expiration. Then percuss anteriorly on each side, noting the apparent size and position of the gastric air bubble ("magenblase") on the left, and the upper and lower limits of hepatic dullness on the right. Pulmonary or pleural disease at the base of the right thorax may invalidate the latter observations. The size of the area of gastric tympany (Traube's semilunar space) depends upon the contents of the stomach. It will be depressed if there is a large pericardial effusion or left pleural effusion; consolidation of the left lower lobe of the lung will not do this. Enlargement of the left lobe of the liver or of the spleen occasionally displaces the tympanitic area downward. If a mass has been felt during palpation, particular attention should be paid to the percussion note at that point. Any solid structure such as a distended bladder, enlarged uterus or an ovarian or uterine tumor will yield a dull or flat percussion note.

AUSCULTATION *is FoR peristalic sounds*

Auscultation is used primarily to determine the presence and characteristics of peristaltic sounds. If abdominal disease is present or suspected, *auscultation should follow inspection* and precede palpation and percussion.

Peristalsis. In a normal abdomen there is always a certain amount of activity that produces gurgling or bubbling sounds of variable pitch, intensity and frequency; experience will be required to enable you to determine what is normal and what is abnormal. Hyperactive peristalsis is present when there is irritation of the gastrointestinal mucosa; it may also be due to disturbances of the autonomic nervous system. With partial obstruction, or before and shortly after complete obstruction, peristalsis is also increased; the typically high-pitched tinkling sounds are sometimes called "fighting peristalsis." When muscular fatigue forces the bowel to give up the fight, peristaltic sounds become infrequent or disappear. With peritoneal irritation or infection of any *appendies* type there is diminution or absence of peristalsis; the return of bowel activity after laparotomy, Dr. Deaver[4] used to tell us, is "music to the surgeon's ears." Incidentally, it also brings comfort to the patient as he expels flatus or feces. Paralytic ileus may also occur during the course of extra-abdominal disease such as severe pneumonia.

Other Sounds. Occasionally one hears a friction over the liver or spleen; infection or infarction can lead to localized areas of peritoneal irritation. A murmur may be heard in the midline over the abdominal aorta; it is of little diagnostic significance. With severe pulmonary emphysema, the heart sounds may be heard nowhere except in the epigastric region. During the latter months of pregnancy the fetal heart sounds are usually audible at some point, and a systolic placental hum or souffle may be present.

PALPATION OF SPECIFIC ABDOMINAL VISCERA

(or masses)

When the preliminary observations have been completed, palpation of deeper structures and of specific organs should be attempted. The hand may be tilted slightly so that the fingers depress the abdominal

---

[4] John B. Deaver, Philadelphia surgeon, 1855–1931.

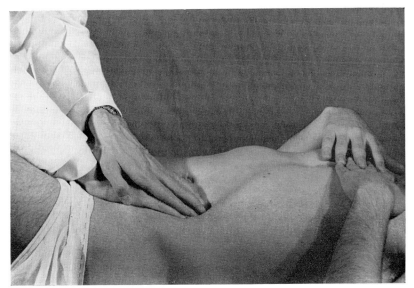

Fig. 198. Palpation with hands superimposed. The left hand supplies the pressure; the right hand is relaxed to improve tactile sensation.

wall. Occasionally the hands are superimposed; the upper one makes pressure while the lower one remains relaxed for more accurate outlining of structures (Fig. 198).

Whenever a mass is felt within the abdomen certain characteristics must be determined and recorded. These include position, size, shape, contour, consistency and sensitivity, and whether the mass moves with respiration, can be moved by the examiner, or is apparently fixed to the abdominal wall or to structures deep in the abdomen. The anatomic site of the abdominal organs must be remembered, but wide variations may be physiologic. The size and shape are subject to much less variation. Certain healthy organs are often palpable in a normal person if the abdominal wall is thin and well relaxed; the liver, kidneys, cecum, descending colon, abdominal aorta and lumbar spine fall into this category. Organs such as the gallbladder, stomach, small intestine, transverse colon and spleen cannot be outlined unless they are diseased or abnormally distended or enlarged.

The Liver

With quiet respiration, most of a normal-sized liver lies under the ribs. The portion extending below the costal margin is largely covered by the rectus muscle; this makes accurate palpation difficult. If these muscles are small and flabby, the liver may be felt somewhat indistinctly beneath them. However, the liver descends with inspiration and may be felt below the ribs in the right upper quadrant and epigastrium when the person takes a deep breath.

Procedure.   Stand or sit at the right side of the patient. Bimanual palpation is usually employed; slip your left hand between the patient and the mattress at or just below the costal margin, with the fingers lateral to the main mass of the spinal muscles. The patient usually tries to cooperate by arching his back or rolling somewhat to his left. When he relaxes and resumes his former position place your right hand flat on the anterior abdominal wall. Some examiners prefer to have the fingers parallel to the costal margin and a centimeter or two below it; others place the fingers in the vertical axis of the body just lateral to the rectus muscle. As the patient inhales slowly and somewhat more deeply than usual, press your left hand upward while gently depressing the right hand and moving it slightly toward the ribs; too much pressure will produce tensing of the abdominal muscles. At or near the end of inspiration the fingers of the right hand may be forced upward by the liver, or slip over the edge of it. If an edge is not felt, deeper palpation should be attempted. To do this, maintain pressure with the right hand as the patient exhales; the muscles will relax somewhat and the abdominal wall is more easily depressed. Keep the right hand in this position during the next inspiration; repeat the procedure during the next few breaths if necessary. Even a relatively muscular abdominal wall can be depressed a surprising distance in this manner.

If there is reason to suspect that the liver is enlarged, palpation should be started at a lower point; occasionally the liver will extend downward to the umbilicus or lower. In such cases it is best to start in the right lower quadrant and work upward until the edge or a definite mass is felt.

Alternate Procedure.   In doubtful cases it may be desirable to move somewhat toward the patient's shoulder, place the palm of one hand on the lower thorax, hook the fingers around or actually behind the costal margin and maintain this position as the patient inhales (Fig. 200).

Palpable Liver Edge.   An edge that is palpable below the costal margin just at the end of inspiration does not necessarily mean that the liver is actually enlarged; 25 per cent of healthy male medical students were found to have this. Moreover, the liver may be depressed by effusion in the right pleural cavity or by pulmonary emphysema. The physical signs found on examination of the lungs and the upper limit of hepatic dullness, as previously determined, will have to be taken into consideration before enlargement of the liver is diagnosed. Also, in a thin visceroptotic person, or one with severe cachexia, the liver may

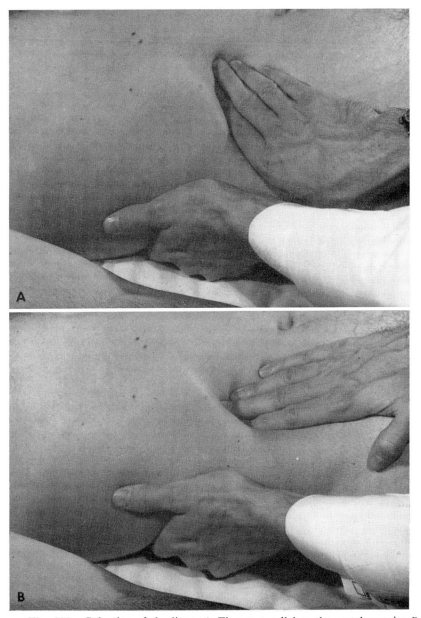

Fig. 199. Palpation of the liver. *A*, Fingers parallel to the costal margin; *B*, fingers in vertical axis of the body. The left hand is making pressure upward to displace the liver toward the palpating fingertips.

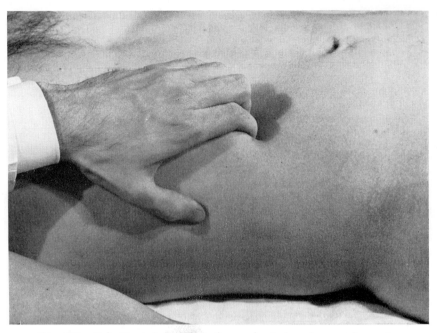

Fig. 200. Palpation of the liver; fingers hooked under costal margin.

be rotated so that one portion dips down while another rises; this may simulate hepatomegaly.

Whenever the liver is felt, its characteristics should be described. A normal liver edge is fairly sharp, smooth and moderately firm but not hard. Pressing against it or flipping the fingers over the edge will give the patient an uncomfortable sensation but no actual pain. With inflammatory disease or with congestion due to acute circulatory failure the liver is usually tender. Palpation produces pain and the patient may "catch his breath" or suddenly stop inhaling as the edge strikes your finger. With primary carcinoma the liver is usually smooth; metastatic nodules produce varying degrees of irregularity, depending upon their size. Syphilis may produce a disproportionate enlargement of the left lobe of the liver or an irregularly lobulated liver (hepar lobatum). Riedel's[5] lobe is an anatomical variant, a tongue-like projection of liver tissue in the right upper quadrant which may be mistaken for a distended gallbladder, an abnormally situated right kidney or a tumor of some type.

Gallbladder.   Normally the gallbladder is not palpable, but with obstruction of the cystic or common duct it may become sufficiently distended to produce a rounded or pear-shaped fluctuant mass below the liver edge. If infection is also present (*acute cholecystitis*) tenderness

[5] Bernhard Moritz Carl Ludwig Riedel, surgeon in Jena, 1846–1916.

will be obvious and muscular rigidity may prevent palpation of the mass. In rare instances a gallbladder filled with stones will be felt as a hard mass just below the liver edge.

The Spleen

The spleen is situated laterally or posterolaterally under the ribs on the left. Various methods are advocated for palpation of the spleen; experience alone will enable you to determine which one you find most satisfactory.

Procedure. The one which the author prefers is performed with the examiner standing or seated at the left side of the patient, whose head is supported by a pillow and whose thighs and legs are flexed to provide maximal abdominal relaxation. The right hand is slipped beneath the lower ribs with the tips of the fingers lateral to the spinal muscles. The left hand is used for palpation, which is performed as in examination of the liver. As the patient inhales deeply, pressure is exerted with the right hand to force the spleen forward and slightly mesially,

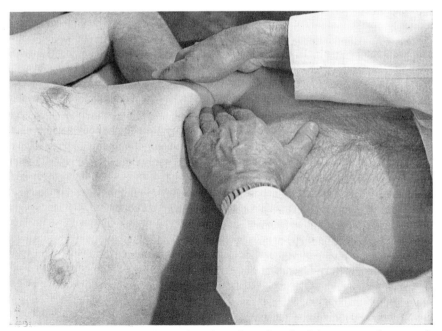

Fig. 201. Palpation of the spleen from the right side of the patient. The patient's left arm is under the lower ribs, aiding in the forward displacement of the spleen by the examiner's right hand.

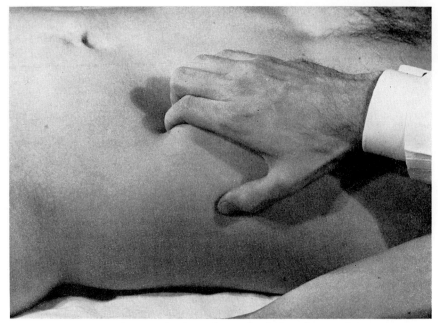

Fig. 202.   Palpation of spleen; fingers hooked under costal margin.

while gentle pressure is made with the left fingers as they search for an edge.

A second method is favored by some. Stand at the right of the patient; reach over and place one hand under the ribs; use the other hand for palpation (Fig. 201). This has the disadvantage that the examiner is in an uncomfortable or strained position, which tends to detract from the accuracy of his observations.

A third procedure, which is occasionally helpful, is to stand near the patient's left shoulder, placing the palm on the lower part of the thorax and hooking the fingers under the costal margin as the patient inhales deeply (Fig. 202).

A spleen of normal size is not palpable unless it has been displaced by depression of the left leaf of the diaphragm or by intra-abdominal disease in the splenic area. With slight enlargement, only the tip will be felt at the end of inspiration. With moderate enlargement it is usually possible to feel an indentation or notch on the mesial edge; this helps to differentiate such a mass from an enlarged kidney. With massive enlargement the spleen may extend downward to the pelvic brim or over into the right side of the abdomen. Needless to say, if there is a mass in the upper abdomen on the left side, palpation should be carried out at successively lower levels and mesially until an edge has been found, if possible.

If severe emphysema is present the spleen may not be felt through the anterior abdominal wall, but farther laterally; it does not move forward as the costal cage flares.

Splenic Enlargement. This occurs in a number of diseases and may be important in suggesting or substantiating a diagnosis. Slight enlargement is present in some acute infectious diseases including typhoid, brucellosis, miliary tuberculosis, septicemia and subacute bacterial endocarditis. It may also be the first sign of various blood dyscrasias. Moderate enlargement is usually indicative of leukemia, infectious mononucleosis or hemolytic anemia. A markedly enlarged spleen suggests chronic myelogenous leukemia, myeloid metaplasia, thalassemia major, Banti's[6] syndrome or a metabolic disturbance such as Gaucher's[7] disease or Niemann-Pick[8] disease. Occasionally splenomegaly is due to impaired circulation, especially in the portal system, to lymphoma or metastatic carcinoma, or to an exotic disease such as malaria or kala-azar.

The Kidneys

Anatomically the right kidney is lower than the left, and in a thin person it is often possible to feel the tip or even the lower third or more of it. Occasionally the kidney descends so low that the fingers can be insinuated above the upper pole and one can grasp the entire organ between the two hands. Less frequently this is possible on the left side.

Procedure. The position of the patient and the technique for palpating the kidneys is much the same as that for palpating the liver or spleen, except that deeper penetration by the exploring hand is necessary. Although the kidneys tend to be forced down by the diaphragm during inspiration, too much pressure exerted by the hand on the anterior abdominal wall can prevent this; there may be only a vague sensation of a mass touching the fingers. It is preferable to apply only slight or moderate pressure during inspiration and then to increase this just as expiration starts. In this way a kidney can descend and become trapped between the two hands; then a mass will be felt to slip upward as the patient exhales. If either kidney is palpable its characteristics should be determined and described.

Fist Percussion. Percussion in the region of the costovertebral angle is used to elicit renal or perirenal tenderness. The patient should be sitting or standing; the blow should be of moderate intensity.

[6] Guido Banti, Italian pathologist, 1852–1925.
[7] Phillipe Charles Ernest Gaucher, French physician, 1854–1918.
[8] Albert Niemann, German pediatrician, 1880–1921; Ludwig Pick, German physician, 1868–1935.

Abnormalities.   Enlargement is usually due to hydronephrosis, malignancy or polycystic disease. A large kidney that does not move with respiration should be considered malignant. Severe tenderness, either anteriorly or in the costovertebral area, suggests renal or perirenal infection. A perinephric abscess may present as a vague mass in the renal area; no definite edge will be felt and tenderness or rigidity will be conspicuous.

The Colon

The cecum and a portion of the descending colon are often palpable; other segments are not felt unless diseased or abnormally distended.

Procedure.   The hand should be placed on the abdominal wall at right angles to the course of the segment being sought, with the fingertips beyond the mesial border. Moderately firm pressure with the fingers is then made in the direction of the lateral abdominal wall. In the cecal region a soft mass will usually be felt. Gas, liquids or semisolid fecal material will permit indentation of the mass; a gurgle will often be heard. Infection or a tumor will produce a firmer mass.

The descending colon should be sought in the left lower quadrant as it courses over the pelvic brim. Ordinarily it is about two centimeters in diameter, fairly firm and only moderately sensitive, but may be larger if diseased or distended.

ASCITES

Ascites in an abnormal collection of fluid other than blood in the peritoneal cavity. It is usually a transudate; occasionally it is an inflammatory exudate. The most common cause is interference with the return of blood from the area below the diaphragm due to right-sided heart failure, to constrictive pericarditis, to high obstruction of the inferior vena cava or to cirrhosis or some other type of hepatic disease. Ascites may also occur in nephritis, especially with the nephrotic syndrome (Fig. 203), or in other conditions accompanied by fluid retention. With a solid ovarian tumor there may be ascites plus hydrothorax (Meigs'[9] syndrome); removal of the growth results in rapid disappearance of all of the fluid. Peritoneal carcinomatosis is often accompanied by ascites, as is chronic infection, especially tuberculosis. Acute infection rarely

[9] Joe Vincent Meigs, Boston surgeon, 1892–1963.

results in any massive amount of free fluid; loculated collections more commonly occur.

The physical signs depend upon the amount of free fluid. Less than a liter is rarely demonstrable in an adult. A somewhat larger amount may be detected if the patient assumes the knee-chest or knee-elbow position, which favors gravitation of the fluid to the epigastric or peri-umbilical regions. An effusion of moderate size will produce bulging in the flanks when the patient is recumbent; there may be little disten-tion of the anterior abdominal wall. If he stands, the lower part of the abdomen will become protuberant; this must not be confused with relaxed muscles and visceroptosis ("potbelly"). With massive ascites there may be 10 liters or more of free fluid. The abdomen is globular, the skin is tense and glistening, the umbilicus usually protrudes and hernial sacs may bulge from hydrostatic pressure. Examination of the thorax has already shown that the diaphragm is high, with little or no excur-sion, and that the heart is displaced upward.

A fluid wave is the most important diagnostic sign; this can be dem-onstrated with a moderate or massive effusion. With the patient supine, place the palm and fingers of one hand on the flank; with the fingertips of the other hand strike the opposite flank sharply. The fluid wave set in motion by the percussing hand will be felt distinctly by the palpating hand. To eliminate the transmission of the impulse by the abdominal wall itself it is customary to have an assistant or the patient exert firm

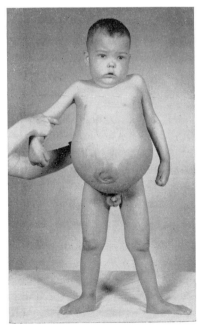

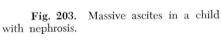

Fig. 203. Massive ascites in a child with nephrosis.

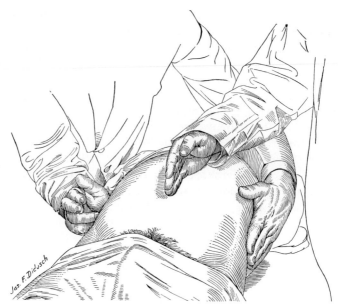

Fig. 204. Demonstration of a fluid wave. (Dunphy, J. E., and Botsford, T. W.: Physical Examination of the Surgical Patient. 3rd ed. Philadelphia, W. B. Saunders Co., 1964.)

pressure with the edge of his hand in the midline (Fig. 204). With experience, equally reliable information can be obtained without such aid; even a very light tap will be transmitted promptly through the fluid and be distinctly felt over the opposite flank. The impulse transmitted through the abdominal wall arrives later.

A second sign is the presence of *shifting dullness;* this is most helpful when moderate ascites is present. Free fluid gravitates to the most dependent regions; gas-filled loops of intestine float above this. With the patient supine the percussion note in the flanks will be dull or flat; around the umbilicus the note will be tympanitic (*coronal tympany*). Percuss the upper limit of dullness in each flank and mark these points; have the patient turn on one side and repeat the percussion. If in doubt, have him lie on the opposite side and again percuss the level of dullness. With *massive* ascites the mesentery may be too short to permit loops of intestine to approach the abdominal wall; the entire abdomen will yield a dull or flat percussion note and no shift is demonstrable.

Ascites must be differentiated from distention due to gas (*tympanites; meteorism*), a large ovarian cyst or obesity. With tympanites there may be tremendous distention but the percussion note will be tympanitic over the entire abdomen. A large ovarian cyst may transmit an impulse much like the fluid wave of ascites. However, the intestines are displaced laterally and backward; instead of dullness in the flanks the note will be tympanitic, and no coronal tympany will be demonstrable. Extreme obesity may be very difficult to differentiate from ascites, but in general, if the person is not in circulatory failure, ascites is not commonly seen in an obese person; most of the conditions that produce it are essentially wasting diseases. Abdominal x-rays may be of some assistance in such cases.

Ballottement. It is often important to know whether the liver or other organs are enlarged and if there are masses lurking under the fluid. With massive ascites the usual methods of examination may be of little value; the various structures glide away from the palpating hand. In such cases ballottement may be helpful. The fingers are kept fully extended and jabbed in toward the organ or area being examined. Momentarily a firm structure may be felt, quite unlike the surrounding fluid; then it bobs away. If this can be demonstrated more than once it is justifiable to conclude that some solid organ is present in that area.

Another method uses both hands, as in palpating for the liver or spleen. A sudden thrust by the hand held posteriorly may bounce the organ up against the anterior abdominal wall.

HERNIA

A hernia is a protrusion of a loop of bowel or portion of an organ or tissue through an abnormal opening. Those hernias that can be iden-

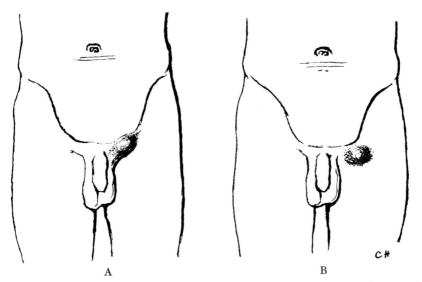

Fig. 205. *A*, Inguinal and *B*, femoral hernias, compared. Note that the femoral hernia is placed more laterally. (After Bailey, H.: Physical Signs in Clinical Surgery. 12th ed. Bristol, John Wright & Sons, Ltd., 1954.)

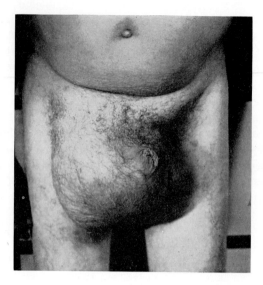

Fig. 206. Large incarcerated right inguinal hernia.

tified by inspection and palpation of the abdomen are inguinal, femoral, umbilical or ventral, depending upon the site of the defect.

Inguinal Hernia. This is by far the most common type, especially in males; the right side is afflicted more often than the left. The hernia may be either direct or indirect. A direct inguinal hernia protrudes through the abdominal wall at a point mesial to the deep epigastric artery and bulges out at the external inguinal ring. A direct hernia as a rule is not very large and does not enter the scrotum. An indirect inguinal hernia may be complete or incomplete. A complete hernia passes through the internal ring, traverses the inguinal canal anterior to the deep epigastric artery and emerges through the external ring. It may then extend downward into the scrotum (scrotal hernia). An incomplete indirect inguinal hernia is one that has not emerged through the external ring, but lies in the inguinal canal.

Femoral Hernia. This extends into the femoral canal mesial to the vessels and presents on the anteromedial surface of the thigh just below Poupart's ligament. A woman is more liable to develop a femoral hernia than an inguinal one.

Umbilical Hernia. A congenital umbilical hernia is a fairly common finding in infants; this usually disappears spontaneously during the first few years of life. In an adult with an acquired umbilical hernia the opening is usually paraumbilical, just below or above the umbilicus. A huge herniation may also develop from pressure of ascitic fluid.

Ventral Hernia. This hernia protrudes through a weak spot in the abdominal wall; the most common sites are through the linea alba and laterally along the linea semilunaris. A small epigastric hernia that contains only peritoneal fat or omentum (*epiplocele*) may give rise to periodic or persistent pain that may simulate abdominal disease. An incisional hernia results from weakness of the abdominal wall following operation, especially if prolonged drainage was required, or healing was otherwise delayed. The sac tends to be adherent to the scar; it may reach considerable size.

Although the hernial sac commonly contains loops of small intestine, other tissues may be present such as peritoneal fat, omentum, cecum, sigmoid colon or an ovary. If the contents of the sac can be slipped back into the abdomen the hernia is reducible; if not, it is irreducible or incarcerated (Fig. 206). If circulation to the tissues is impaired, congestion, edema or gangrene may follow (*strangulation*); signs of intestinal obstruction will appear if the sac contains a loop of bowel.

Procedure. It is sometimes easier to see a hernia than to feel it; coughing or straining will produce a sudden increase in the size of the mass, or a bulge where there was none before. Often it will not be

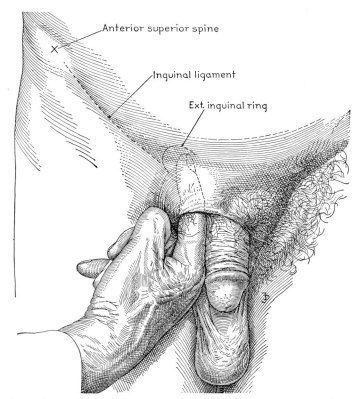

Fig. 207. Technique of invagination of the scrotum to permit thorough palpation of the inguinal canal. (Dunphy, J. E., and Botsford, T. W.: Physical Examination of the Surgical Patient. 3rd ed. Philadelphia, W. B. Saunders Co., 1964.)

seen except at such time if the patient is recumbent; the structures drop back into the abdomen. Whenever possible the patient should be examined recumbent and erect, and an attempt should be made to determine the site and the size of the opening.

To palpate for a small or incomplete inguinal hernia in a man, pick up a fold of skin on the right side of the scrotum with the little finger and invaginate this upward along the spermatic cord until the finger reaches the external ring (Fig. 207). A rough approximation of the size of the ring can be made; often the finger can enter this orifice. Then the patient should bear down or cough. With an indirect inguinal hernia the cough impulse will be felt as pressure against the fingertip; a direct inguinal hernia will press against the side of the finger. When a large hernia is present it is often possible to insert the finger through the external ring and up the inguinal canal, and thus determine the size of the internal ring. The left side is then examined in the same manner.

In women the inguinal canals are much smaller and contain only the round ligaments. A hernia is usually small; in rare instances it may extend down into the labium majus.

Other Hernias.   Herniation may occur upward through the diaphragm, especially at the esophageal hiatus (hiatal hernia). This may give rise to vague symptoms attributed to cardiac or gastrointestinal disease. Intra-abdominal herniation may also occur through other normal or acquired openings such as the duodenojejunal recess (Treitz's[10] hernia) or the foramen of Winslow.[11] X-ray and other studies are needed to establish the presence of such lesions.

[10] Wenzel Treitz, Austrian physician, 1819–72.
[11] Jakob Benignus Winslow, Danish anatomist working in Paris, 1669–1760.

XVII

The Male Genitalia

Inspection and palpation are the two procedures used in the routine examination of the male genitalia; endoscopic, radiologic and various laboratory studies are useful in confirming or supplementing the initial observations. Inspection should not be limited to the genitalia alone; it should include such things as the amount and distribution of the pubic hair or the presence of dermatophytosis of the skin of the upper thigh adjacent to the scrotum.

THE PENIS

Size and Development

During infancy and childhood the genitalia grow very slowly. At puberty there should be a rapid increase in size, as production of androgenic hormone begins. In an adult the average length of the penis is about 15 cm. when flaccid, but many variations occur. The size bears no constant relation to the size or habitus of the individual.

Hypogonadism. If for any reason testicular development is completely lacking, or if castration is performed before the age of puberty, there will be little or no development of the genitalia or of the secondary sexual characteristics. Frölich's syndrome (p. 39) is one example of this. If there is partial or incomplete development of the testes at puberty, masculinization will be roughly proportional to the amount of functioning tissue. Orchiectomy or total destruction of the testes after puberty results in a gradual decrease in the secondary sexual characteristics but libido and potentia may persist for some time.

Hypogonadism is also classified as primary or secondary. The primary form is usually due to a destructive disease such as mumps, tuberculosis or syphilis, or to severe trauma. It is also seen with unde-

317

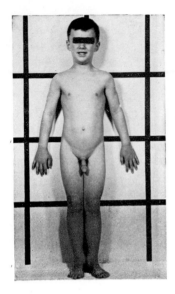

Fig. 208. Probable adrenogenital syndrome in a child 3 years and 11 months old. Note size of penis and pubic hair. Urinary 17-ketosteroid excretion, 16 mg. per 24 hours (normal for adult male). (Courtesy of Dr. Fred Harvie.)

scended testes or following surgical castration. The secondary form is generally due to a deficiency of anterior pituitary gonadotropic hormone; occasionally it accompanies severe hypothyroidism. The testes may be capable of development but the stimulus is lacking, or they may develop initially and then undergo involution.

Hypergonadism. This results from premature or excessive stimulation of the testes by gonadotropic hormones. A disturbance of pituitary function or a lesion in the suprasellar region is usually responsible; in rare instances it is attributable to an adrenocortical masculinizing tumor (Fig. 208). There is precocious development of the genitalia, with deepening of the voice, increased muscular development and hirsutism of the male type.

Congenital Anomalies

Hypospadias. In this congenital malformation the urethral opening is on the under side of a short penis at some point along the course of the anterior urethra.

Epispadias. In this rare condition the urethra opens on the dorsum of the penis; it is often accompanied by exstrophy of the bladder.

Lesions of the Penis

Phimosis. A very small orifice or the presence of adhesions between the prepuce and glans prevents retraction of the foreskin. Inadequate cleansing may lead to infection of the glans (*balanitis*). Whenever possible, the prepuce must be completely retracted to permit adequate inspection of the entire organ.

Paraphimosis.   This develops when a tight or inflamed prepuce is retracted and becomes caught behind the corona. This constriction leads to edema of the glans and compromises its blood supply; prompt surgical intervention is usually required.

Urethritis.   Gonorrhea is the most common cause; a number of other organisms may also invade the urethra. If no pus is seen at the meatus, gentle stripping of the urethra from the base to the glans may produce secretions for bacteriologic study.

Syphilis.   The penis is the most common site for a primary syphilitic lesion (chancre). There is a painless, indurated, shallow, indolent ulcer with a sharply defined border, covered with a small amount of serous exudate. Slow painless enlargement of the inguinal lymph nodes occurs later. When the chancre heals, only a small thin scar may remain. Demonstration of *Treponema pallidum* is required to confirm the diagnosis of syphilis. Since the introduction of systemic antimicrobial agents, medication given for some other infection may alter the development of the chancre; more extensive laboratory studies are then needed to prove or disprove the presence of syphilis.

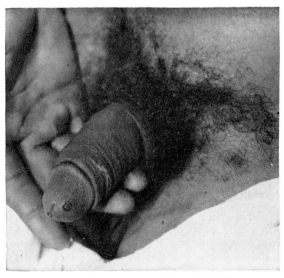

Fig. 209.   Primary syphilis demonstrated by darkfield examination. The lesion on the glans is relatively insignificant, but there is a firm satellite lymph node. (Cecil, R. L., and Conn, H. F.: The Specialties in General Practice. 3rd ed. Philadelphia, W. B. Saunders Co., 1964.)

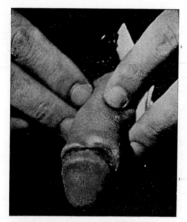

Fig. 210. Highly characteristic induration of the prepuce (double chancre). On drawing back the foreskin, this induration "flops" back in almost diagnostic fashion. (Stokes, H. J., Beerman, H., and Ingraham, N. R., Jr.: Modern Clinical Syphilology. 3rd ed. Philadelphia, W. B. Saunders Co., 1944.)

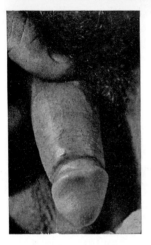

Fig. 211. Slightly scaling papule with faint induration—all there was to this patient's chancre. Such lesions, if they attract the patient's attention at all, are usually interpreted as "chafes" or "hair cuts." The induration is barely perceptible. Such lesions may also follow the application of irritants to slight abrasions. (Stokes, H. J., Beerman, H., and Ingraham, N. R., Jr.: Modern Clinical Syphilology. 3rd ed. Philadelphia, W. B. Saunders Co., 1944.)

Chancroid.   This is sometimes called a soft chancre, as opposed to the hard (indurated) syphilitic lesion. It is a localized venereal disease caused by *Haemophilus ducreyi*.[1] Superficial or deep irregular painful ulcers develop; purulent material may cover the base. The inguinal lymph nodes become enlarged and tender, and may suppurate. Chancre and chancroid can develop simultaneously from a single exposure or repeated exposures; syphilis must always be ruled out even though *H. ducreyi* has been found in the ulcer.

Lymphogranuloma Venereum.   This virus disease is also known as *lymphogranuloma inguinale, lymphopathia venereum* and *climatic bubo*. Small vesicles or shallow painless ulcers first appear; these may be overlooked, ignored or considered to be a "hair cut." Later the regional lymph nodes enlarge and are painful; if they suppurate they tend to heal spontaneously. In women especially there may be involve-

[1] Augusto Ducrey, Italian dermatologist, 1860–1940.

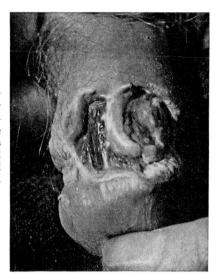

Fig. 212. Chancroid, proved by absence of spirochetes, positive Ducrey streptobacillus smear and negative follow-up for syphilis. There is a gangrenous type of chancre which may closely simulate this lesion. (Stokes, H. J., Beerman, H., and Ingraham, N. R., Jr.: Modern Clinical Syphilology. 3rd ed. Philadelphia, W. B. Saunders Co., 1944.)

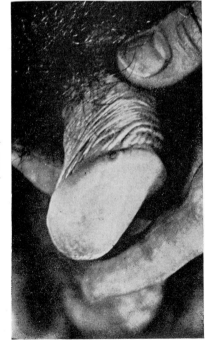

Fig. 213. Primary lesion of lymphogranuloma venereum. (Stokes, H. J., Beerman, H., and Ingraham, N. R., Jr.: Modern Clinical Syphilology. 3rd ed. Philadelphia, W. B. Saunders Co., 1944.)

ment of the perirectal structures leading to stricture formation; in men, elephantiasis of the genitalia has been reported.

Granuloma Inguinale.   Known also as *granuloma venereum,* this disease is caused by *Donovania granulomatis*—the Donovan[2] body. A sharply defined papule develops on the penis, scrotum or adjacent skin surface; later this becomes an indolent ulcer that slowly enlarges. Healing may occur at one point while ulceration progresses at another. The inguinal lymph nodes may be slightly enlarged but do not ulcerate.

Condyloma Acuminatum (Venereal Wart).   These benign papillomatous overgrowths of tissue occur on the glans, the prepuce, the scrotum and in the perianal area. They are usually associated with poor hygiene.

Carcinoma.   The glans, coronal sulcus and prepuce are the three common sites of epidermoid carcinoma; circumcision performed early in life seems to prevent this. Much less frequently the shaft of the penis is involved. Epidermoid carcinoma begins as a thickened area which gradually enlarges and may ulcerate; biopsy is necessary to differentiate such an ulcer from chancre, chancroid or other ulcerating lesions. The inguinal nodes become involved later; they are firm or hard but rarely suppurate unless infection is superimposed.

THE SCROTUM AND TESTES

Size and Development

During infancy and childhood the scrotum and the testes are very small; at puberty there is a rapid increase in size. A normal testis in an adult is a slightly flattened ellipsoid structure with average measurements of 4 to 5 cm. in length, 2.5 to 3 cm. in breadth and 2 cm. in thickness; considerable variation in size may be physiologic.

The scrotum is a pear-shaped sac with a median furrow and partition; the left side is usually larger than the right. Transversely curved folds of muscle and skin permit it to expand or contract with changes of temperature or from other stimuli. The skin is more deeply pigmented than that of adjacent areas. Local warmth, moisture and friction may result in maceration, or render the skin susceptible to fungus infection or eczematoid changes. Sebaceous cysts are prone to develop here, and also small hemangiomas which are frequently seen in association with "caviar tongue" (p. 106).

---

[2] Charles Donovan, Irish physician who spent many years in India; born 1863. The Donovan body should not be confused with Leishman-Donovan bodies, the cause of kala-azar. These were jointly described with Sir William Boss Leishman, British Army surgeon who also worked in India, 1865–1926.

Edema of the scrotum may be tremendous in circulatory failure or other diseases leading to anasarca, or following trauma. The penis may be engulfed by the massive scrotum, or if the penis also is edematous the meatus may be almost invisible.

Palpation

This is performed with the thumb and fingers. A normal testis is smooth, firm, resilient and freely movable within the scrotum. Compression produces a typical sickening pain unless sensation has been lost; this may occur with tabes dorsalis or other neurologic diseases.

Anatomically, the epididymis is a highly convoluted portion of the spermatic duct. It is composed of the enlarged upper pole (globus major), the body and the lower pole or globus minor. It is softer in consistency than a normal testis, but it should be palpable over the upper and lower poles of the testis and along the posterolateral border.

The spermatic cord should be palpated from the upper pole of the testis to the external inguinal ring. It is a soft, somewhat irregular structure within which you should be able to feel the much firmer vas deferens.

Two testes of approximately the same size and consistency should be present in the scotum. If there is a marked difference in size or in consistency the cause for this should be determined. If only one can be located, the other may never have entered the scrotum or it may have been removed surgically.

Congenital Anomalies

Cryptorchidism. Early in fetal life the testes are intra-abdominal; they should descend through the inguinal canals and down into the scrotum shortly before birth. If for any reason one or both of the testes fail to descend, it may cause trouble later. Often the testis is palpable in the inguinal canal; such a testis may descend normally at puberty. At times the testis never reaches the internal ring; such an abdominal testis is more prone to become malignant than is a normally situated one

Lesions

The epididymis is the most common site of infection (*epididymitis*); the testis may also be involved (*orchitis*). This can be due to mumps or other systemic infection; tuberculosis and syphilitic infection still occur occasionally. More commonly it is a result of untreated or inadequately treated gonorrhea.

Enlargement of one testis is usually due to a neoplastic lesion; the gland becomes firm or hard and may be irregular or nodular in outline.

Atrophy, either unilateral or bilateral, may follow postpubertal mumps orchitis; it can also result from impairment of circulation following inguinal herniorraphy or from direct trauma. Hepatic cirrhosis and certain abnormalities of other endocrine glands may also result in atrophy. In later life the testes gradually approach retirement and become smaller and softer.

Hydrocele.   This is an accumulation of fluid in the tunica vaginalis of the testis; it may be congenital or acquired. The latter may develop rapidly after trauma or infection, but in most instances it develops slowly and for no demonstrable reason. A hydrocele is translucent unless the fluid is very purulent or bloody or unless marked thickening of the tunica has occurred. In a suitably darkened area (or under a blanket) hold a flashlight behind that side of the scrotum; you should see a pink glow with a dark area (the testis) within it. This must not be confused with a loop of bowel that has entered the scrotum.

Varicocele.   This denotes enlargement and tortuosity of the veins of the left pampiniform plexus; it rarely develops on the right side. It is most easily visible and palpable with the patient erect; when he is recumbent the veins tend to empty. The left side of the scrotum will be considerably larger than the right, and a mass of wormlike veins will be felt. In rare instances varicocele is due to compression or invasion of the renal or spermatic vein; ordinarily it has no medical significance but may produce a dull ache or dragging sensation locally.

Hernia.   An inguinal hernia can gradually force its way down the canal and eventually appear in the scrotum, where it may be mistaken for a hydrocele, varicocele or other local lesion (see Fig. 206, p. 314). With the patient recumbent, the loop of bowel can usually be restored to its normal intra-abdominal site; the presence of peristaltic sounds or of tympany on percussion may also aid in the differential diagnosis.

THE PROSTATE AND SEMINAL VESICLES

Physiologically these constitute a part of the male genital system; however, digital examination of these structures will be discussed as a part of the rectal examination (p. 350).

XVIII

The Female Genitalia

Pelvic examination is performed to determine the presence of abnormalities of the female genital tract. It consists of two procedures: inspection and palpation. Because certain laboratory tests are frequently initiated at the time of the examination they will also be described briefly.

The history is often an extremely important factor in gynecologic diagnosis; coupled with the findings on pelvic examination it may direct specific diagnostic and therapeutic measures when physical findings alone would have been inconclusive.

Preparation of the Patient.   The patient should void before the examination. If vaginal discharge is a problem, she should not have douched during the preceding 24 hours. A nurse or other female assistant should prepare the patient and remain in attendance; if this is impossible the mother, husband, a relative or a friend may be used as a substitute to afford legal protection to the examining physician.

Position of the Patient.   The lithotomy position is the one most frequently used. The patient lies on her back with her thighs and legs flexed and abducted; whenever possible the legs or feet are supported in stirrups (Fig. 214). For Sims'[1] position the patient ordinarily lies on her left side with her left arm and hand behind her (Fig. 215). The left thigh is flexed moderately for comfort; the right thigh is acutely flexed and the right knee rests on the table. The knee-chest position can also be used (Fig. 216). This has the advantage that as the labia are separated the vagina fills with air; an unobstructed view of the vagina and cervix is obtained.

THE EXTERNAL GENITALIA

With the patient's thighs adequately abducted, inspect the mons

[1] J. Marion Sims, New York gynecologist, 1813–83.

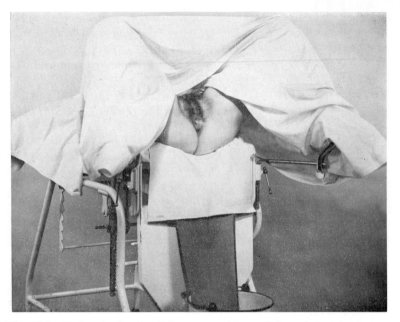

Fig. 214.   Patient in the dorsolithotomy position and draped for examination.

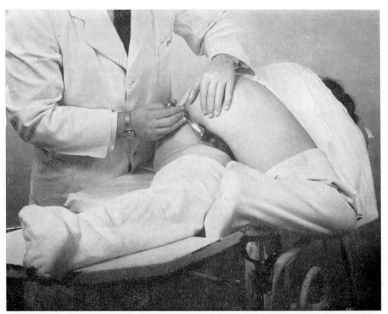

Fig. 215.   Patient in Sims' position. Notice that the right thigh is flexed; the left thigh is almost straight.

veneris, the labia majora and minora, the clitoris, Bartholin's[2] glands, the perineal body, the fourchette and the vestibule. With the labia separated, the urethral meatus, the hymen and the introitus can be seen.

Mons Veneris.   This is a subcutaneous fat pad lying over the symphysis pubis and usually partially concealed by a thick growth of hair. Note the distribution, amount and texture of the hair, the presence of any skin lesions and the amount of subcutaneous fat; then confirm these findings by palpation.

Labia Majora.   The labia majora, located on either side of the introitus, extend from the mons anteriorly to the perineal body posteriorly. They are folds of fatty tissue covered by integument containing numerous hair follicles and sebaceous glands. Visible or palpable swelling or a mass may be due to hernia or hydrocele of the canal of Nuck,[3] trauma (hematoma) or edema. An ulcer may indicate the presence of carcinoma, chancroid, syphilis, granuloma inguinale or other infection.

Labia Minora (Nymphae).   When the labia majora are separated, the labia minora are seen; they are covered with more delicate pink hairless skin. Anteriorly each labium divides into a lateral and a medial portion. The lateral divisions unite above the clitoris to form the prepuce; the medial limbs join below the clitoris and form its

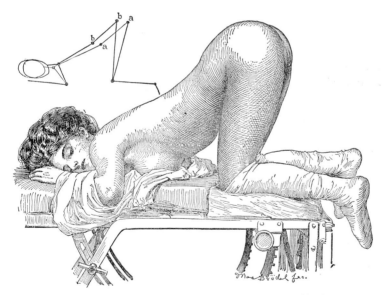

Fig. 216.   The knee-chest position. This position is invaluable for examining the bladder and uterus, the vagina and its contents and also the rectum. (Wharton, L. R.: Gynecology. 2nd ed. Philadelphia, W. B. Saunders Co., 1947.)

[2] Caspar Bartholin, Jr., Danish anatomist, 1655–1738.
[3] Anton Nuck, Dutch anatomist, 1650–92.

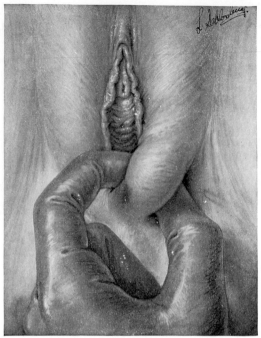

Fig. 217.   Palpation of the left Bartholin gland to determine whether there is thickening or tenderness, or whether pus can be expressed from it. (Wharton, L. R.: Gynecology. 2nd ed. Philadelphia, W. B. Saunders Co., 1947.)

frenum. Posteriorly the labia minora merge with the labia majora to form the fourchette. Abnormalities of the labia minora are rare but infection or malignant changes can occur.

Clitoris.   The clitoris, located below the mons at the apex of the merging labia minora, is a firm cord of erectile tissue about 5 mm. in diameter and 2 to 2.5 cm. long. Tenderness or abnormal fixation of the prepuce should be determined. Hypertophy of the clitoris is found with certain endocrine disturbances or may occasionally be due to masturbation. An ulcer of the clitoris must be considered malignant until that possibility has been eliminated.

Bartholin's Glands.   These lie beneath the fascia of the lower third of the vagina; their ducts open just lateral to the vaginal introitus at the lower pole of the labia minora. Normally they are neither visible nor palpable but compression of that area may express a tiny drop of clear mucus from the duct. When inflamed, the gland enlarges and may be tender and fluctuant (Fig. 217). The opening of its duct becomes unusually prominent and reddened, and purulent material may exude or be expressed from the orifice of the duct.

Perineal Body.   This is the wedge of soft tissue covered by hairless skin that lies between the rectum and the distal vagina. In nulliparous women the skin is thin, pink and soft; in parous women it is scarred by healed lacerations. Such tears incurred during parturition frequently shorten the perineal body, decrease its tone, result in separation of the lower portion of the labia and produce a gaping introitus. If the laceration involves only the mucosa and superficial tissues of the perineal body (first-degree laceration) it is unimportant. A second-degree laceration involves the fascia and superficial muscles; this weakens the support of the genital tract and may give rise to a "heavy" sensation or chronic pain. A third-degree laceration involves the rectal sphincter and usually results in poor bowel control or fecal incontinence.

Vestibule. The vestibule, the elliptical entrance to the vagina itself, lies between the labia minora; it contains the external opening of the urethra and the hymen or the remnants thereof.

Urethral Meatus. This is directly below the clitoris; normally it is 2 to 3 mm. in diameter, is flush with the surrounding tissues, and of the same color. Prolapse of the urethral mucosa may follow a tear incurred during childbirth; this mucosa is redder than the adjacent skin. With urethritis the meatus is red; pus may be expressed by gently stroking the urethral floor toward the meatus with the index finger (Fig.

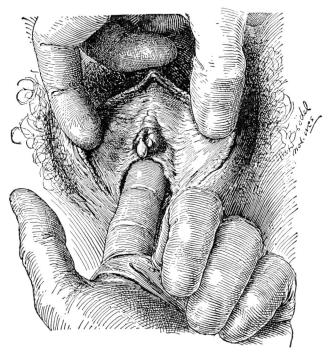

Fig. 218. Method of expressing pus from the urethra by gently stroking the index finger toward the meatus. (Wharton, L. R.: Gynecology. 2nd ed. Philadelphia, W. B. Saunders Co., 1947.)

218). Any secretions so obtained should be examined bacteriologically. A *urethral caruncle* is a bright red polypoid tumor appearing at the meatus; it is usually extremely tender and may be premalignant.

Skene's[4] glands lie in the wall of the urethra; the ducts open on the posterior wall just inside the meatus. Normally they are not visible but with atrophy of the surrounding tissues, or in the presence of infection, two pinpoint openings may be seen. Gentle pressure on one or both sides of the urethra may cause a small drop of pus to appear.

Hymen.   The hymen separates the external genitalia from the vagina. When the labia are spread apart it will be seen as a circular fold of skin and subcutaneous tissue of variable prominence and with one or more openings. In rare instances there is no opening (imperforate hymen); this can lead to complications with the onset of menstruation. The size of the hymenal orifice determines whether or not digital examination of the vagina can be done. With intercourse, the continuity of the hymen is generally destroyed; in parous women the hymenal remnants (*carunculae myrtiformes*) are seen as small individual skin tabs surrounding the introitus.

Palpation is necessary to supplement inspection. The resistance of the hymen varies from that of a piece of thin rubber to that of normal skin. Evaluation of this resistance is especially important in a premarital examination, to determine whether stretching, incision or excision of the hymen is indicated or required.

Senile Changes.   Atrophy of the vulvar structures is physiologic in the postmenopausal woman; the skin becomes dry, thin and shrunken and there is loss of subcutaneous fat. Exaggeration of these changes, with the appearance of leathery or parchment-like skin, is known as *kraurosis vulvae;* there may also be pale or white areas (leukoplakia). These changes are often considered as premalignant; the examination should be repeated at frequent intervals.

THE VAGINA AND CERVIX

Inspection

In the following discussion it will be assumed that the patient has a marital introitus; examination of a virgin requires special precautions and should rarely be undertaken.

A speculum is needed for adequate inspection of the vagina and cervix. Various types and sizes are available, but a bivalve speculum of the Graves type or some modification of this is the most popular.

[4] Alexander J. C. Skene, American gynecologist, 1838–1900.

It has become practically a routine procedure to obtain secretions for cytologic study at the time of the initial pelvic examination and at intervals thereafter (p. 341). In such cases the usual lubricant should not be used, but the speculum can be moistened with water to permit easier insertion. Separate the labia and depress the perineum with the left hand; introduce the speculum with the right hand (Fig. 219). The blades must be closed and held in an oblique position to minimize pressure on the meatus or the urethra (Fig. 220). When the instrument has been completely inserted, rotate the handle downward to the vertical position and gently open the blades (Fig. 221). The vaginal vault will be visible, and usually the cervix. When slides of the secretions have been prepared, resume inspection as you slowly withdraw the speculum.

The Cervix. The cervix is generally directed posteriorly, but in about 20 per cent of normal women it points downward or anteriorly. It may be from 2 to 4 cm. in length and 2 to 3 cm. in diameter, and is covered with squamous epithelium. During pregnancy the cervix enlarges somewhat and has a dusky cyanotic hue. With endocrine dysfunction the cervix may be small in diameter but elongated. Atrophy of variable degree occurs after the menopause.

The *external os* is a small round or slightly oval dimple in a nulli-

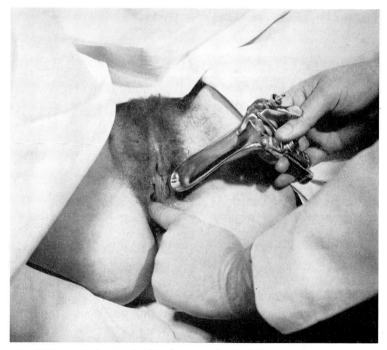

Fig. 219. Introducing the bivalve speculum. First step: Depress the perineum to give room for the speculum to be introduced.

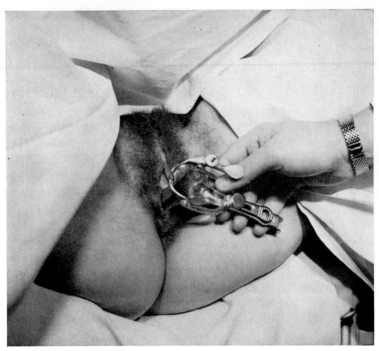

Fig. 220.   Introducing the speculum. It has been passed part way in. Notice the oblique position, which prevents pressure on the meatus.

parous woman; stretching and lacerations accompanying childbirth lead to scarring that produces a larger slitlike or irregularly stellate os.

A congenital defect may result in reduplication of the cervix, or it may be completely absent; absence may also be due to a surgical procedure.

An *erosion* is a cherry-red lesion of variable size at the external os; it is due to replacement of the normal squamous cells by an outgrowth of columnar epithelium from the cervical canal. Often it is congenital. With extensive laceration, the mucosa of the endocervix may protrude and be visible at the external os; this is known as *eversion.*

Acute infection will produce inflammatory changes in the cervix; mucopurulent discharge may exude from the os. *Nabothian*[5] *follicles* are retention cysts and suggest chronic infection; they are small raised areas a few millimeters in diameter, which appear pale or slightly blue in color.

A chancre may develop on the cervix; since it is usually asymptomatic it can give rise to one or many penile lesions.

Polyps are usually small, bright red and pedunculated; they may arise either from the exocervix or from tissues in the endocervical canal.

Carcinoma of the cervix in its early stages cannot be detected on

[5] Martin Naboth, Saxon anatomist, 1675–1721.

physical examination; only cytologic study and biopsy are of diagnostic value in the preinvasive stage (*carcinoma in situ*). A more advanced lesion may resemble a cervical erosion, or ulceration and necrosis may be present. When far advanced a large, fungating, friable mass may be present; this bleeds readily when manipulated. Cancer in the cervical canal or in the uterus itself will be completely invisible. A history of blood-tinged or bloody discharge occurring between periods or after the menopause means that cancer is the cause until that possibility has been ruled out.

The Vagina.   After the cervix has been inspected, examine the vagina as you slowly withdraw the speculum while rotating it somewhat around its long axis; this will permit visualization of all areas.

During the years of ovarian activity, the moderately distended vagina will appear as a corrugated tube with a pink, smooth and slightly glistening surface. A moderate amount of colorless or white mucus will be present. When ovarian stimulation ceases, either naturally or as a result of surgery or irradiation, there is atrophy and thinning of the vaginal wall, the rugae disappear and the secretions decrease.

Vaginitis.   Although various organisms may cause vaginitis, the two most common and most troublesome ones are *Tichomonas vaginalis*

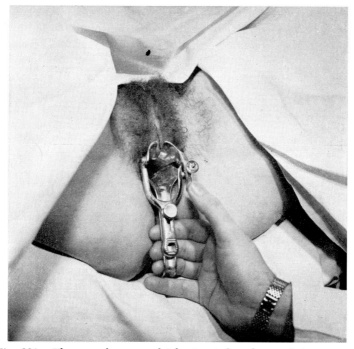

Fig. 221.   The speculum completely inserted and turned into position for opening.

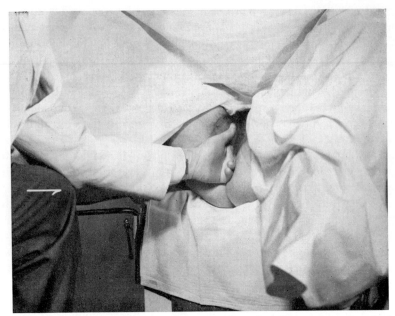

Fig. 222. Position of the examiner. Note how the elbow rests against the knee to allow complete relaxation of the examining hand.

and *Candida albicans.* Trichomonads produce a thin, watery, frothy discharge with a characteristic odor. With monilial vaginitis (*C. albicans*) the secretions are thick and contain small clumps that have been likened to particles of cottage cheese. These tend to adhere to the vaginal wall and if forcibly removed, a punctuate red spot may be seen. Monilial infection frequently involves the vulva, producing intense pruritus; it is particularly troublesome during pregnancy or in uncontrolled diabetes mellitus.

Palpation

Palpation of the internal pelvic organs is usually performed after inspection; sometimes the order is reversed. Palpation of the external genitalia has already been discussed. Ordinarily it is possible to insert two fingers without causing discomfort, but if inspection has disclosed obvious abnormalities this should be done very gently, or one finger alone may be used.

Position of the Examiner.   You may stand either in front of the patient or to one side, and use either your left hand or your right hand. If you are right-handed you will probably find it advantageous to learn to use your left hand for palpation; this leaves your more highly skilled right hand free for handling instruments. Resting the elbow on a firm support such as your iliac crest or knee will relax the arm and hand and improve perception (Fig. 222).

Procedure. The size, sensitivity and musculature of the perineal body is first determined (Fig. 223). Lacerations resulting from numerous deliveries may have reduced this to a fraction of its former size, with resulting weakness of the pelvic floor. Abnormal sensitivity, with consequent muscular spasm, may be a cause of difficult or painful intercourse (*dyspareunia*).

With deeper penetration the cervix will be encountered and the findings of inspection can be verified. You should also determine the consistency; in a normal cervix this has been described as similar to that of the tip of the nose. Pregnancy or a uterine tumor may soften the cervix; chronic inflammation or a tumor in the cervix itself may decrease its resiliency.

Mobility of the cervix should also be tested by attempting to displace it in various directions; this should be painless. If pressure in any direction is definitely painful rather than slightly or moderately uncomfortable, inflammatory disease of the uterus or adjacent structures may be present. Total immobility of the cervix (fixation) occurs with pelvic malignancy and with various inflammatory or benign processes.

After any other abnormalities noted on inspection have been pal-

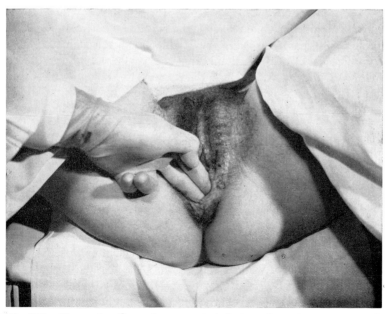

Fig. 223. Depressing the perineum posteriorly to estimate its resistance to backward pressure.

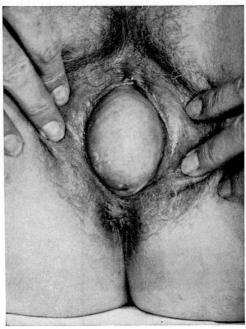

Fig. 224. A large cystocele; patient straining slightly. (Curtis, A. H., and Huffman, J. W.: Textbook of Gynecology. 6th ed. Philadelphia, W. B. Saunders Co., 1950.)

pated, the degree of relaxation of the vaginal walls should be determind. In a nullipara the walls are pliable but firm; each vaginal delivery produces a little relaxation. Press the perineal body and posterior vaginal wall downward and ask the patient to "bear down" ("cough"; "strain"; "try to move your bowels"). This increases the intra-abdominal pressure and may produce bulging of the anterior wall. Then make pressure anteriorly and repeat the maneuver to determine relaxation of the posterior vaginal wall. In doubtful cases, and especially if the patient is unable to cooperate successfully, it may be necessary to repeat this procedure with the patient standing.

Abnormal relaxation of the posterior urethral wall distal to the bladder sphincter and of the anterior vaginal wall is called a *urethrocele*. This is usually accompanied by some degree of embarrassing urinary incontinence when the patient coughs, sneezes or otherwise raises intra-abdominal pressure (stress incontinence). Relaxation of the superior portion of the anterior vaginal wall permits the bladder to bulge downward and backward (*cystocele*) (Fig. 224). Usually the two coexist (*cystourethrocele*). Relaxation of the posterior vaginal wall permits the rectum to bulge forward (*rectocele*). This must be differentiated from an *enterocele* or *cul-de-sac hernia,* which extends down into an enlarged

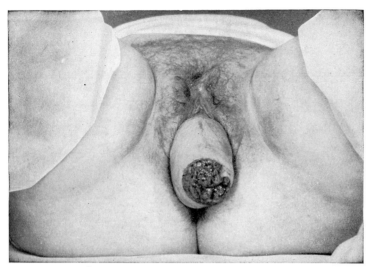

Fig. 225.   Procidentia uteri; decubitus ulcer. (Curtis, A. H., and Huffman, J. W.: Textbook of Gynecology. 6th ed. Philadelphia, W. B. Saunders Co., 1950.)

pouch of Douglas[6] between the vagina and the rectum. It can be felt high in the vagina, and can be outlined most easily by rectovaginal examination. For this, the index finger is inserted into the vagina and the middle finger into the rectum. It then becomes apparent that there is a mass lying between these two structures and separating them. Other abnormal masses may also be palpable by this procedure. A severe degree of relaxation may allow the vaginal wall to bulge through the introitus and present as a soft tumor mass outside the labia.

Descensus Uteri.   In some instances the entire uterus may slide down the vaginal canal. Relaxation of the round ligaments, which normally limit retroversion, first occurs and allows the uterus to assume a position parallel to the vagina. With loss of elasticity and tensile strength of other supporting tissues, the intra-abdominal pressure plus gravity initiate the gradual descent of the entire uterus. If the cervix presents at the introitus there is first-degree descensus; if outside the introitus, it is second-degree. When the entire uterus is outside the introitus, third-degree prolapse or procidentia uteri is present (Fig. 225).

Bimanual Examination

The right hand is now used to apply pressure to the lower abdominal wall. This will enable you to palpate and outline more accurately the pelvic organs nestling between the right hand and the gloved fingers

[6] James Douglas, Scottish anatomist who did most of his work in London, 1675–1742. His studies on the peritoneum were published in 1730.

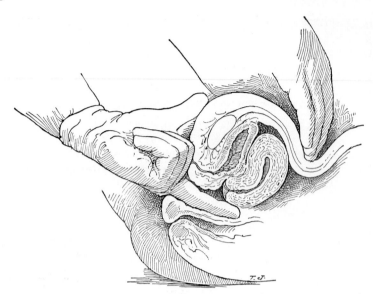

Fig. 226. Bimanual vaginal examination. Vaginal examination in infants and children is difficult and yields less information than rectal examination, which is performed in the same manner except that the examining finger of the left hand is inserted into the rectum. (Curtis, A. H., and Huffman, J. W.: Textbook of Gynecology. 6th ed. Philadelphia, W. B. Saunders Co., 1950.)

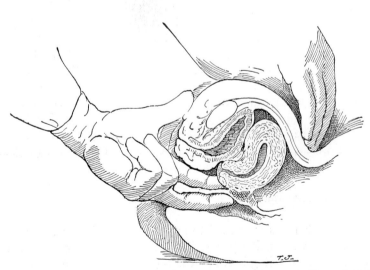

Fig. 227. Rectovagino-abdominal examination. (Curtis, A. H., and Huffman, J. W.: Textbook of Gynecology. 6th ed. Philadelphia, W. B. Saunders Co., 1950.)

in the vagina (Fig. 226). When searching for the uterus, start in the midline below the umbilicus and direct the pressure toward the lower sacral region. Gradually move your right hand toward the symphysis pubis until a mass is felt between the two hands, or until the pubic arch is reached. To examine the adnexal areas, pressure is made in the right and left lower quadrants lateral to the uterine corpus.

An alternate procedure is to put on a clean glove and insert one finger into the rectum, rather than into the vagina. This is the method of choice in some instances, and of necessity when examining a virgin or a child. To avoid upsetting or confusing the patient, you should tell her that you are now going to examine the rectum.

A third method is to insert the index finger into the vagina and the middle finger into the rectum (rectovaginal examination). This can also be combined with abdominal pressure if indicated.

The amount of information gained by either of these procedures will be roughly proportional to the amount of cooperation and the degree of muscular relaxation obtained and inversely proportional to the thickness of the abdominal wall.

THE UTERUS

Size and Shape.   At birth the uterus is about 3 cm. long; over half of this is the cervical segment. It enlarges slowly until the menarche; then there is fairly rapid growth until the adult size is reached. The normal uterus in an adult is a somewhat pear-shaped hollow muscular organ about 4 cm. broad, 2.5 cm. thick and 7 cm. long; the lower 2.5 cm. comprises the cylindrical cervical segment. After one or more pregnancies the uterus enlarges by about 1 cm. in each dimension but the cervical segment becomes relatively shorter. Postmenopausal involution produces a slow, moderate decrease in size.

Hypoplasia may result from a congenital defect or from an endocrine disorder. Enlargement of the uterus is most frequently due to pregnancy; it remains fairly smooth in outline but may be somewhat asymmetrical. Solitary or multiple benign tumors are the usual cause of enlargement of a nongravid uterus; these are usually *leiomyomas* (myomas; uterine fibroids). Carcinoma of the corpus rarely produces definitely palpable enlargement until the process is far advanced.

Position.   The cervical segment is moderately flexible and will permit the axis of the corpus to lie at an angle from the direction of the lower cervical canal. The corpus therefore may be *anteflexed* or *retroflexed* in relation to the cervix. Moreover, the entire uterus may change position and be *anteverted* or *retroverted*. Lateral displacement of any great degree is uncommon; it is usually due to pressure from a pelvic tumor or to traction by adhesions following pelvic inflammation.

The corpus is tilted forward and rests on the upper surface of the urinary bladder in about 80 per cent of women; in 20 per cent it will lie posteriorly against the rectum or in some intermediate position. Retroversion is frequently congenital; it may also follow repeated pregnancies and be due to relaxation of the supporting structures.

Motion. The normal uterus can be moved a moderate amount in any direction without producing pain. Limitation of motion may be due to acute or chronic inflammatory disease, a benign tumor or cancer. Severe pain on movement is almost invariably due to acute infection of some type.

ADNEXAE

Palpation of the fallopian[7] tubes and the ovaries should be attempted. With the external hand, make pressure on the anterolateral abdominal wall downward and toward the midline. With the intravaginal fingers, palpate the tissues between the two hands in a systematic manner. If an abnormality is felt it may be desirable to alter the position of the external hand so that the mass can be palpated by the finger tips of both hands. Each side must be examined carefully and thoroughly.

A normal fallopian tube is rarely palpable. Acute inflammation (*salpingitis*) is usually due to gonorrhea; the tube may be enlarged and very tender. The end stage may be a soft cystic mass (*hydrosalpinx*) near the lateral or posterolateral uterine wall; this may be mistaken for enlargement of the uterus. An ectopic (tubal) pregnancy will also give rise to a very tender mass lateral to the uterus; amenorrhea and other signs suggesting pregnancy may be present. Primary malignancy of the tube is rare.

A normal ovary is an elusive, somewhat flattened and slightly irregular oval structure 2 to 3 cm. in diameter; it lies from one to several centimeters lateral to the uterus. It is movable, relatively soft in consistency and slightly to moderately sensitive.

Enlargement of an ovary may be due to inflammation (*oöphoritis*) or to a benign or malignant lesion. Multiple benign cysts may develop or a solitary cyst of tremendous size; the latter is occasionally misdiagnosed as ascites. In rare instances a benign ovarian fibroma or other lesion actually does result in the development of ascites and hydrothorax (Meigs' syndrome), both of which promptly disappear when the tumor

[7] Gabriello Fallopio (also Fallopius), Italian anatomist, 1523–1562.

is removed. Neoplastic lesions may be cystic or solid; any solid ovarian tumor must be considered malignant until proved otherwise.

Endometriosis.   This is a non-neoplastic disease in which there are cysts on the peritoneum that are lined by endometrial tissue and filled with blood (chocolate cysts). They tend to increase in size and become tender with each menstrual period, and to recede with the menopause. Although histologically benign, they may become large enough to interfere mechanically with the function of the intestinal tract.

SPECIAL TESTS

Certain simple diagnostic procedures are easily performed and should constitute a part of every complete gynecologic examination. Other more complicated studies are not a part of the routine examination and are done only when indicated.

Hanging-drop Preparation.   This is used to identify trichomonads and monilia. Whenever possible the specially designed slide should be used; this has a shallow depression on one surface. If not available, an ordinary slide with coverslip can be used.

When trichomonas vaginitis is suspected, obtain secretions by aspiration or with a cotton-tipped applicator moistened with isotonic sodium chloride solution. Transfer the secretions, further diluted with the saline solution if necessary, to the coverglass and examine microscopically for the typical pear-shaped motile flagellate with an undulating membrane.

To identify monilia, dilute the secretions with a small amount of 10 per cent potassium hydroxide solution and look for mycelia and conida. Smears stained with various bacteriologic stains may be helpful if the direct smear is not diagnostic.

Bacteriology.   When purulent secretions are present, smears should be prepared and examined; Gram[8] staining is preferred. Acute infection is usually due to N. gonorrhoeae; with chronic infection a variety of organisms may be found. Culture of the secretions is also desirable for identification of these organisms; it is mandatory if there are any legal factors involved.

Exfoliative Cytology.   The desirability of preparing slides for cytologic study by the Papanicolaou[9] technique ("Pap smear") is well known to the laity; every student should know how to prepare these. A long pipet is used to aspirate secretions from the posterior fornix of the vagina. A small drop is placed on a slide and spread out so that

[8] Hans Christian Joachim Gram, Danish physician, 1853–1938.
[9] George N. Papanicolaou, Greek anatomist working in the United States, 1883–1962.

a *very thin* smear results; this is immediately placed in a special fixative solution. With a suitable spatula or other instrument secretions are scraped from the cervical os and a second slide is prepared. The staining and interpretation of these must be done by a person who has had special training in this field.

XIX

The Anus and Rectum

Although examination of the anus and rectum is of great importance, it is omitted all too frequently because of false modesty on the part of the patient or for esthetic reasons. Without it, no examination can be considered complete unless the patient is gravely ill with some disease unrelated to the gastrointestinal tract. In such cases the examination should be done at a more propitious time; an unsuspected lesion of great importance may be found in this area. Ideally, proctosigmoidoscopy should be a part of the examination of all older persons and of any person with gastrointestinal symptoms or signs, but this requires special training and many physicians lack the skill and equipment to do this in the office.

Preparation of the Patient.   No special preparation is required for the routine examination, but it is helpful if the patient can defecate so that the rectum will be empty. Occasionally it may be desirable or essential to use enemas or suppositories to insure complete evacuation.

Position of the Patient.   This may be influenced by the physical condition of the patient or by the site of some suspected lesion. To feel a mass high in the bowel it is customary to have a man stand, flex the trunk at the hips and lean over the bed, examining table or other convenient support. This position is also generally preferred for palpation of the prostate. If the patient leans forward and squats somewhat the increased intra-abdominal pressure will tend to force the colon and other structures toward the anus. For women, the knee-chest, lateral Sims or lithotomy position may be used. The latter is especially useful when bimanual palpation is to be performed. These positions have been described in the preceding chapter (p. 325).

343

INSPECTION

The Anal Region.   Look for skin lesions, scars or abnormalities of any type on the buttocks and perineum, in the gluteal cleft and in the anal region itself. Pilonidal disease occurs in the gluteal cleft, usually in a very hirsute brunet; it is much more common in males than in females. One or more draining sinuses may be present in this area, or there may be infection with the characteristic signs of inflammation. An anal fistula ordinarily opens in the perianal region. Sebaceous cysts, condyloma acuminata, leukoplakia and syphilitic condylomas (*condyloma lata*) may also develop here.

Excoriated macerated skin is often seen with *pruritus ani;* it may be secondary to disease in the anal canal or to redundant folds of skin at the anal margin (skin tags), which are difficult to keep clean. The latter commonly represent the end stage of thrombosed small external hemorrhoids. Fungus infection also occurs here. Occasionally the skin is abnormally dry and may have superficial fissures.

An external hemorrhoid may not be conspicuous or even noticed unless the patient strains or "bears down." If thrombosis occurs, a very tender, glistening, edematous, bluish mass will be seen at the anus. Internal hemorrhoids may also protude after defecation or with straining; there may be a single vessel or a cluster of them. With gentle pressure these dilated veins again enter the anal canal unless they become thrombosed.

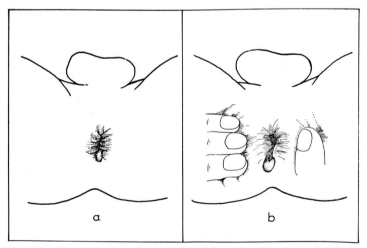

Fig. 228.   Demonstration of a typical anal fissure. *a,* "Sentinel pile." *b,* By gently separating the anal verge the fissure marked by the externally presenting nubbin of edematous skin is readily brought into view. (Child in Cecil, R. L., and Conn, H. F.: The Specialities in General Practice. 3rd ed. Philadelphia, W. B. Saunders Co., 1964.)

An edematous tag of skin (*sentinel pile*) may be present, usually in the midline and posteriorly (Fig. 228). This marks the outer limit of an anal fissure, which can be visualized as a longitudinal slit in the anal wall if the buttocks are spread apart as the patient strains. A fistula is painful; injudicious palpation may cause spasm of the sphincter muscles and aggravate the pain.

Occasionally there may be prolapse of hypertrophied anal papillae, of the rectal mucosa or even the entire wall of the rectum; the latter two can be recognized by the circumferential folds of the mucous membrane. These conditions usually require surgical correction.

PALPATION

Before you start the digital examination, explain to the patient what you are going to do. Lubricate the gloved index finger and make gentle pressure on the anus. Not infrequently this will produce reflex contraction of the corrugator cutis ani and of the sphincter muscles; wait until this relaxes or ask the patient to bear down slightly. Then insert the finger slowly, rotating it so that all areas of the anal canal are palpated, but avoid unnecessary pressure on any sensitive spot. When full penetration has been achieved and the finger is in the rectum, flex it slightly to bring it in contact with the wall of the rectum, then partially withdraw it. Rotate the hand somewhat and repeat this stroking movement until you have palpated the anterior, posterior and both lateral walls and the adjacent structures. After withdrawing the finger, examine any fecal material clinging to the glove and perform a guaiac test on it for occult blood.

The Anal Canal

In an adult, the anal canal is about 2.5 cm. long. The first centimeter is covered with skin and is encircled by the external sphincter muscle. This portion is supplied by nerves from the sacral plexus; any disease in this area will be very painful and may result in referred pain with wide radiation. A slight depression can often be felt just above the external sphincter; this anorectal groove (*pectinate line; white line*) marks the division between the external and internal hemorrhoidal veins and the nerve supply. Above this the innervation comes mainly from the sympathetics; lesions of the upper portion of the anal canal or of the rectum produce little or no pain. In this area the mucosa contains a

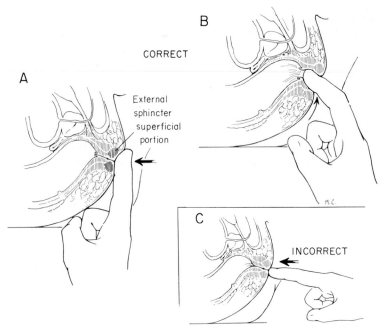

Fig. 229. *A,* Before introducing the finger into the anal canal, the sphincter should be relaxed by gentle pressure with the palmar surface of the fingertip. *B,* The finger is then inserted into the anal canal. *C,* Incorrect method of anal digital examination. (Dunphy, J. E., and Botsford, T. W.: Physical Examination of the Surgical Patient. 3rd ed. Philadelphia, W. B. Saunders Co., 1964.)

number of vertical folds (*columns of Morgagni*[1]) with small semicircular valve-like folds connecting the bases of these columns; these cups (anal crypts) tend to collect feces and become infected. The upper limit of the anal canal is easily recognized laterally and posteriorly; the finger slips through the constricting components of the levator ani muscle and enters the capacious rectum.

Spasm of the sphincter muscle is not uncommon and is usually of psychogenic origin; occasionally it is due to an inflammatory lesion such as a fissure. A stricture may be present due to scar formation resulting from a surgical procedure, trauma or an infection such as lymphogranuloma venereum or colitis. Fibrosis of the sphincter muscles in the elderly may constrict the anal canal and can be a factor in producing bowel disturbances, fecal retention and impaction. A neoplasm of the anus can produce partial obstruction; a mass should be palpable in the wall and extending to the underlying tissues.

[1] Giovanni Battista Morgagni, Italian anatomist and pathologist, 1682–1771. Considered the founder of pathologic anatomy, his work was not published until he was 79.

Abnormal relaxation of the muscles results in a patulous sphincter. This suggests neurologic disease when it cannot be attributed to some trauma; in women, such relaxation is usually due to parturition.

The Rectum

The rectum is a tube, largely extraperitoneal, about 12.5 cm. in length; when distended it may be 6 cm. or more in diameter. It is somewhat sacculated in outline; the lowest portion is called the rectal ampulla. These saccules are produced by the rectal valves, usually 2 or 3 in number. These are folds in the wall, about 2.5 cm. apart, each of which runs somewhat more than half way around the bowel. They project like transverse shelves into the lumen when it is distended, alternately on the left and right, but sag down when the rectum is empty.

ANAL AND RECTAL LESIONS

Hemorrhoids.   External hemorrhoids develop in the veins below the pectinate line; they can usually be diagnosed by inspection. Internal

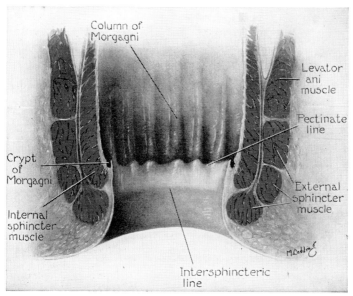

Fig. 230.   Relationship of muscles to anal and rectal mucosa. (Dunphy, J. E., and Botsford, T. W.: Physical Examination of the Surgical Patient. 3rd ed. Philadelphia, W. B. Saunders Co., 1964.)

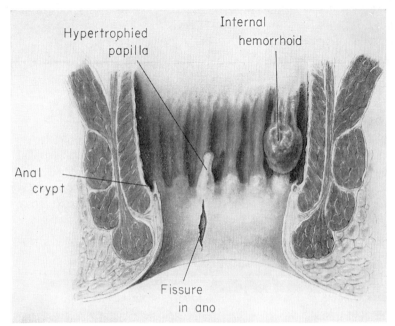

Hypertrophied papilla

Internal hemorrhoid

Anal crypt

Fissure in ano

Fig. 231. Composite drawing of some common anorectal lesions. (Dunphy, J. E., and Botsford, T. W.: Physical Examination of the Surgical Patient. 3rd ed. Philadelphia, W. B. Saunders Co., 1964.)

hemorrhoids arise higher in the canal; unless prolapsed, they are not visible. They are sometimes palpable as thickened longitudinal folds bulging into the anal canal that seem to disappear on pressure and enlarge if the patient strains. Anoscopic examination is usually necessary to differentiate these from the normal columns of Morgagni, or from hypertrophy or infection of these. Internal hemorrhoids may result from direct interference with the circulation by conditions such as pregnancy, ovarian or prostatic enlargement or chronic constipation. Indirectly they may be produced by increased pressure in the veins resulting from unrelated disease elsewhere such as cardiac failure, or from intermittent pressure accompanying chronic cough or repeated lifting of heavy objects. They may also result from chronic irritation, infection or congestion of the anal wall.

Internal hemorrhoids are more prone to bleed than are the external type. Slight bleeding, if it persists for months, can produce anemia of moderate severity. With severe bleeding the person usually sees his doctor promptly.

Anal Fistula (Fistula in Ano).   Infection of the anal wall spreads to the perianal region, then tends to open back into the anal canal or through the skin near the anus. If an opening is present in the skin of the posterior half of the anal region, look again; one often finds two or more openings in such cases. The internal orifice may be palpable as a small firm nodule projecting slightly into the lumen; induration of the surrounding tissues can sometimes be felt if the area is gently palpated between the thumb externally and the index finger in the canal.

Ischiorectal Abscess.   This is produced by infection that spreads outward from the anus or rectum and does not open externally. A bulge may be felt by thumb-and-finger palpation; tenderness and pain on defecation accompanied by fever and other constitutional symptoms will be present.

Anal Polyp.   A small nodule may be palpable at or near the upper margin of the anal canal. This probably represents the end-stage of a thrombosed internal hemorrhoid, with fibrosis and organization.

In the rectum, a variable amount of fecal material may be felt. This may be soft, firm, scybalous or a single massive concretion (fecal impaction). The latter is not uncommon in elderly or bedridden patients, or after the administration of various drugs that interfere with peristalsis; sometimes it is composed largely of barium sulfate given for gastrointestinal radiography. Foreign bodies of various sizes and shapes may also be found. Stricture or stenosis can follow infection of any type; lymphogranuloma venereum is a common cause. An adenomatous *polyp* may be sessile or pedunculated; the latter is freely movable and is easily mistaken for feces. Sometimes numerous polyps are present; malignant degeneration may occur in these. Carcinoma of the rectum usually develops within reach of the examining finger; it may be a localized elevated nodule or it may encircle the entire rectum. Other submucous tumors occasionally develop and are more easily felt than seen. Any abnormally firm or hard area in the rectal wall calls for further study.

PERIRECTAL LESIONS

Pelvic or intraperitoneal disease unrelated to the rectum can sometimes be suspected or diagnosed by palpation. Tenderness high in the rectum may be due to appendicitis if on the right, diverticulitis of the colon on the left, or pelvic inflammatory disease of some other type. Abdominal carcinoma or endometriosis may produce a nodular ridge anteriorly at the site of reflection of the peritoneum (Blumer's shelf). Thickening or induration of the broad ligaments may also be palpable, as well as other abnormalities of the female pelvic organs.

ANOSCOPY AND PROCTOSIGMOIDOSCOPY

One or both of these procedures should be done whenever any abnormality of the anal canal or rectum has been discovered on inspection or palpation, or when there is a history of change in bowel habits or of rectal bleeding. Over half of all carcinomas of the large bowel develop within the area visible through the standard 25 cm. sigmoidoscope. Direct inspection and biopsy of any suspicious area is the most accurate diagnostic procedure; radiographic studies are of limited value in this area, especially if the lesion is small. However, these procedures do not constitute a part of the routine physical examination; the details will not be discussed here.

PROSTATE AND SEMINAL VESICLES

Anatomically the prostate is an appendage of the urinary tract; physiologically it is concerned with procreation. For practical reasons it is first examined by palpation through the wall of the rectum; cystoscopy and other procedures may be needed for definitive diagnosis of prostatic lesions.

The Prostate

Size and Shape.   The prostate is roughly conical in shape, with its apex down and the base upward against the surface of the bladder. It is traversed by the urethra and penetrated by the ejaculatory ducts as they open into the urethra. The posterior surface lies close to the rectum just above the anal canal, and is easily felt. The size is variable; average dimensions for a young adult would be 2.5 to 3.5 cm. from apex to base and 3.5 to 4.5 cm. transversely at the broadest point.

On palpation, two symmetrical lateral lobes separated by a median furrow should be obvious. The outline is smooth and regular; the consistency is firm yet somewhat resilient. The entire prostate can be displaced a short distance laterally or anteriorly by pressure. The median lobe cannot be felt by rectal examination.

Alterations in Size.   Hypoplasia of the prostate is present in endocrine disturbances that delay or restrict general sexual development. In a normal male, *benign prostatic hypertrophy* of variable degree occurs with advancing age. If only the lateral lobes are involved the consequence may not be serious unless they become huge enough to bulge into the rectum and interfere with defecation. When the middle lobe is involved, as it frequently is, an increasing degree of urethral obstruction develops. Difficulty in starting or stopping the urinary flow, a small feeble stream or dribbling and incontinence from overdistention of the bladder are common symptoms. Increased pressure in the bladder can produce changes in the bladder wall, the ureters, the renal pelves and eventually in the renal parenchyma.

Prostatitis. With acute prostatitis the gland is enlarged, tender and softer than normal. There is pain on urination, and often on defecation. Purulent secretions may be obtained by *gently* stroking each lateral lobe from the upper outer portion downward toward the midline. With abscess formation one area is abnormally sensitive and larger than anticipated.

Chronic prostatitis may produce no change that can be palpated, but often the gland is somewhat enlarged and spongy in consistency. In some instances areas of fibrosis produce an irregular, nodular or lobulated gland that may suggest carcinoma, but fixation rarely occurs. Examination of secretions obtained by massage is necessary to establish the diagnosis of chronic prostatitis.

Calculus. A superficially situated prostatic calculus is occasionally palpable; this is a small, stony-hard, sharply demarcated nodule. It must not be mistaken for carcinoma.

Carcinoma. Early in the disease a small hard area may be palpable; as this enlarges the gland becomes asymmetrical or nodular and immobile. Microscopic examination is often necessary to differentiate this from chronic prostatitis.

Seminal Vesicles

The seminal vesicles are sacculated appendages of the vasa deferentia that extend upward and outward from the upper limit of the prostate. Each is about 5 cm. long and is a somewhat convoluted tube that is too soft to be palpable if normal. When acutely inflamed, a tender cord or sac may be felt. Carcinoma of the prostate occasionally extends into the seminal vesicles; they become firm or hard.

XX

The Extremities

Not only are there disease processes with manifestations in the extremities alone, but also many systemic disorders produce definite and easily recognizable changes there. A systematic detailed examination will require only a short time. Inspection and palpation are the important procedures; percussion and auscultation are rarely needed. The examination of the musculoskeletal system is discussed in Chapter XXI; neurologic disorders are described in Chapter XXII.

THE UPPER EXTREMITIES

The Fingers and Hands

Size and Shape. The hands and feet should be proportional to the stature and general build of the patient, except that during adolescence they may temporarily outgrow the rest of the skeleton. Abnormally large hands in an adult may be indicative of acromegaly (Fig. 232), especially if they have gradually increased in size. In myxedema the hands appear broad and puffy (Fig. 233). In hypopituitarism they may be narrow with long tapered fingers. Unilateral enlargement may be congenital; it may also follow an abnormal arteriovenous communication or an aneurysm of a peripheral artery. Hypogenesis or agenesis is occasionally present. The explanation for traumatic deformities or for the absence of a portion or all of one or more fingers should have been recorded in the history. Congenital abnormalities such as webbing (*syndactylia*) or supernumerary digits are occasionally seen.

The Skin. This may give a clue to the general nature of the person's occupation or activities. The laborer or mechanic will have thickened, toil-worn, scarred or stained skin with calluses; the office

352

worker will not. The palms deserve special attention. Anemia will produce pallor; if the normal creases or "lines" are equally pale, the hemoglobin is very low. With polycythemia the palms are unduly red or reddish-purple in color. In chronic liver disease the thenar and hypothenar areas are often much redder than the rest of the palm; this is called the liver palm or sometimes the "primate palm," from its resemblance to the palms of our supposed arboreal ancestors.

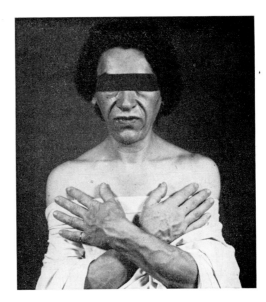

Fig. 232. Acromegaly. Note size of the head and face and the "spade hands." (Courtesy of Dr. F. Curtis Dohan.)

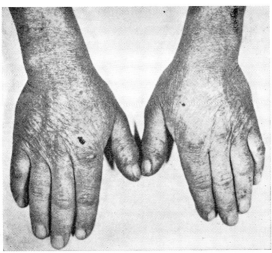

Fig. 233. The hands in myxedema. Note that they are broad and that the skin is dry and wrinkled. (From the service of Dr. William G. Leaman, Jr., Philadelphia General Hospital.)

The Nails.   The finger nails should always be inspected. Biting of the nails (*onychophagia*) is usually a sign of emotional disturbances. Excessive curvature (*parrot-beaking*) has already been mentioned; flattening or concavity (*koilonychia; spoon nails*) may be present with idiopathic microcytic anemia. The color of the nail bed may be suggestive of anemia, polycythemia or cyanosis. Small linear "splinter" hemorrhages may appear in subacute bacterial endocarditis; they should not be confused with hemorrhage due to minor trauma. Transverse ridges may be the result of a recent illness. White spots (*leukonychia*) indicate imperfect nail growth. Discoloration may be due to occupational exposure to chemicals or to local applications. Infection under the nail is usually due to fungi; infection around the nail (*paronychia*) is generally bacterial in origin. The capillary pulse has been described (p. 277).

Abnormal Movements.   These may be visible or palpable or may become evident if the patient can cooperate. With hyperthyroidism a fine tremor is often present. This can be seen more easily if a piece of paper is placed on the hand when the patient extends his arm; it is easily felt by pressing against the fingertips. This fine rhythmic tremor should not be confused with the coarser jerky movements seen in "nervous" people or in various neurologic diseases. In paralysis agitans (Parkinson's disease) the fingers are restless and one or both hands may exhibit "pill-rolling" movements; the thumb is rubbed back and forth across the tips of the fingers. These purposeless movements decrease or disappear with voluntary activity. In multiple sclerosis (disseminated sclerosis) the reverse is true; a tremor appears with voluntary movement (*intention tremor*). The presence of intention tremor, staccato or scanning speech and nystagmus (Charcot's[1] triad) is very suggestive of multiple sclerosis. With high fever or delirium and in moribund patients one may see repeated picking at the bedclothes or gown (*carphology*). In hepatic failure, and occasionally in other diseases, a *liver flap* may be demonstrable. When the patient holds the arms extended, with the palms down and the fingers spread apart, there are peculiar intermittent jerky flexion-extension movements and often a fine tremor of the fingers. Choreiform movements occur in Sydenham's[2] chorea, Huntington's[3] chorea and occasionally in other diseases; these are spasmodic jerks or twitches that recur at irregular intervals.

Temperature and Moisture.   The relative temperature and moisture are determined by palpation. Cold, dry hands are present in wasting diseases and circulatory disorders and after chilling. Cool or cold, moist, "clammy" hands are usually indicative of emotional strain, but are also present is vasomotor or vascular disturbances or in shock. With fever, the hands are usually hot and dry; occasionally they are warm and moist

[1] Jean Martin Charcot, French neurologist, 1825–93.
[2] Thomas Sydenham, English physician, 1624–89.
[3] George Sumner Huntington, American physician, 1862–1927.

if the temperature is falling. Slightly warm, moist hands are normal in children; in an adult this suggests hyperthyroidism, especially if the skin seems thin and soft. In myxedema the hands are usually cool and dry, and the skin feels coarse and thickened.

Clubbing.   Clubbing of the fingers is occasionally present. The tips of the fingers become bulbous and the nails show abnormally increased curvature both transversely and longitudinally (Fig. 234). This should not be confused with simple curvature or parrot-beaking of the nails, which is not uncommon. A more important feature is the change in the angle between the soft tissue at the base of the nail and the nail itself. As shown in Figure 235, this is normally about 160 degrees. With clubbing, this angle becomes progressively greater as the degree of clubbing increases. To avoid error, disregard the dorsal view of the fingers; look at them from the palmar surface and from the sides. If the angle is definitely increased, if the terminal phalanx is definitely broader and thicker than the middle phalanx, and if the nail is abnormally curved or beaked, clubbing is present.

Clubbing of the fingers was described by Hippocrates and has aroused interest ever since then. The cause is still unknown, but clubbing immediately suggests disturbances in tissue oxygenation. It is not uncommon in congenital heart disease or with acute or chronic pulmonary disease such as bronchiectasis, empyema, lung abscess, emphysema or bronchogenic carcinoma. It has also been found in other diseases such as polycythemia, subacute bacterial endocarditis, chronic hepatic dis-

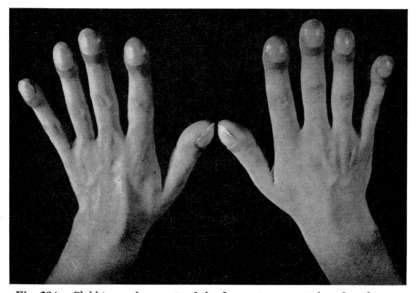

Fig. 234. Clubbing and cyanosis of the fingers in congenital cardiac disease.

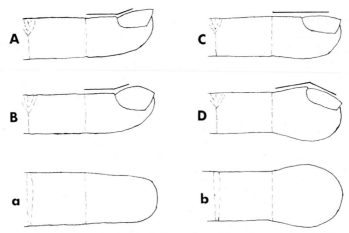

Fig. 235.   Clubbing. *A*, Normal flat nail. *B*, Normal curved nail. The angle in
each case is about 160°. *C*, Early clubbing. *D*, Severe clubbing. Viewed from the palmar
surface, the terminal phalanx normally is narrower than the middle phalanx (*a*). With
clubbing, it becomes definitely broader (*b*).

ease, chronic diarrhea and ulcerative colitis. Occasionally it seems to be
congenital or familial. Unilateral clubbing may occur with vascular
anomalies leading to anoxia of the hand or fingers. When one digit alone
seems involved, trauma or nerve injury must be ruled out.

Hypertrophic Pulmonary Osteoarthropathy.   Some authors believe that this is merely a more advanced stage of clubbing; others consider it a distinctly different entity. The distal ends of the radii, ulnae,
tibiae, fibulae or bones of the hands or wrists become enlarged by
periosteal proliferation and new bone growth; usually this is bilateral
and symmetrical (Fig. 236). Occasionally other bones are involved.
There may be pain around the joints, soft tissue swelling and decreased
mobility of the joints that can be mistaken for arthritis. Occasionally
the onset is fairly acute, further heightening the resemblance to arthritis. In many of these patients the underlying factor seems to be a
previously unrecognized bronchogenic carcinoma or other intrathoracic
mass lesion. In some instances surgical intervention has been followed
by regression of the arthropathy.

Arthritis.   Rheumatoid arthritis (arthritis deformans; atrophic
arthritis) damages or destroys the joint; subsequent fibrosis or new bone
formation results in deformity with impaired movement or actual fixation (*ankylosis*) of the involved joint. In the fingers the earliest and
most obvious changes occur in the proximal interphalangeal joints; the
involvement is usually bilateral and often it is symmetrical (Fig. 237).
In the later stages other joints of the fingers may be involved; the
interosseous muscles atrophy and ulnar deviation of the fingers is common (Fig. 238).

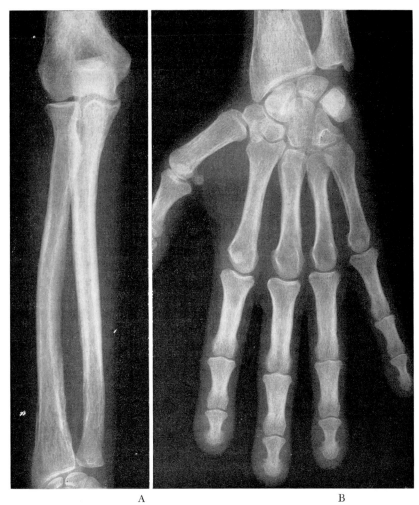

A   B

Fig. 236.   Hypertrophic pulmonary osteoarthropathy in a patient with lung abscess. A, Soft tissue clubbing at finger tips and periosteal proliferation along the
borders of the fifth metacarpal. B, Similar changes in the radius and ulna. (Courtesy
of Dr. E. P. Pendergrass.)

Generally the disease is not confined to the hands; widespread joint
changes will develop and the person may be crippled by them.

Heberden's[4] **Nodes.**   These are knoblike bony outgrowths at the
terminal interphalangeal joints; they are more common in women than
in men (Fig. 239). They may be the first manifestation of osteoarthritis
(hypertrophic arthritis; degenerative arthritis) but usually they are of

[4] William Heberden, British physician, 1710–1801. King George III and Dr.
Samuel Johnson, the author, were two of his famous patients. The lucid description
which has perpetuated his name required only 79 words.

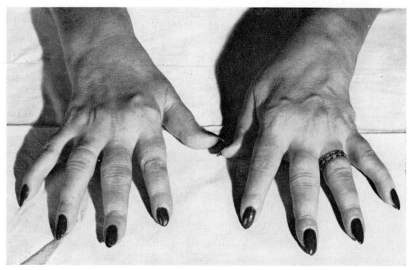

Fig. 237. Rheumatoid arthritis; early changes. There is symmetrical fusiform swelling of the proximal interphalangeal joints, especially noticeable in the middle fingers. (Courtesy of Dr. Joseph L. Hollander.)

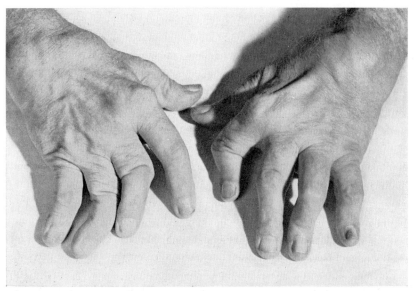

Fig. 238. Rheumatoid arthritis; far advanced. There is distortion of the joints, fixation of the left fourth proximal interphalangeal joint and marked ulnar deviation of the fingers, especially prominent in the left index finger and the third, fourth and fifth fingers of the right hand. (Courtesy of Dr. Joseph L. Hollander.)

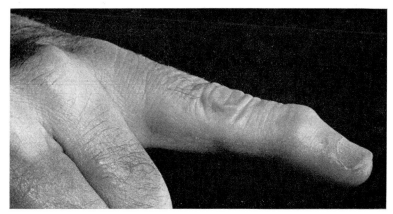

Fig. 239. Heberden's nodes. These may be unsightly but rarely interfere with normal joint movement.

no clinical significance. These excrescences may be unsightly but not painful; they rarely interfere with normal joint movement.

Gout. This may occasionally involve the hands but is much more common in the feet. In the early acute stage the affected joint is hot, swollen, bluish-red, extremely painful and exquisitely tender. After repeated attacks, or in mild chronic gout, the joint may be somewhat enlarged and motion is restricted; this can be mistaken for rheumatoid arthritis. Nodules composed of urate crystals (tophi) may be present; the skin overlying such deposits may break down and chalky material will exude (Fig. 240).

Osler's Nodes. These are small, painful reddish or bluish spots in the pulp of the fingertips. They are usually associated with bacterial endocarditis and are thought to be due to bacterial emboli. They may be more apparent to the patient than to the examiner.

Raynaud's[5] Disease. This occurs predominantly in women; it is characterized by paroxysmal spasm of digital arteries and arterioles, usually bilateral and symmetrical, which is precipitated by chilling or emotional stress. The affected areas become numb or painful and white or occasionally cyanotic; the line of demarcation is sharp. When the spasm is relieved, reactive hyperemia with burning and redness follows. Between attacks the hands appear normal but may be cold and moist. The toes occasionally show similar changes. In doubtful cases it may be helpful to immerse the hand in ice water for a few minutes; this will produce the typical symptoms.

Similar changes may appear with Buerger's[6] disease (p. 366), sclero-

[5] Maurice Raynaud, French physician, 1834–81.
[6] Leo Buerger, New York physician, 1879–1943.

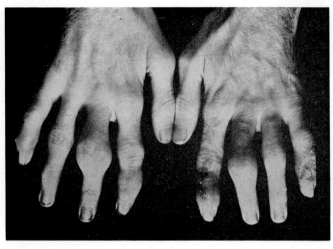

Fig. 240. Chronic gout. Swelling of proximal interphalangeal joints and areas of infection in the overlying skin.

derma, sickle cell disease, ergotism, cervical rib or scalenus anticus syndrome, nerve injury due to continued improper use of crutches, or trauma incident to prolonged use of a vibrating tool such as a pneumatic hammer. When some definite etiologic factor can be established the term "Raynaud's phenomenon" is used.

Scleroderma. This may begin in the fingers and later appear in other areas. Initially there is edema and cellular infiltration followed by proliferation of connective tissue, changes in the collagen, and atrophy. The skin is smooth and waxlike in appearance. It is firmly adherent to the deeper tissues, and motility of the joints is decreased.

Dupuytren's[7] Contracture. This results from an abnormal thickening and shrinking of the palmar fascia along the course of the flexor tendons of one or more fingers, usually the fourth or fifth. Slowly progressive flexion deformity results. A firm ridge can be felt over the involved tendons.

Volkman's[8] Contracture. This is produced by interference with the blood supply, usually in the region of the elbow, by damage or destruction of the median or ulnar nerve, by syringomyelia or by progressive muscular atrophy. The wrist and fingers are flexed; claw hand results.

Trousseau's[9] Sign. This may be demonstrable in tetany. The wrist and metacarpo-phalangeal joints are flexed; the interphalangeal joints are extended; the finger tips are drawn together and the thumb is adducted into the palm. Compression of the arm, manually or with

[7] Baron Guillaume Dupuytren, French surgeon, 1778–1835.
[8] Richard von Volkman, German surgeon, 1830–89.
[9] Armand Trousseau, French physician, 1801–67.

a sphygmomanometer cuff to decrease blood flow, may be needed to elicit this sign. Tetany may be due to hypocalcemia secondary to hypo-parathyroidism; it can also occur with acid-base imbalance from chloride loss, excessive ingestion of alkalies or hyperventilation.

The Wrists

The general contour, symmetry and motility should be noted. Rheu-matoid arthritis may produce various degrees of deformity and limita-tion of motion; usually this is bilateral. Unilateral deformity may follow unsatisfactory reduction of a fracture of one of the carpal bones or of the distal end of the radius (Colles'[10] fracture). An abnormal twitching of muscles and tendons in the region of the wrist (*subsultus tendinum*) may occur in conjunction with carphology and is of similar grave import. Occasionally a ganglion (p. 381) will be present on the dorsal surface of the wrist. Palpation of the radial and ulnar arteries has been dis-cussed (p. 47).

The Arms

The size, shape and symmetry of the forearms, elbows and arms should be compared and any abnormalities investigated. In a right-handed person the right arm may show greater muscular development; this should not be confused with atrophy of the left arm due to neuro-logic disorders or to limited use following injury or joint disease.

Vessels. The superficial veins may be prominent in a thin person but almost invisible in an obese one. Distended veins in one arm only are usually indicative of obstruction distal to the superior vena cava. In an elderly arteriosclerotic patient the brachial arteries may be tor-tuous and writhe under the skin with each heartbeat, producing the "brachial dance."

Edema. This may be present in one or both arms, but is much more commonly found in the legs. In the absence of generalized edema one should look for signs of localized vascular obstruction. *Lymphedema* is due to interference with lymphatic drainage; it is seen most commonly after radical mastectomy and may be related to the removal of the axillary lymph nodes. Red streaks are visible when lymphatic channels are infected (*lymphangitis*); the primary site is usually apparent.

Lymph Nodes. Palpation for epitrochlear and axillary nodes is essential. The epitrochlear nodes are located immediately above the medial condyle of the humerus; normally they cannot be felt (Fig. 241).

[10] Abraham Colles, Irish surgeon, 1773–1843.

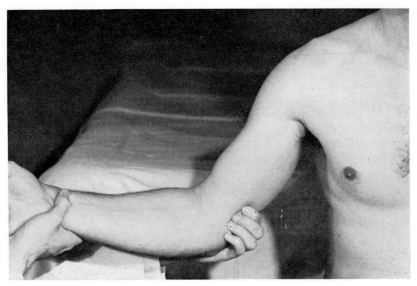

Fig. 241. Palpation for epitrochlear nodes. The forearm is moderately flexed; the palpating fingers are exploring the region immediately above the medial condyle of the humerus.

They may become enlarged and palpable with infection in the hand or forearm, in secondary syphilis or in leukemia or other diseases of the lymphoid tissue. The axilla should be palpated with the arm at the side and then abducted (Fig. 90, p. 140). The examining fingers press upward and against the chest wall first; one or more nodes may be palpable. With the arm abducted the axillary fascia is tensed and superficial nodes may be more easily felt against this. If a node is felt, determine its size, consistency, tenderness and mobility; if several are present, note whether they are discrete or matted together.

THE LOWER EXTREMITIES

The same general procedure should be followed, starting with the toes and feet and ending at the groin. Since the lower extremities must bear weight when a person is upright, they are subject to greater stress and are more prone to show abnormalities. Whenever possible it is advisable to examine the patient both erect and recumbent. This is especially important if the patient has circulatory or vascular disease or has difficulty in walking for any reason.

Size and Shape.   The size and shape are usually proportional to the general build, muscular development and nutritional status of the individual. Occasionally an obese adult will have relatively little fat in the lower extremities, which may then appear abnormally thin. Conversely and especially in women, the trunk may be normal in contour but the thighs will be very large. Atrophy may be unilateral or bilateral; it is usually due to poliomyelitis or other neurologic disease. If one extremity appears larger than the other, measure the circumference of each leg or thigh at corresponding levels.

The shape of one or both legs may be altered by abnormalities of the joints or by bone disease such as an old fracture, rickets, syphilis or osteitis deformans (Paget's disease). In the latter two, forward bowing with the production of saber shins is commonly seen.

The Skin. In addition to the usual generalized dermatologic diseases, the legs may be the site of stasis dermatitis. This results from impaired venous blood flow. The skin over the lower third of the leg, and occasionally the dorsum of the foot, becomes thickened and scaly, and brown or reddish in color. Itching is common; scratch marks may be present; ulcers are prone to develop.

Edema. This is the most common cause of enlargement of the lower extremities. It may be limited to the feet or ankles, or it may involve the entire leg. To demonstrate pitting edema, make *moderately firm* pressure with the fingers over the area and maintain this for ten or fifteen seconds to allow the interstitial fluid to be displaced. A definite indentation will be palpable and visible when the fingers are removed (Fig. 242). The depth of the depression will be roughly proportional to the amount of swelling present. If the tissue feels soft and pits easily, the process is usually of fairly recent origin; chronic edema leads to induration and tissue changes that decrease the mobility of the fluid.

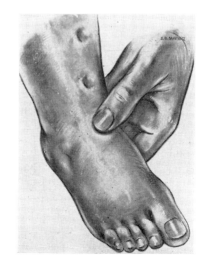

Fig. 242. Pitting edema of foot and leg.

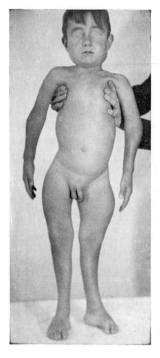

Fig. 243. Refractory rickets. Physical deformities in a 10-year-old boy in whom the disease had been active since the end of the first year of life. There is reduction of stature and deformities of the arms, legs, feet and chest. Enlargement at the wrists, elbows and knees can also be seen. (Howorth, M. B.: Textbook of Orthopedics. Philadelphia, W. B. Saunders Co., 1952.)

Bilateral edema is seen most frequently with congestive heart failure; it also occurs with nephritis or nephrosis. It may be due to compression of the iliacs or the inferior vena cava by ascitic fluid, by a gravid or myomatous uterus, or by some other pelvic or abdominal mass. Thrombosis or varicosities of the larger veins can also lead to edema. Since contraction of the muscles plays an important role in the return of blood from the lower extremities, prolonged immobilization may produce slight or moderate edema. Edema due to obstruction of the lymphatic channels is occasionally seen.

Unilateral edema is almost invariably due to some disease of the veins or lymphatics, or to vasomotor changes secondary to hemiplegia or other neurologic disorder.

When an edematous patient is kept in bed, the swelling of the legs may disappear very rapidly. Rest and the horizontal position not only facilitate the resorption of fluid, but also lead to redistribution of it. The feet and ankles may appear almost normal, but the back of the thighs, the buttocks and the sacral area become edematous. This facilitates the development of bed sores (*decubitus ulcers*); such areas should be examined daily if the patient is confined to bed.

Arteries.   Palpation of the arteries of the feet is mandatory. The *dorsalis pedis* artery usually lies in the space between the first and second metatarsal bones; if it is not felt there, explore the adjacent areas.

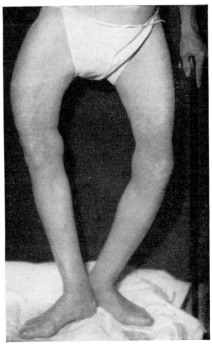

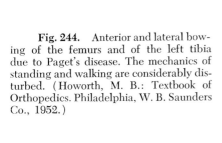

Fig. 244. Anterior and lateral bowing of the femurs and of the left tibia due to Paget's disease. The mechanics of standing and walking are considerably disturbed. (Howorth, M. B.: Textbook of Orthopedics. Philadelphia, W. B. Saunders Co., 1952.)

The *posterior tibial* artery lies between the posterior aspect of the internal malleolus and the mesial side of the Achilles[11] tendon; it is more accessible when the foot is dorsiflexed. Determine not only the general characteristics of the arterial wall and of the pulsations, but compare the pulses in the two feet. Occasionally these arteries will not be palpable if there is tremendous edema or myxedema; more commonly these pulses disappear because of severe arteriosclerosis.

If the dorsalis pedis and posterior tibial pulses are not palpable, check the popliteal artery. To do this it is best to have the patient lie prone. Raise the foot with one hand until the leg is at an angle of 30 to 45 degrees; palpate the popliteal space with your other hand (Fig. 245). If no pulsation can be felt, the femoral artery should be sought just below Poupart's ligament, midway between the anterior superior iliac spine and the symphysis pubis.

Arteriosclerosis. This is more common in males and especially in elderly men with diabetes. Often the first symptom is *intermittent claudication*. After walking a relatively short distance the person gets a "cramp" in the calf muscles of one or both legs and has to slow up or stop. Examination at that time will show that the muscle is not firm

[11] Achilles, Greek hero of the Trojan war. He was invulnerable except in the region of the tendo calcaneus. Paris, the Trojan playboy, scored a bull's-eye there; infection ended Achilles' life.

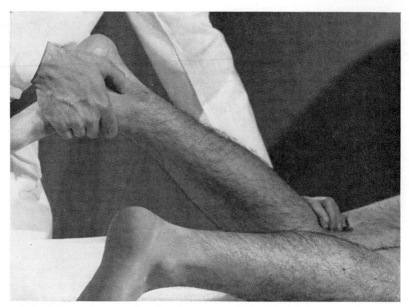

Fig. 245. Palpation of popliteal artery. With the patient prone, the leg is flexed to an angle of 30 degrees or more. The popliteal artery should be palpable in the area bounded by the internal condyle of the femur and the inner head of the gastrocnemius mesially, and the external condyle and outer head of the gastrocnemius laterally.

and contracted, as with true spasm; it is soft, relaxed and incapable of contracting. With rest, the tissue anoxia is relieved and for a short time the person can again walk comfortably. In the later stages abnormal coldness, cyanosis or extreme pallor of the toes and feet will be present. Ischemic ulcers or gangrene may ultimately develop.

Thromboangiitis Obliterans (Buerger's Disease). Whether or not this clinical syndrome so fully described by Buerger in 1908 should actually be considered a distinct disease entity is a moot question, but the general picture is seen frequently, whatever one wishes to call it. The process begins in early adult life and is much more common in males. At least 50 per cent of those afflicted are said to be Russian or Polish Jews; almost without exception they are cigarette smokers. Initially, the smaller arteries slowly become occluded; the veins may also be involved. Pathologically there are inflammatory lesions of the vessel wall with thrombosis and obliteration of the lumen. When the foot is elevated, pallor is usually pronounced; when it is dependent, increased redness or cyanosis may appear. Episodes of acute angiitis or of migratory phlebitis may alternate with periods of apparent quiescence; gradually the process spreads to the larger vessels. Ischemic necrosis, gangrene or ulcers may develop in the toes; in extreme cases the patient may lose one or both feet, or even a leg. The upper extremities may be involved, but usually the disease is less severe there and appears later.

Arterial Embolism.   A thrombus in the left atrium, left ventricle or aorta may break loose and lodge in any artery. Large emboli tend to be swept along to the bifurcation of the aorta or to one of the iliac or femoral arteries. There will be agonizing pain in one or both legs, absence of all pulses peripheral to the embolus, and intense pallor; gangrene may then begin in the toes and extend proximally. Similar complications will develop if a clot lodges in other arteries.

Veins.   Because the great saphenous veins are the longest in the body and are subjected to the greatest hydrostatic pressure, they are the ones most liable to develop varicosities. The small saphenous veins are much less frequently involved; sometimes both systems are affected. The intercommunicating veins that connect these two may also develop varicosities. Both systems also anastomose with the deep veins through *venae perforantes,* which pierce the deep fascia. Normally the superficial veins drain upward or to the deep system through the communicating veins. Incompetent valves that allow reversal of the direction of blood flow are the main cause of eventual segmental or widespread dilatation and tortuosity of the veins, especially in women.

Although huge varicosities may be obvious when the patient is recumbent, smaller ones may be overlooked unless the patient stands; examine all aspects of both legs. In some persons a thick layer of fat may obscure moderate-sized varicosities, but these can be found by palpation.

A number of tests have been described to determine the competency of the valves in these venous systems; the Trendelenburg (Brodie-

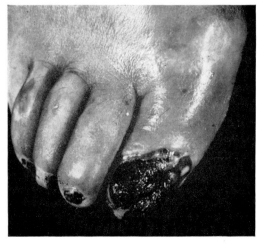

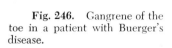
Fig. 246.   Gangrene of the toe in a patient with Buerger's disease.

Trendelenburg[12]) is a simple test for screening purposes. With the patient supine, elevate the leg; the superficial veins should collapse. With the fingers (or thumb) compress the vein at the saphenous opening, or place a tourniquet moderately tightly around the thigh as high as possible. Then have the patient stand, while pressure is maintained. If the veins fill fairly promptly from below upward, the valves in the communicating veins are incompetent. If there is little or no visible filling in 30 seconds, release the compression; rapid filling from above downward is indicative of incompetency of the valves in the superficial veins only. If the veins begin to fill from below, but distend rapidly when the pressure is released, both systems have incompetent valves.

Since varicose veins lead to gradually increasing stasis of blood, a moderate degree of edema with dermatitis and pigmentation or even ulceration is not an uncommon complication.

Thrombophlebitis.   This is inflammation (*-itis*) of a vein (*phlebos*) that accompanies or leads to local changes in the blood clotting mechanism with formation of a clot or *thrombus*. It occurs most commonly in the legs, especially in damaged dilated varicose veins, but it may develop in any vein. It may follow a minor insult such as venipuncture; it is not rare as a sequel of procedures such as angiography or cardiac catheterization, or following a prolonged intravenous infusion. Most commonly it develops without any definite local trauma; congestive heart failure, obesity, general debility, infection elsewhere or the postpartum or postoperative state are some of the possible contributory factors.

With involvement of a superficial vein the pain is rarely severe and the symptoms are relatively mild. The skin over the involved segment is red and tenderness is present. Localized edema develops but the entire leg is seldom affected. When a deep vein is involved the pain tends to be more severe, edema is greater, and malaise, fever and leukocytosis are commonly present. If the veins of the calf are involved, Homans'[13] sign may be demonstrable. With the patient supine, lift the knee several inches from the bed and flex the leg, then sharply dorsiflex the foot. This will elicit or aggravate pain in the calf. When the veins of the thigh are involved firm pressure on the inner side toward the femur will cause pain.

Phlebothrombosis.   Pathologically, this denotes a vein filled with thrombus but without actual inflammation of the vessel wall. It is prone to develop in elderly persons in whom there is circulatory stasis, as with prolonged bed rest for conditions such as myocardial infarction, a major operation or immobilization of a fractured leg. The clot forms

[12] Benjamin Brodie, British surgeon (1783–1862), probably deserves the credit; he described this test in 1846. However, Friedrich Trendelenburg, a German surgeon (1844–1925), was the one who popularized this maneuver.
[13] John Homans, Boston surgeon, 1877–1954.

slowly; pain is rarely present. Since initially the inflammatory reaction is absent, the thrombus is only slightly adherent to the vessel wall and is easily dislodged; pulmonary embolism is often the first indication of such a process. If this does not occur, the clot itself causes irritation, resulting in reactive phenomena in the wall of the vein; clinically it may then be difficult to differentiate this from thrombophlebitis. The presence of Homans' sign, slight tenderness along the course of a vein, minimal edema and unequal filling of the veins of the feet may be the only findings; even these may be deceptive because bilateral involvement is not uncommon. Pain can sometimes be elicited by inflating a sphygmomanometer cuff wrapped around the suspected area. Normally this procedure is not painful until the pressure rises to 180 mm. of mercury. The test is considered positive if the patient complains bitterly of pain at some pressure below 150 mm. of mercury.

In uncomplicated thrombophlebitis or phlebothrombosis the clot is slowly organized. Recanalization may occur during this period, but often the involved segment of the vein is reduced to a firm fibrotic cord. In either case, the circulation is impaired and a further burden is placed on the collateral veins. These in turn may dilate and eventually become varicose, thus setting the stage for repeated episodes of thrombosis.

Cutaneous Ulcers.   These are much more common on the feet and legs than on any other body surface. They may result from impairment of arterial or of venous blood flow. With diabetic arteriosclerosis the ischemia tends to be most severe in the distal areas. A minor injury such as a carelessly trimmed toenail or pressure from a poorly fitted shoe initiates the process; gangrene soon develops. The ulcer is usually deep, and osteomyelitis of the underlying bone may follow. Such a person often loses one toe after another; before the introduction of antimicrobial drugs to control the infection that is almost invariably present, high amputation was usually required. An arteriosclerotic ulcer may also develop in other areas exposed to trauma, such as the skin over the lower shin or lateral malleolus. Such an ulcer is deep and penetrates the fascia; gangrene of the toes is liable to follow.

Impaired venous circulation can also lead to ulceration. When varicose veins are present the edematous skin becomes vulnerable to trauma, infection and ulceration. A varicose ulcer is shallow, with irregular shelving edges that may show a thin blue margin of growing epithelium; it is rarely more than 3 cm. in diameter. It occurs in the lower third of the leg, more commonly on the mesial aspect, and is relatively painless unless a nerve is involved in the scar tissue as it heals. Stasis dermatitis with pigmentation is almost invariably present around the ulcer.

Ulceration may also occur after venous thrombosis, in much the same distribution as varicose ulcers. Such an ulcer is deep and is cov-

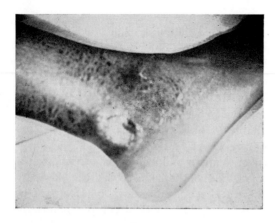

Fig. 247. Leg ulcer in sickle cell anemia.

ered by a thick, tenacious grayish slough. If untreated it continues to enlarge and may threaten to encircle the leg. Skin pigmentation is usually absent, but pain is a prominent feature.

Ulcers occasionally develop in a paralyzed leg or in one that is immobilized by severe bone or joint disease such as arthritis. Blood dyscrasias, especially sickle cell anemia, may also be accompanied by leg ulcers (Fig. 247).

XXI

The Musculoskeletal System

Physical examination of the musculoskeletal system is performed largely by inspection and palpation. The object is to determine the condition of voluntary muscles, joints and bones. If an abnormality is found, radiography or other special procedures may be needed to establish the diagnosis.

A diseased joint may give rise to secondary alterations in the musculature; conversely, muscle disease can alter the function and movement of a joint. Therefore it is necessary to determine the range of active and of passive motion in a joint. If active motion alone is limited, the muscles are at fault. In this chapter, determination of the integrity or status of the major joints will be considered first; the procedures for testing muscles will be discussed later.

EXAMINATION OF THE JOINTS

General Procedures

The first step should be a quick inspection of all of the important joints, looking for enlargement, abnormal contour or other signs suggestive of orthopedic disease. Each joint is then examined in detail.

The range of active motion is first determined. (Normal values will be given as various joints are discussed.) Whenever limitation of motion is found, the approximate range should be recorded. For precise measurement a goniometer is necessary; with this device it is possible to measure exact angles and the number of degrees through which movement is possible.

Whenever the full range of active motion seems decreased, passive movement should be tested. Determine the degree of flexion, extension

371

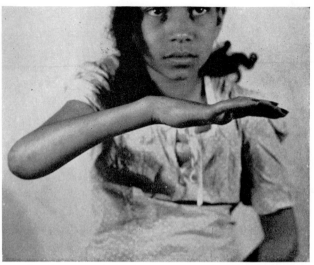

Fig. 248.   Early ulnar nerve palsy following supracondylar fracture of humerus.

or rotation that can be achieved, but do this carefully and gently to avoid unnecessary pain. With muscular weakness (paresis) or paralysis, the range of passive motion may be entirely normal even when active motion is absent.

If there is limitation of both active and passive movement, try to establish whether this is due to intrinsic joint disease or to some extra-articular cause. Look for redness, swelling, hypertrophy, atrophy, abnormal contour or other evidence of disease or injury in the joint itself and in the periarticular structures. Acute inflammation will give rise to pain even when the joint is at rest; movement will aggravate this. Overgrowth of bone or cartilage may suddenly inhibit further movement, with or without pain. With complete fusion of the bones (*ankylosis*) there is no movement at the joint. With thickening of the periarticular tissues, pain and limitation of motion may decrease with activity.

Muscular spasm may produce pain and resistance to active or passive motion; at some point the person's threshold of pain will halt further movement. Muscle contractures may be painless but result in an abnormal position of the extremity at rest and limitation of active and passive movement.

Shortening or atrophy of a limb can result in altered function of a joint or may lead to actual joint changes. Accurate measurements from appropriate points should be made to determine such changes. The length of the upper extremity is usually measured from the acromium to the styloid process. In the lower extremity, measure from the umbilicus or from the anterior superior spine of the ilium to the internal malleolus. The circumference of the limbs can be compared by measuring each at a point that is some definite distance above or below a bony landmark.

The changes distal to a diseased joint may be more striking than the local signs. For example, a fracture or dislocation of the elbow may produce only minor loss of movement of the joint, but coincident injury to the ulnar, the median or the radial nerve may result in weakness or deformities in the hand.

Some of the more common processes involving joints are rheumatoid arthritis, osteoarthritis (degenerative joint disease; hypertrophic arthritis), tuberculous or nontuberculous infection and changes due to trauma, fracture or dislocation with resulting scarring of the joint or of the capsular structures.

The Shoulder Joint

This is a ball-and-socket joint. The shallowness of the glenoid cavity permits a greater variety and degree of movement than is found in any other joint. The humerus can be abducted laterally, swung forward and

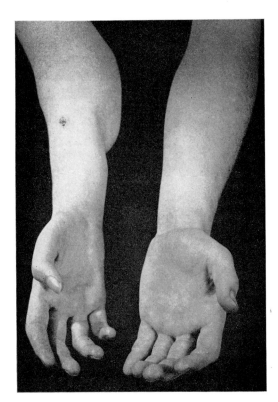

Fig. 249. Volkmann's ischemic contracture following fracture of both bones of the right forearm.

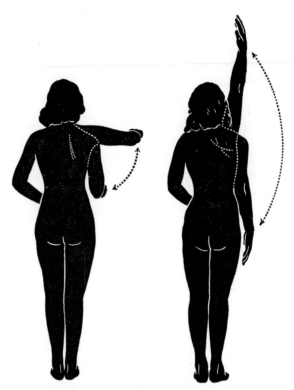

Fig. 250. Scapulohumeral rhythm. The scapula begins rotating during the initiation of arm abduction movement. (Colonna, P. C.: Regional Orthopedic Surgery. Philadelphia, W. B. Saunders Co., 1950.)

backward and rotated externally and internally. However, much of the motion that seems to occur in the shoulder involves more than the scapulohumeral articulation alone; movements at the sternoclavicular and acromioclavicular joints and of the scapula on the thoracic wall all play a part. These movements are rhythmic, not separate motions; they are called scapulohumeral rhythm.

Normal Function.   To determine the mobility of the shoulder joint itself, have the patient stand or sit with his arms hanging loosely at his sides, then flex his elbows to 90 degrees. Stand behind him, place your hands on his shoulders and press firmly in the acromioclavicular region to eliminate movement there. Test extension and flexion by asking him to keep his forearms horizontal and move his elbows as far backward as possible, then forward. A normal range from the vertical line should be 30 degrees or more backward (extension) and 90 degrees forward. With the arm in its original position (elbow bent) test external rotation by seeing how far laterally he can swing his hands; then ask him to bring the hands together (internal rotation). Next, test abduction by having him swing the arms outward without moving the scapulae; the arms should be horizontal. Now have him raise the forearms until they are vertical; test rotation in abduction by swinging the hands backward, then forward; the total arc should be about 180 degrees.

To test scapulothoracic movement, remove your hands, ask him to straighten his elbows and then swing his arms laterally up over his head; the range of motion should be 180 degrees. When the arm is completely elevated, about one-third of the movement occurs in the scapulothoracic region.

The normal range of movement, and especially of rotation, is much greater in children than in elderly persons. With unilateral disease the two sides can be compared; with bilateral involvement experience will help you decide whether the range of motion is normal or decreased. If there is impairment of active motion, determine the range of passive motion that can be achieved without causing undue pain.

Two other simple tests may be helpful. Have the patient cross his arms behind his back with the forearms horizontal; this involves extension and internal rotation. Then have him lock his fingers behind his head with the forearms forming a straight line; this tests abduction and

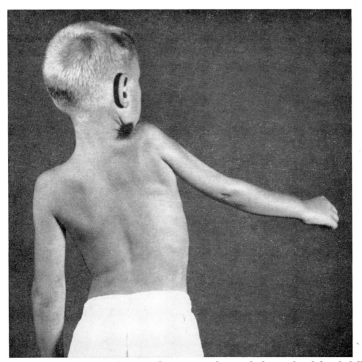

Fig. 251.   Loss of abduction due to paralysis of the right deltoid following poliomyelitis.

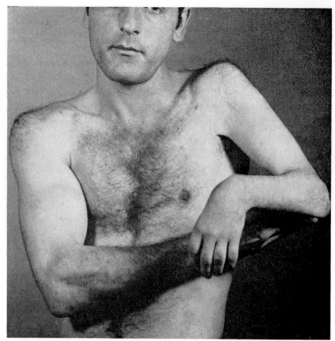

Fig. 252.   Brachial plexus birth injury, left, with paralysis (Erb's paralysis).

external rotation. These are the movements most limited by disease or injury about the shoulder joint, especially ligamentous tears and the so-called subdeltoid bursitis.

Abnormalities.   Abduction and external or internal rotation may be limited either by intra-articular or by extra-articular disease. Limitation of flexion and extension is generally due to intra-articular disease. The most common intra-articular diseases of the shoulder joint are rheumatoid arthritis, osteoarthritis and lesions due to trauma, especially fracture in the region of the surgical neck or dislocation of the head of the humerus. Limitation of active motion may also be due to disease of the muscles themselves, or to weakness or complete paralysis secondary to altered innervation such as that seen following poliomyelitis, for example, or in Erb's paralysis (Erb-Duchenne[1] paralysis; obstetric paralysis). The latter is due to stretching or tearing of fibers of the brachial plexus during difficult delivery.

Normal function may be impaired when there is injury to other components of the shoulder girdle. Fracture of a clavicle will result in point tenderness over the fracture site and altered alignment or overriding of the proximal and distal fragments. Sternoclavicular separation can be suspected if the inner end of the clavicle appears unusually prom-

[1] Wilhelm Heinrich Erb, Heidelberg physician, 1840–1921; Guillaume Benjamin Amand Duchenne, French neurologist, 1806–75.

inent; pain on pressure and preternatural mobility will confirm the suspicion. With acromioclavicular separation there will be pain on pressure, abnormal prominence of the acromium and increased deformity if the arm is pulled downward.

The Elbow Joint

This complex joint permits flexion and extension movements of the forearm (hinge type) and also rotation of the radius and ulna.

The *carrying angle* should first be observed. Have the patient stand or sit facing you, allowing his arms to hang naturally at his sides with the forearms fully extended and rotated so that the palms are forward. The forearm will not be in a straight line with the arm; the angle will be about 160 to 170 degrees, with the forearm deviating away from the body. Normally, this angulation is greater in women than in men. Unilateral alteration of the carrying angle is usually the result of fracture or other injury of the humerus or of an epiphysis in this area. If the forearm deviates outward more than normal, *cubitus valgus* is present; if it deviates less than normal or actually turns inward there is *cubitus varus.*

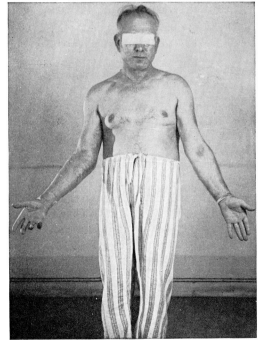

Fig. 253. Right cubitus valgus deformity and ulnar palsy following old elbow fracture. (Colonna, P. C.: Regional Orthopedic Surgery. Philadelphia, W. B. Saunders Co., 1950.)

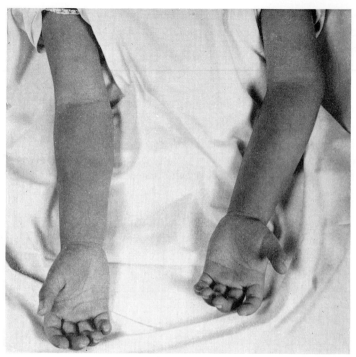

Fig. 254. Cubitus varus, left, following supracondylar fracture.

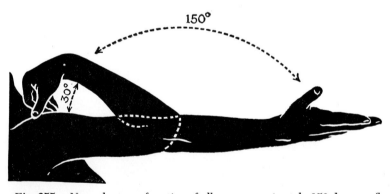

Fig. 255. Normal range of motion of elbow: approximately 150 degrees; flexion to 30 degrees, extension to 180 degrees. (Colonna, P. C.: Regional Orthopedic Surgery. Philadelphia, W. B. Saunders Co., 1950.)

Normal Function.   Test flexion and extension; the forearm should extend to 180 degrees and flex to about 30 degrees. Any limitation or inequality of movement should be recorded and the probable cause noted. Pronation and supination of the forearm are then observed. Have the patient sit with his elbows flexed to a right angle and the forearms resting on some level surface such as a table, the arms of a chair, or on his own thighs if necessary. If he holds a pencil or other small object in his hand it will be easier to estimate the range of motion. Ask him to pronate and supinate the forearm as much as possible without moving the position of the elbow or arm; abduction or rotation at the shoulder joint will increase the apparent range of motion. The normal arc is about 150 degrees.

Abnormalities.   Limitation of supination and pronation may be due to any disease in or about the elbow joint, especially those that affect either the head of the radius or the capitellum. It can also be due to anything that alters the normal size, shape or relationship of the radius and ulna, such as excess callus formation or malposition of frag-ments following fracture. Limitation of flexion and extension may be the result of any type of joint disease.

The Wrist Joint

The wrist or radiocarpal joint involves the distal end of the radius and the carpus; the lower end of the ulna is separated from the wrist joint itself by a triangular cartilage.

Normal Function.   Flexion, extension and lateral deviation of the hand occur here. The range between full extension (dorsiflexion) and palmar flexion is from 150 to 160 degrees. Radial and ulnar deviation

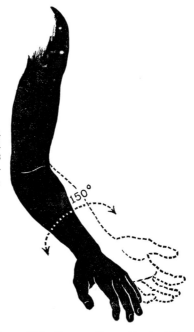

Fig. 256.   The elbow should be held at a right angle while the forearm is pronated and supinated. The total range of normal rotation is approximately 150 degrees. (Colonna, P. C.: Regional Orthopedic Surgery. Philadelphia, W. B. Saunders Co., 1950.)

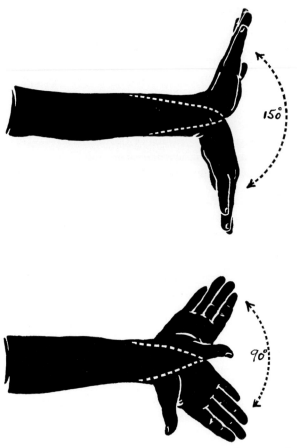

Fig. 257. *Upper,* Range of normal dorsal and palmar flexion at the wrist joint. *Lower,* Normal range of radial and ulnar deviation at the wrist in young adults. (Colonna, P. C.: Regional Orthopedic Surgery. Philadelphia, W. B. Saunders Co., 1950.)

of the metacarpals is usually possible over a range of 75 degrees or more, with ulnar deviation greater than radial. Ulnar deviation is greater and radial deviation less if the palms are up (forward) rather than down, and *vice versa.*

Abnormalities.   Trauma is very common; this is usually incurred when the person falls and attempts to protect himself by his outstretched dorsiflexed hand. A Colles' fracture of the lower end of the radius produces the "dinner fork" deformity due to dorsal displacement of the distal fragment. Fracture of the carpal scaphoid or epiphyseal separation of the lower end of the radius (in children) can follow similar accidents. Rheumatoid arthritis, osteoarthritis and various bacterial infections may also involve the wrist joint.

Irritation, injury or infection of tendon sheaths (*tenosynovitis*) will

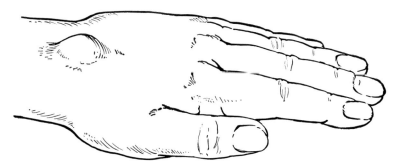

Fig. 258. Common location of ganglia. (Colonna, P. C.: Regional Orthopedic Surgery. Philadelphia, W. B. Saunders Co., 1950.)

produce pain and limitation of motion, even though the joint surfaces are not involved. A common site for this is over the radius about 5 cm. above the wrist joint; at this point the superficial extensor tendons cross over the deep extensor tendons. Chronic or repeated irritation or inflammation can lead eventually to stenosis of the sheath, producing stenosing tenosynovitis or tenovaginitis (tendovaginitis). Involvement of the common sheath of the abductor pollicis longus and extensor pollicis brevis at the radial styloid process is known as Quervain's[2] disease. This is much more common in women than in men; it is often attributed to excessive use of the thumb in the never-ending household chores.

Degeneration of connective tissue in the joint capsule can result in a cystlike swelling known as a *ganglion*. Although ganglia can occur elsewhere, the most common site is on the dorsum of the wrist over the scaphoid-lunate articulation (Fig. 258). When the wrist is flexed the swelling becomes more prominent and very tense; with extension, it may disappear completely. In some cases repeated trauma seems to be an underlying etiologic factor.

Compression of the median nerve between the carpal bones and the transverse carpal ligament (*carpal tunnel syndrome*) produces progressive weakness and loss of fine movements in the distribution of that nerve. Attacks of pain, tingling, numbness or a "swollen" sensation follow excessive movements of the wrist. Atrophy of the radial portion of the thenar eminence may develop.

The Hands and Fingers

The interphalangeal hinge joints of the fingers permit flexion and extension of the phalanges; in addition, the metacarpophalangeal joints allow slight ulnar and radial deviation of the fingers.

Normal Function. The metacarpophalangeal joints allow the

[2] Fritz de Quervain, Swiss surgeon, 1868–1940.

proximal phalanges to be extended to 180 degrees or slightly more, flexed to 90 degrees and deviated through an arc of about 30 degrees (radial-ulnar). At the interphalangeal joints there should be full extension (180 degrees), with flexion at the proximal joints to 90 degrees or more, and somewhat less at the distal articulations.

Movement of the thumb is much more complex; the metacarpal bone plays an important part in abduction, adduction and apposition. With abduction, the thumb should be at an angle of about 90 degrees from the forefinger; when apposed it should lie on the palm of the hand. Flexion at the metacarpophalangeal and the interphalangeal joint is usually less than 90 degrees; extension to 180 degrees or more should be possible.

Abnormalities.   Rheumatoid arthritis often involves the proximal interphalangeal joints initially, producing the typical fusiform swelling; other joints may be involved later in the disease. In far-advanced cases excessive ulnar deviation of the phalanges and even of the metacarpals is not uncommon (Fig. 238, p. 358). Dislocations and sprains are common, especially in athletes; slight pain, swelling and limitation of motion may persist for a long time. Repeated injuries can lead to permanent deformity or limitation of motion. On the dorsum of the hand the metacarpal bones are very superficially situated. A fracture can often be diagnosed clinically; localized tenderness and pain, deformity and swelling are the important clues. Fracture of a phalanx usually results from trauma. Sometimes the symptoms are slight and the individual ignores them; the resulting deformity may be the only residual sign. Heberden's nodes have been mentioned (p. 357).

The Hip Joint

This is a ball-and-socket joint; the head of the femur fits into the acetabulum, a deep cup-shaped socket. A wide range of motion is possible, but when testing movement you must make certain that the pelvis and lumbar spine remain in a fixed position so that they do not participate. Since the hip is a weight-bearing joint, part of the examination should include observation of the patient as he stands and walks, wearing no more than a loin cloth if feasible.

Then have the patient lie on his back on a firm mattress or examining table. With each limb at an angle of 90 degrees to a line joining the anterior superior iliac spines, compare their length and size; measure corresponding areas if there is any inequality. If there is a deformity on one side, the normal limb must be placed in a similar position before measuring length. Also, with normal hip joints both extremities will rest flat on the table. If there is flexion deformity of one hip, the opposite thigh should be flexed to the same position; this eliminates compensatory tilting of the pelvis, which might result in an incorrect measurement.

Normal Function. Have the patient flex one leg as far as possible with the knee bent; the opposite leg must remain flat on the table. The thigh and trunk should form an angle of 60 degrees or less. The degree of abduction and adduction are then determined with reference to the line joining the anterior superior spines; the total arc is about 90 degrees. Then flex the thigh and the leg to 90 degrees each and determine external and internal rotation by swinging the foot and leg to the right and to the left. External rotation is usually slight; internal rotation may be from 60 to 90 degrees.

Have the patient turn over and lie prone. Place one hand on the pelvis and test for extension of the thigh by seeing how high the knee can be raised before the pelvis begins to move. Then flex the leg to 90 degrees; determine external and internal rotation with the thigh

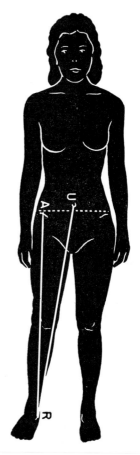

Fig. 259. Routine methods for measuring length of lower extremity. R-A, Anterior superior spine to internal malleolus. R-U, Umbilicus to internal malleolus. If the hip joint is not freely movable, the normal limb must be placed in a similar position before the measurements are compared. (Colonna, P. C.: Regional Orthopedic Surgery. Philadelphia, W. B. Saunders Co., 1950.)

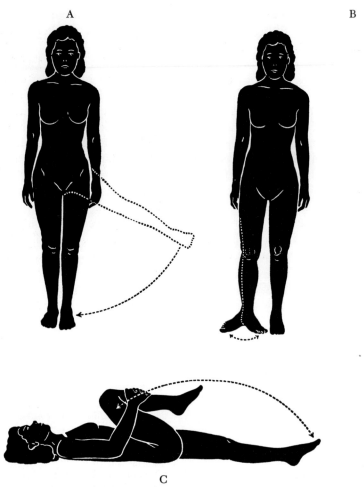

Fig. 260.   Normal range of movement of the hip in a young adult: *A*, abduction and adduction; *B*, internal and external rotation; *C*, flexion and extension. (Colonna, P. C.: Regional Orthopedic Surgery. Philadelphia, W. B. Saunders Co., 1950.)

extended by swinging the leg and foot from side to side. The normal range is about 135 degrees.

   Abnormalities.   Congenital dislocation or subluxation of the hip is difficult to diagnose in the newborn, but should be recognized within two months after birth. With the infant supine and the knees flexed, the thighs are flexed to a right angle and then gradually abducted. If either thigh cannot be abducted 40 degrees or more, subluxation should be suspected.

   Osteochondritis of the hip (Perthes'[3] disease) is most common between the ages of four and nine years. Pain in the hip or knee, a

   [3] George Clements Perthes, German surgeon, 1869–1927.

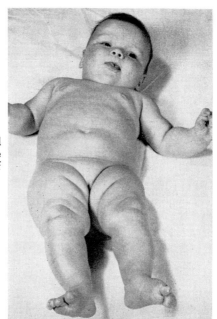

Fig. 261. Infant with congenital dislocation of left hip. Shortening of the leg, eversion of the foot and asymmetry of the skin creases is apparent.

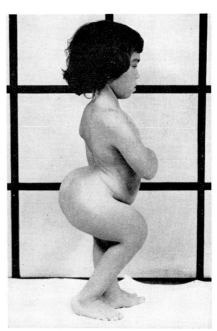

Fig. 262. Bilateral congenital dislocation of hips. Note marked increase in lumbar lordosis and protuberant abdomen.

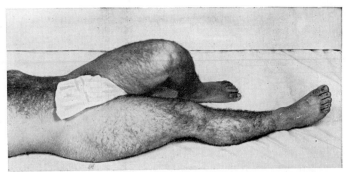

Fig. 263.   Position of flexion, adduction and internal rotation characteristic of posterior dislocation of the hip. (Colonna, P. C.: Regional Orthopedic Surgery. Philadelphia, W. B. Saunders Co., 1950.)

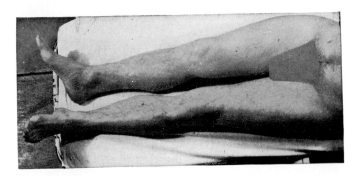

Fig. 264.   Characteristic position of right leg with fracture of the femoral neck. Shortening and external rotation are obvious. The patient is lying on a mat on the floor. (Colonna, P. C.: Regional Orthopedic Surgery. Philadelphia, W. B. Saunders Co., 1950.)

slight limp, limitation of motion of the hip joint and slight muscle spasm or atrophy are usually present. During adolescence the capitular epiphysis of the femur may be partially or completely displaced, often following slight trauma. There may be mild pain in the hip and knee, and a slight limp develops. Adduction may be increased, but other movements are generally decreased. If proper treatment is not instituted, bony union may occur and result in a decrease in the angle between the neck and the shaft; this is known as *coxa vara.* Tuberculosis of the hip may occur at any age, but predominantly it is a disease that starts during childhood.

Dislocation of the hip may result from trauma. It may be a simple dislocation or there may also be a fracture of the posterior lip of the acetabulum. Pain is severe; the thigh is flexed and adducted; muscle spasm is obvious and attempted motion in any direction causes excruciating pain.

Arthritis of the hip may also develop at any age; it may be rheumatoid or degenerative in type. The physical signs and degree of impairment of motion will depend upon the duration and severity of the disease.

Fracture of the hip is most common in older persons; it may be intertrochanteric or involve the neck of the femur. Shortening and external rotation of the limb are usually obvious, but in either type the bone fragments may be driven together (*impacted*) and deformity may be minimal or absent. Whenever an elderly person falls or sustains a serious bump and has pain in the region of the hip, fracture must be suspected and x-ray studies should be made at once.

The Knee Joint

This is the largest hinge-type joint, but its strength and stability depend to a great extent upon powerful ligaments and muscles that reinforce it. The most important ligaments are the internal collateral, the external collateral and the anterior and posterior cruciate.

For adequate examination of the knee the entire extremity must be bare; disease of the knee often results in disuse atrophy of the quadriceps or other muscles. Whenever possible the patient should be examined while walking, standing, sitting, lying supine and then lying prone.

In most persons, when the knees are fully extended each leg and thigh form a practically straight line; occasionally the line is curved or angled. With *genu valgum* (knock-knee) the leg angles outward; with the knee joints touching, the internal malleoli are separated by several centimeters. The opposite deformity is called *genu varum* (bow legs); with the feet side by side, the knees are widely separated. With *genu recurvatum* there is hyperextension of the knee joints; flexion is often limited in severe cases. These deformities may be idiopathic, due to relaxation of the ligaments or due to metabolic disorders such as rickets. A unilateral alteration is often traumatic.

Normal Function. The normal range of motion is somewhat less than 180 degrees, from full extension to the point at which the joint itself or contact of the calf muscles with the thigh prevents further flexion. Although flexion and extension are the primary movements, a slight amount of rotation can be elicited when the knee is flexed; this disappears with full extension. With the leg flexed to an angle of 90 degrees, the malleoli can be rotated through an angle of 15 to 30 degrees.

After flexion, extension and rotation have been measured, the ligamentous stability of the joint should be determined. To test the internal collateral ligament, extend the leg, brace the lower thigh or knee with

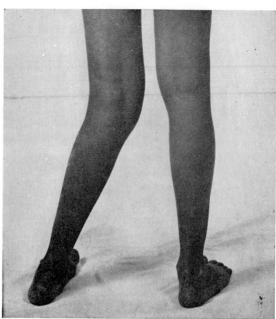

Fig. 265. Marked left genu valgum (knock-knee), secondary to epiphyseal damage.

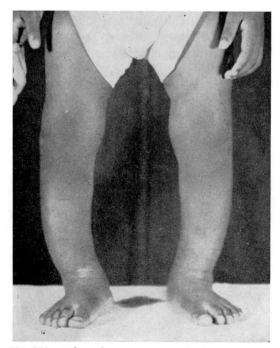

Fig. 266. Bilateral genu varum (bow legs), rachitic.

one hand and attempt to abduct the leg. The external collateral ligament is then tested by reversing the movements and attempting to adduct the leg. If movement of more than a few degrees is possible, the ligament examined must be relaxed or torn. The cruciate ligaments are tested with the patient seated or lying supine with the knee flexed so that the leg forms an angle of 90 degrees with the thigh. Immobilize the foot and attempt to displace the head of the tibia backward, then forward. Excessive forward motion indicates relaxation or a tear in the anterior cruciate ligament; excessive backward mobility, damage to the posterior ligament.

Abnormalities. Injuries of the knee joint itself or of the supporting structures are not uncommon. Discoloration may be obvious if the trauma is recent; swelling may persist for a long time. Excess fluid (*hydrarthrosis*) will often accumulate within 6 to 12 hours after an injury; very rapid accumulation suggests bleeding into the joint space (*hemarthrosis*). Acute infection will produce purulent fluid (*pyarthrosis*), with local or constitutional signs of infection.

With the leg extended, excess fluid will obliterate the hollow areas on either side of the patella; larger amounts will cause these areas to bulge, and give rise to a crescent of swelling above the patella. To confirm the presence of fluid rather than fat, edema or other changes in the tissues, place one hand around the thigh proximal to the patella and press downward and distally to displace the fluid from the suprapatellar pouch into the knee joint itself. Then depress the patella sharply

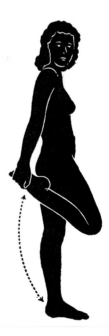

Fig. 267. Normal range of knee motion in the young adult. (Colonna, P. C.: Regional Orthopedic Surgery. Philadelphia, W. B. Saunders Co., 1950.)

with one finger; a tap will be felt as it strikes the underlying bone (*patellar tap*). If the effusion is small it may be necessary to place the hands above and below the patella and tap with one index finger to elicit this sign.

Either of the cartilaginous menisci may also be injured or torn if the leg is violently twisted while the knee is flexed and weight-bearing. It is a common injury in athletes. In some cases so-called "locking" of the joint will occur immediately or subsequently. Actually the joint is not locked; the leg can be flexed but full extension is suddenly checked.

The knee is also subject to damage by various specific and non-specific types of arthritis and by bone tumors. The latter may cause pain and swelling but rarely interfere with joint function until they invade the joint surface or enlarge sufficiently to interfere with motion.

Bursae.   Several bursae are present around the joint and may become distended with fluid if repeatedly traumatized. The prepatellar bursa lies between the skin and the patella; swelling of it is commonly called "housemaid's knee." The infrapatellar bursa lies between the distal portion of the ligamentum patellae and the tibia. When enlarged it bulges on either side of the ligament. Infrapatellar bursitis can usually be attributed to prolonged pressure on this area and is seen in workmen whose trade requires long periods of kneeling. It is often called "clergy-man's knee."

In the popliteal space the semimembranous bursa may enlarge and produce a somewhat mesially situated bulge; this is most easily seen and felt when the leg is extended, but it remains constant in size when the leg is flexed. Baker's[4] cyst is a swelling somewhat similar in appearance but centrally located; it is a pressure diverticulum of the synovial membrane through a hiatus in the capsule. With the leg fully extended the sac is tense; with flexion it becomes much smaller or disappears.

The Ankle Joint

This is a hinge joint formed by the articulation of the distal end of the tibia and fibula with the astragalus. Inversion (adduction) and eversion (abduction) of the foot are functions of the subastragalar and midtarsal joints, but for convenience in testing they will be considered at this point. Whenever possible the patient should be allowed to stand and walk; a deformity not apparent when he is at rest may become obvious with weight-bearing.

Normal Function.   The primary movements of the ankle joint are dorsiflexion to about 75 degrees and plantar flexion to about 140

[4] William Morrant Baker, British surgeon, 1839–96.

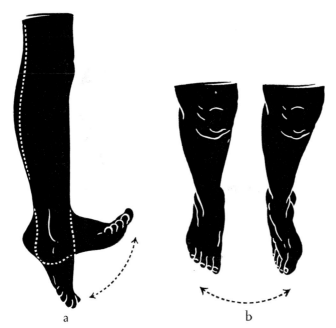

a   b

Fig. 268.   *a*, Normal degree of dorsal and plantar flexion; *b*, eversion and inversion. (Colonna, P. C.: Regional Orthopedic Surgery. Philadelphia, W. B. Saunders Co., 1950.)

degrees. To test for mobility of the subastragalar joints, grasp the leg above the ankle with one hand and the heel with the other; test for inversion and eversion. Motion should be possible through an arc of 60 degrees or more (Fig. 268).

Abnormalities.   Like that of the knee, the stability of the ankle joint depends largely upon ligaments. A slight misstep or twist may be enough to tear one or more of these; such sprains are relatively frequent and range from mild to very severe. There will be pain, tenderness and swelling. Ecchymosis may be visible soon after the injury but later it may be concealed by edema of the overlying tissues.

The most common type is the inversion sprain; the foot turns in and puts sudden excessive strain on the lateral ligaments. If the force is great enough there may be a fracture of the fibula (Pott's[5] fracture) with backward displacement of the ankle joint. An injury due to eversion is less commonly seen; it produces similar changes over the internal malleolus and adjacent tissues.

Rheumatoid arthritis frequently involves the ankles, making walking painful, difficult or hazardous; other types of joint disease may also occur here.

[5] Percival Pott, London surgeon, 1714–88. His literary works were started while he was confined to bed with such a fracture.

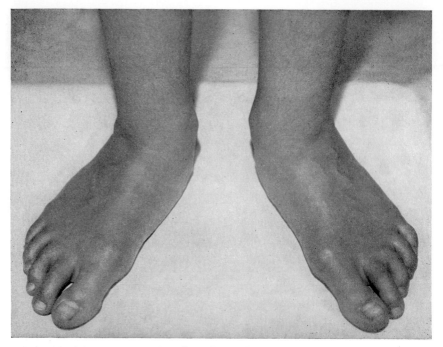

Fig. 269.   Bilateral pes planus (flat feet).

The Foot

A slight degree of motion occurs in the midtarsal and tarsometa-
tarsal joints. Grasp the heel firmly with one hand and the metatarsal
region of the foot with the other. Test inversion, eversion, dorsiflexion
and plantar flexion.

Normal Function.   Although some degree of motion is normal,
it is difficult to determine the exact articulation involved.

Abnormalities.   In addition to the usual diseases that involve
joints, the foot may have anatomic variants: flatfoot or clubfoot.

The Arches.   The normal foot has two arches: the longitudinal
or medial and the transverse or metatarsal. Either or both of these may
be altered in one foot or both. A variety of abnormalities of the bones
or muscles of the foot, leg or thigh can produce the abnormality commonly called flatfoot (*pes planus*) (Fig. 269).

To study the arches, have the patient stand normally with his feet
bare. Observe the medial arch and look for eversion of the foot. Then
slip a finger under each arch; estimate the space between the foot and
the floor and compare the two sides. If the patient is not ambulatory,
a rough estimate of the status of the arches can be obtained by pressing
against the sole with a flat object such as a book. Examine the feet

again with the patient seated or the pressure removed. A flatfoot due to relaxation will have an apparently normal arch when it is not bearing weight; the rigid flatfoot, more commonly in elderly persons, will show little change. Unilateral changes are often the result of trauma or disease of the foot. An abnormally high longitudinal arch (*pes cavus*) will throw more weight on the heads of the metatarsal bones and thus produce symptoms.

Relaxation or other abnormalities of the metatarsal arch can produce pain (*metatarsalgia*); this may be diffuse or sharply localized to the inferior aspect of one metatarsal head. A plantar callus or a corn (*heloma*) may be seen; the latter indicates pressure over a limited area and is rarely seen if the foot is normal.

Clubfoot. Certain common deformities involve both the ankle (*talus*) and the foot (*pes*) and are therefore called *talipes*, or more commonly, clubfoot. Since the principal movements are dorsiflexion, plantar flexion, inversion and eversion, four major deformities are possible. If the foot is dorsiflexed, the patient tends to put more weight on his heel (*os calcis; calcaneus*); this is talipes calcaneus. If plantar flexion is present the heel is raised, as it is in a horse (*equus*); this is talipes equinus. A foot may also show eversion (valgus) or inversion (varus) deformity. Appropriate combinations of these four positions will describe all of the common deformities. Thus there may be dorsiflexion plus eversion, or talipes calcaneovalgus; similarly there can be

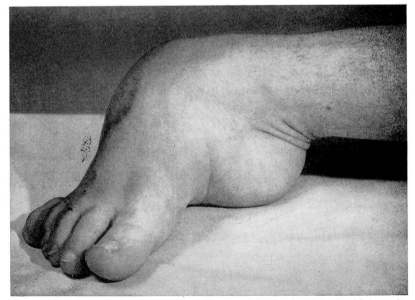

Fig. 270. Marked equinovarus deformity (clubfoot). This should have bee treated in infancy.

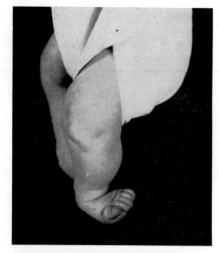

Fig. 271.   Calcaneovalgus (reverse clubfoot).

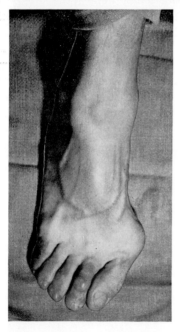

Fig. 272.   Hallux valgus.

talipes calcaneovarus, talipes equinovalgus and talipes equinovarus; the latter is the most common congenital deformity.

The Toes

The patient should now be asked to flex and extend his toes. The range of motion is not great, but any fixation or restriction of movement

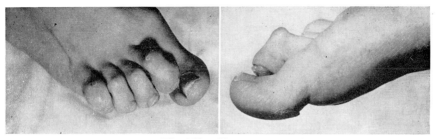

Fig. 273.   Hammer toes.

should be recorded. Loss of mobility may lead to disturbances in walking or pain while standing. Usually several toes are involved, as in arthritis. Lateral deviation of the great toe is not rare (*hallux valgus*); it may be congenital or acquired. The latter form seems to result from prolonged pressure due to shoes that are stylish but too narrow or too pointed. In most instances it is asymptomatic; if pain is present there is probably an accompanying bursitis (*bunion*) or a hammer toe. Gout also seems to prefer the metatarsophalangeal joint of the great toe (*podagra*), but the sudden onset of excruciating pain and tenderness will serve to differentiate this from acute bursitis. An ingrown toenail with or without infection (*paronychia*) will also produce pain.

The second toe, or occasionally one of the others, may show *hammer toe* deformity. The proximal phalanx is dorsiflexed; the distal phalanges are in plantar flexion. The head of the proximal phalanx is repeatedly traumatized and a corn usually develops; there may also be one on the tip of the toe. The deformity is usually bilateral and associated with hallux valgus.

The fifth toe may deviate mediad and overlap the fourth toe or even the dorsum of the foot at the base of that toe. A small bunion can also develop at the fifth metatarsophalangeal joint.

Partial or complete fusion of two toes (*syndactylia*) may be present; the second and third toes are most commonly involved.

The Spine

Whenever possible, the examination should begin with the patient standing and the back bared. A woman should wear an examining gown that can be opened from the neck to the sacrum or lower; a loin cloth can be worn.

Normal Structure.   The spinous process of the seventh cervical vertebra (C-7; vertebra prominens) is visible except in an obese person; the vertebral column should be in a vertical line from this point to the gluteal cleft. If the spinous processes cannot be seen, run a finger down

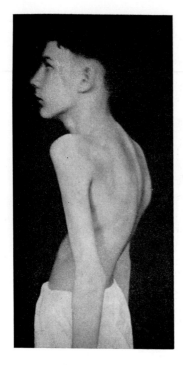

Fig. 274.   Postural thoracic kyphosis (dorsum rotundum) in a poorly developed, malnourished boy.

the back to identify them, and if necessary, mark their locations. The profile of the spine should then be inspected. Normally the cervical spine curves slightly, with the midportion a few centimeters farther forward than the first and seventh vertebrae (*lordosis*). The direction of the curve is reversed in the thoracic spine (*kyphosis*) but lordosis reappears in the lumbar region.

After inspection, palpation should be performed. If you have not already done so, run one finger down the spinous processes to confirm inspection; then palpate the paraspinal muscles for atrophy, spasm or tenderness. Percussion of the spinous processes should also be performed; any undue sensitivity warrants further study for underlying vertebral disease.

Abnormalities of Structure.   The normal lordotic curve of the cervical spine may be altered by injury or disease of the vertebrae, but it is often decreased physiologically in elderly persons. When thoracic kyphosis is increased there may be either a gentle curve or an angular deformity. The former can be postural, especially in adolescents (Fig. 274). In elderly persons it occurs with slow decrease in stature of the vertebral bodies resulting from demineralization (*osteoporosis*) or with pulmonary emphysema. A localized or angular deformity (*gibbus*) is suggestive of a destructive process involving one or more of the vertebral bodies; in children, tuberculosis must always be suspected (Pott's

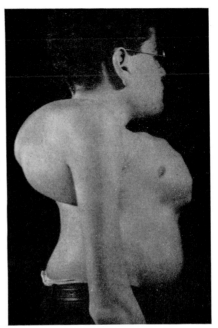

Fig. 275. Tremendous deformity secondary to tuberculosis of thoracic spine.

disease*). Traumatic fracture can occur at any age. In older persons compression fracture of a demineralized vertebra can occur, but metastatic carcinoma, Paget's disease and other destructive processes must be ruled out. The normal lumbar curve may also be altered. Physiologically it is obviously increased during the later months of pregnancy and in obese "potbellied" persons. This change is also seen with rickets, cretinism and spondylolisthesis. In the latter, the fifth lumbar vertebra (or occasionally the fourth) slips forward, producing a localized increase in lordosis.

Scoliosis.   This denotes a lateral deviation from the normal vertical line; it may be a single curve or an S-shaped deformity. Several types are recognized.

FUNCTIONAL SCOLIOSIS (POSTURAL SCOLIOSIS).   A very minor degree of scoliosis is not uncommon and is usually of no significance. Often it seems to result from generally poor posture, especially in children and adolescents. In these cases the spine becomes straight when the person bends forward.

COMPENSATORY SCOLIOSIS.   In the lumbar region especially, this may be due to a difference in the length of the legs. If the length of each leg was not measured, do it now or compare the height of the

---

* Percival Pott, who also described Pott's fracture (p. 391), wrote extensively about the palsy resulting from this spinal deformity, but not about the anatomic or pathologic processes responsible for these vertebral lesions.

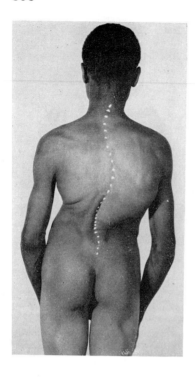

Fig. 276. Idiopathic scoliosis, showing deformity in spine, rib cage and shoulders.

iliac crests. If one is higher, or if one leg has been found to be longer than the other, have the patient raise the opposite heel slightly without bending the knee until the crests are level, or place an object of proper height under the heel to compensate for the difference. The scoliosis should decrease or disappear. Compensatory scoliosis may also be the result of lung disease that has decreased the volume of one hemithorax, or it may be due to an operation such as thoracoplasty or pneumonectomy that has produced a permanent deformity of the thoracic cage. Hip joint disease can also alter the alignment of the spine.

STRUCTURAL SCOLIOSIS.   This is much more important. It is classified as idiopathic, congenital or paralytic. The most common form is idiopathic scoliosis. This develops in adolescence, almost invariably in girls, and can lead to extensive deformity. A double curve is present, giving an "S" or "2" appearance. Rotation of the bodies of the vertebrae also occurs. Eventually the deformity of the trunk may be so great that the heart, lungs and abdominal viscera are compressed and displaced into new positions, making physical and roentgen examination difficult and confusing. This type of scoliosis may decrease but does not disappear when the person bends forward.

In congenital scoliosis there is failure of development of one or more hemivertebrae; the spine has a definite angulation because of this. Paralytic scoliosis is usually a sequel of poliomyelitis; the illness may have been relatively mild and not diagnosed or suspected until the deformity began to be apparent.

Normal Function. Mobility may be determined with the patient standing, or he may be seated on a firm surface. The cervical spine has the greatest range of movement. Nodding of the head tests the atlanto-occipital articulation. Flexion and extension are accomplished mainly by the lower cervical vertebrae; lateral flexion is primarily a function of the midcervical region. The atlanto-axial articulation is the principal site of rotation. Each of these movements should be tested. Have the patient tilt his head forward, backward, to the right and to the left; then have him rotate his head from side to side. Normally the head can be tilted in all directions at least 45 degrees from the resting position, and rotated 45 to 60 degrees to the right and left. If there appears to be limitation or inequality of active motion, determine passive motion by seeing how far the head can be moved in any given direction before resistance is felt. However, if injury or disease of the vertebrae is suspected, extreme caution must be used.

The thoracic and lumbar sections of the spine are conveniently examined as a unit. You will find that motion in the thoracic spine is restricted, mainly by the attached rib cage; also, much of the apparent motion of the lower back actually occurs at the hip joints. Have the patient lean backward, stand erect and then slump forward or attempt

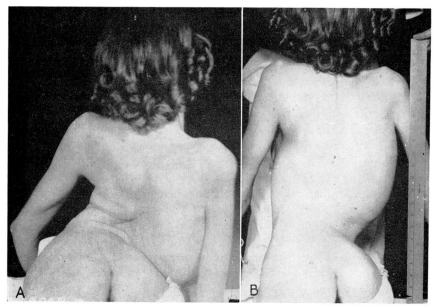

Fig. 277. Marked telescopic action of spine in paralytic scoliosis. A, Sitting; B, with head traction.

to touch the floor without bending his knees. To test lateral flexion, have him slide his left hand as far as possible down the outer aspect of the left thigh; then test the right side. Rotation is determined by having him twist to the right, then to the left, without moving his hips. If the patient is seated, have him attempt to touch the floor on either side and in front without shifting his weight or moving his hips.

Abnormalities of Function. Whenever there is evidence suggesting disease of the vertebrae, the spine should be examined with the patient prone and supine. With lumbosacral disturbances the patient finds that lying supine on the table soon becomes uncomfortable; he will flex his legs and thighs slightly to relax that area. Full flexion of both thighs, however, may aggravate the pain. If sacroiliac disease is suspected, grasp one leg just below the knee, fully flex the hip and knee joints and then attempt to force the knee toward the opposite shoulder without allowing the ipsilateral shoulder to be raised from the table. A marked limitation of motion on one side suggests sacroiliac disease. A further test is to have the patient prone; lift the thigh to hyperextend the hip joint. This will also produce pain on the affected side.

The straight-leg-raising test should then be performed. This is known by various eponyms; each author described minor modifications of the procedure.[6] With the patient supine, grasp the ankle with one hand and slip the other hand between the lumbar spine and the table. Slowly raise the entire extremity without allowing the knee to bend. In a normal person an angle of approximately 90 degrees can be achieved with no pain and no movement in the lumbar spine. Pain, straightening of the normal lumbar curve or limitation of flexion of the thigh will be apparent if there is tension on the sciatic nerve, compression of the nerve roots by a lumbar disk, or shortening of the hamstring muscles. It may be helpful to repeat the test; when pain first appears, sharply dorsiflex the foot. This will further stretch the nerve and increase the pain if there is involvement of the sciatic nerve or roots.

The evaluation of symptoms referred to the spine is often difficult. "Backache" is a common complaint, especially in women. Chronic strain may be due to apparently innocuous but oft-repeated routine household tasks such as lifting the baby out of his play pen, picking up his toys, wiping up the food he spilled, making the beds and wrestling with heavy baskets of laundry. Acute back strain may follow sudden severe stress during bending or twisting movements. In such cases the pain is usually maximal in the tense paraspinal muscles.

Rheumatoid arthritis may involve the spine; this is sometimes called

[6] J. J. Forst, "These de Paris," 1881; Joel E. Goldthwait, Boston surgeon, 1866–1961; Ernest Charles Lasegue, French physician, 1816–83.

Marie-Strümpell[7] or von Bechterew's[8] spondylitis. It begins in the sacro-iliac or lumbar region and tends to spread upward, producing straight-ening of the lumbar curve and then increased thoracic kyphosis. Even-tually the entire spine may be rigid ("poker spine").

With advancing age the vertebral bodies lose stature, especially in the thoracic region; increasing kyphosis and narrowing of the foram-ina result. Osteoarthritic changes may also develop, with lipping or spurs demonstrable by x-ray. Either of these may produce backache of variable severity or compression of nerve trunks.

Rupture of one or more of the intervertebral disks is most common in the lumbar region but can occur at any level. The disk protrudes posteriorly or posterolaterally and impinges upon the spinal cord or a nerve root. Pain is the most frequent complaint; it may be intermittent or constant and may be induced or aggravated by sneezing, coughing or physical exertion. Neurologic signs are usually demonstrable periph-erally, such as analgesia or anesthesia, loss of reflexes or muscular atro-phy. Neurologic disorders resulting from spinal disease are discussed in Chapter XXII.

EXAMINATION OF THE MUSCLES

Many medical, orthopedic and neurologic disorders produce varying degrees of weakness or complete paralysis of individual muscles or of those muscles supplied by a common motor nerve. One of the most common causes of muscular weakness is disuse atrophy, which may follow a fracture or may be due to chronic disease of bones or joints. Other important causes are acute poliomyelitis, myasthenia gravis and the various congenital and acquired muscular atrophies and dystrophies.

Figures 278–317 are modified from those of Daniels, Williams and Worthington. They depict techniques for estimating muscle power in practically all of the important voluntary muscle groups.

The National Foundation for Infantile Paralysis has designed a chart (Fig. 318) listing the various muscle groups. This chart provides space to record in parallel columns the date and result of the initial examination and of each subsequent one. This, or some similar chart, should be used for recording the findings when there is muscular weakness.

[7] Pierre Marie, French neurologist, 1853–1940; Adolf von Strümpell, German neurologist, 1853–1925.

[8] Vladimir Mikhailovich von Bechterew, Russian neurologist, 1857–1927.

Fig. 278.   Fig. 279.

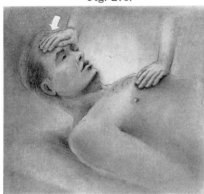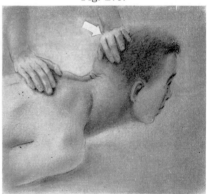

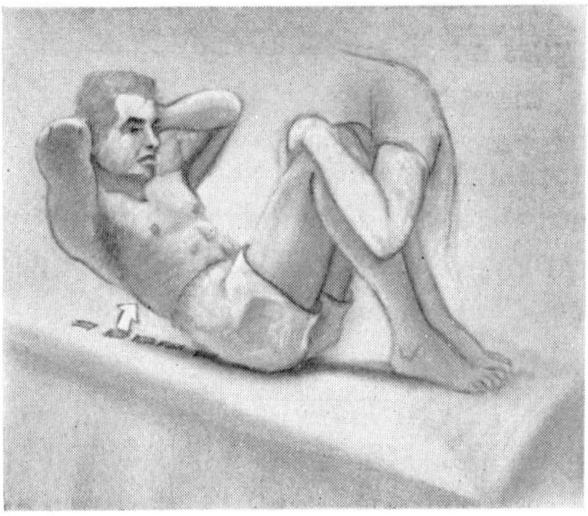

Fig. 280. 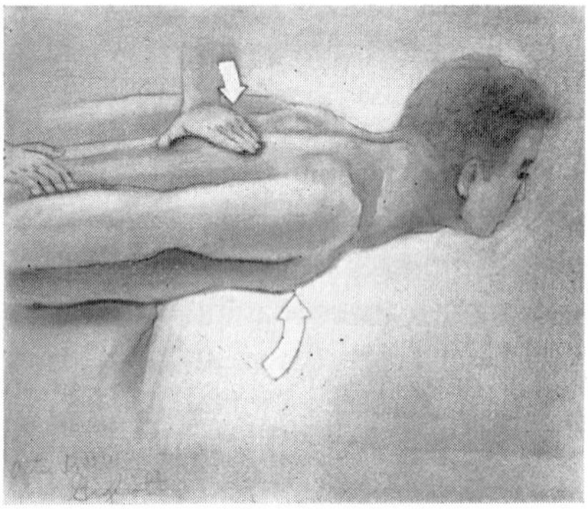   Fig. 281.

Fig. 278.   Flexion of the neck against resistance demonstrates chiefly the strength of the sternocleidomastoid muscles.

Fig. 279.   Extension of the neck against resistance demonstrates the neck extensors.

Fig. 280.   Flexion of the trunk demonstrates the strength of the rectus abdominis muscle.

Fig. 281.   Extension of the trunk demonstrates the power of the sacrospinals.

Fig. 282.   Fig. 283.

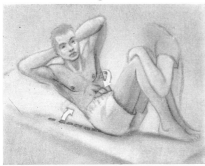 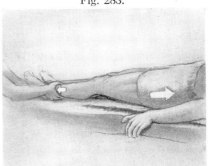

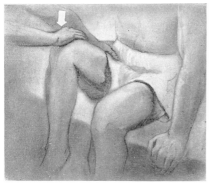

Fig. 284. 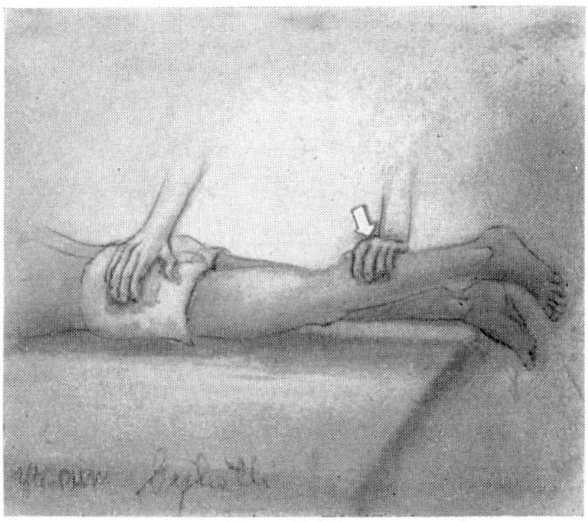   Fig. 285.

Fig. 282.   Rotation of the trunk demonstrates the power of the internal and external obliques.

Fig. 283.   Elevation of the pelvis against resistance demonstrates the power of the quadratus lumborum.

Fig. 284.   Flexion of hip, testing the power of the iliopsoas.

Fig. 285.   Extension of hip, demonstrating the power of the gluteus maximus and hamstrings.

Fig. 286.   Fig. 287.

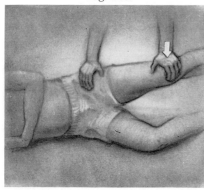
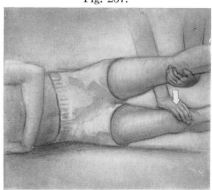

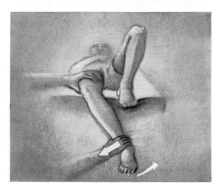
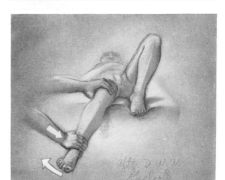

Fig. 288.   Fig. 289.

Fig. 286.   Abduction of hip, demonstrating the power of the gluteus medius and minimus.

Fig. 287.   Adduction of hip, testing the power of the right adductor magnus, longus, brevis and pectineus.

Fig. 288.   External rotation, demonstrating the power of all the external rotators of the hip.

Fig. 289.   Internal rotation, testing the power of the gluteus minimus and tensor fasciae latae.

Fig. 290.

Fig. 291.

Fig. 292.

Fig. 293.

Fig. 290. Flexion of knee, testing the power of the hamstrings.
Fig. 291. Extension of knee, testing the power of the quadriceps.
Fig. 292. Plantar flexion of ankle, demonstrating the power of the posterior leg muscles.
Fig. 293. Dorsiflexion of ankle, demonstrating the power of the anterior leg muscles.

Fig. 294. Fig. 295.

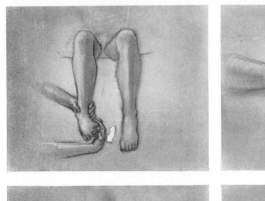 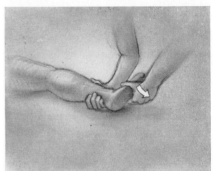

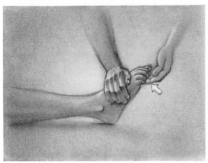 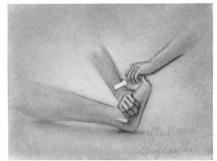

Fig. 296. Fig. 297.

Fig. 294. Inversion of foot, demonstrating the power of anterior and posterior tibials.

Fig. 295. Eversion of foot, showing the power of the peroneals.

Fig. 296. Flexion of toes, testing the power of the toe flexors.

Fig. 297. Extension of toes, showing the power of the toe extensors.

Fig. 298.

Fig. 299.

Fig. 300.

Fig. 301.

Fig. 298. Abduction and upward rotation, demonstrating the power of the serratus anterior.

Fig. 299. Adduction and downward rotation of scapula, testing the power of the rhomboideus.

Fig. 300. Elevation of the scapula, testing the levator scapulae and the upper fibers of the trapezius.

Fig. 301. Depression and adduction of the scapula, demonstrating the power of the lower fibers of the trapezius.

Fig. 302.   Fig. 303.

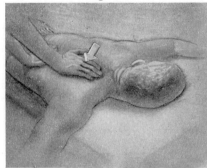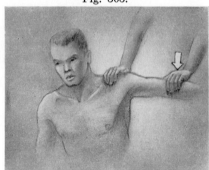

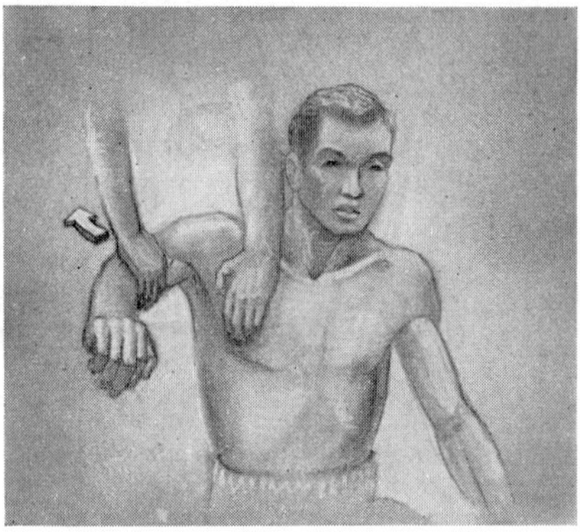

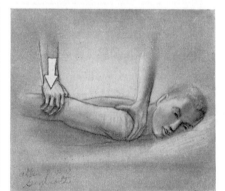

Fig. 304.   Fig. 305.

Fig. 302. Adduction of the scapula demonstrates the middle fibers of the trapezius.

Fig. 303. Abduction of the shoulder, testing the power of the deltoid and supraspinatus.

Fig. 304. Adduction of shoulder, demonstrating the power of the pectoralis major.

Fig. 305. Extension of shoulder, testing the power of the latissimus dorsi and teres major.

Fig. 306.   Fig. 307.

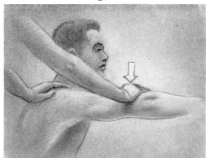 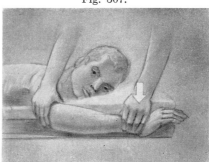

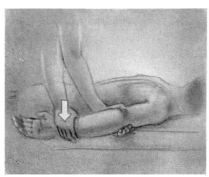

Fig. 308. 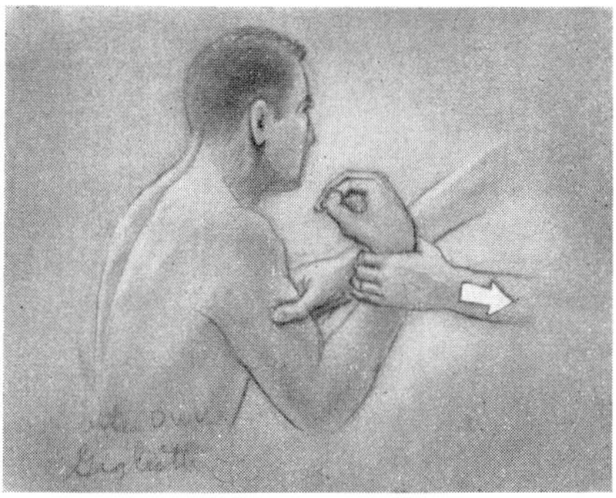   Fig. 309.

Fig. 306. Flexion of the shoulder, demonstrating the power of the anterior fibers of the deltoid and coracobrachialis.

Fig. 307. External rotation of the shoulder, testing the power of the infraspinatus and teres minor.

Fig. 308. Internal rotation of the shoulder, testing the power of the subscapularis.

Fig. 309. Flexion of the elbow, demonstrating the power of the biceps and brachialis.

Fig. 310.

Fig. 311.

Fig. 312.

Fig. 313.

Fig. 310. Extension of elbow, testing the triceps.
Fig. 311. Supination of forearm, testing the biceps and supinator brevis.
Fig. 312. Pronation of forearm, testing the power of the pronator radii teres and pronator quadratus.
Fig. 313. Flexion of wrist, testing the power of the flexor carpi ulnaris.

Fig. 314. Fig. 315.

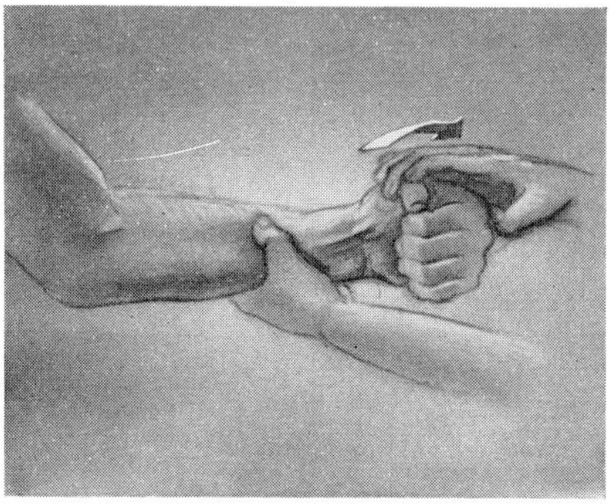

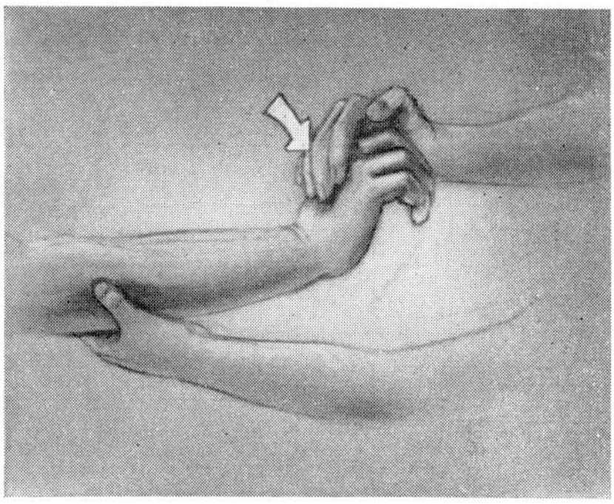

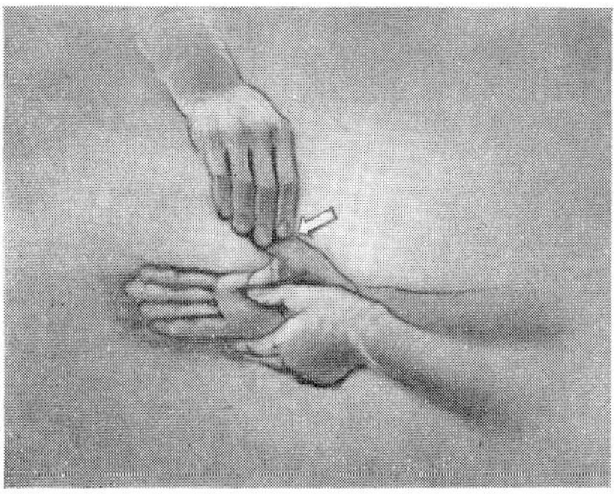

Fig. 316. 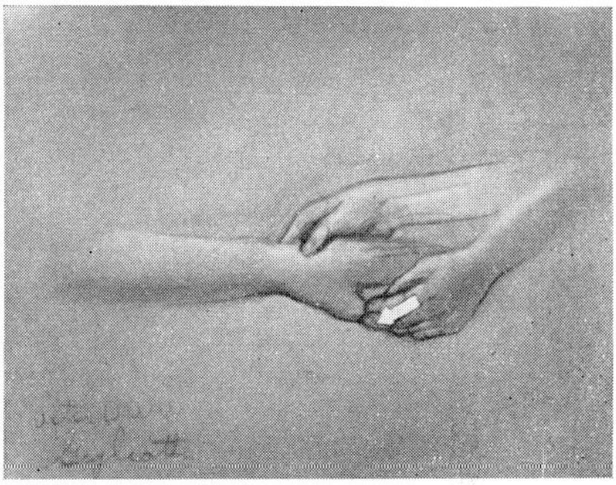 Fig. 317.

Fig. 314. Flexion of wrist, testing the power of flexor carpi radialis.
Fig. 315. Extension of wrist, testing the dorsiflexors of the wrist.
Fig. 316. Abduction of thumb, testing the power of abductor pollicis longus and brevis.
Fig. 317. Adduction of thumb, testing the power of adductor pollicis.

MUSCLE EXAMINATION

Patient's Name_____Chart No._____

Date of Birth_____Name of Institution_____

Date of Onset_____Attending Physician_____M. D.

Diagnosis:

LEFT   RIGHT

				Examiner's Initials					
				Date					
				NECK Flexors	Sternocleidomastoid				
				Extensor group					
				TRUNK Flexors	Rectus abdominis				
				Rt. ext. obl. Lt. int. obl. } Rotators { Lt. ext. obl. Rt. int. obl.					
				Extensors { Thoracic group Lumbar group					
				Pelvic elev.	Quadratus lumb.				
				HIP Flexors	Iliopsoas				
				Extensors	Gluteus maximus				
				Abductors	Gluteus medius				
				Adductor group					
				External rotator group					
				Internal rotator group					
				Sartorius					
				Tensor fasciae latae					
				KNEE Flexors { Biceps femoris Inner hamstrings					
				Extensors	Quadriceps				
				ANKLE Plantar flexors { Gastrocnemius Soleus					
				FOOT Invertors { Tibialis anterior Tibialis posterior					
				Evertors { Peroneus brevis Peroneus longus					
				TOES M. P. flexors	Lumbricales				
				I. P. flexors (1st)	Flex. digit. br.				
				I. P. flexors (2nd)	Flex. digit. l.				
				M. P. extensors { Ext. digit. l. Ext. digit. br.					
				HALLUX M. P. flexor	Flex. hall. br.				
				I. P. flexor	Flex. hall. l.				
				M. P. extensor	Ext. hall. br.				
				I. P. extensor	Ext. hall. l.				

Measurements:

Cannot walk	Date	Speech	
Stands	Date	Swallowing	
Walks unaided	Date	Diaphragm	
Walks with apparatus	Date	Intercostals	

Fig. 318 (a).

Fig. 318. (From Daniels, L., Williams, M., and Worthingham, C.: Muscle Testing. 2nd ed. Philadelphia, W. B. Saunders Co., 1956.)

LEFT   RIGHT

				Examiner's Initials						
				Date						
				SCAPULA	Abductor	Serratus anterior				
					Elevator	Upper trapezius				
					Depressor	Lower trapezius				
					Adductors	{ Middle trapezius { Rhomboids				
				SHOULDER	Flexor	Anterior deltoid				
					Extensors	{ Latissimus dorsi { Teres major				
					Abductor	Middle deltoid				
					Horiz. abd.	Posterior deltoid				
					Horiz. add.	Pectoralis major				
					External rotator group					
					Internal rotator group					
				ELBOW	Flexors	{ Biceps brachii { Brachioradialis				
					Extensor	Triceps				
				FOREARM	Supinator group					
					Pronator group					
				WRIST	Flexors	{ Flex. carpi rad. { Flex. carpi uln.				
					Extensors	{ Ext. carpi rad. l. & br. { Ext. carpi uln.				
				FINGERS	M. P. flexors	Lumbricales				
					I. P. flexors (1st)	Flex. digit. sub.				
					I. P. flexors (2nd)	Flex. digit. prof.				
					M. P. extensor	Ext. digit. com.				
					Adductors	Palmar interossei				
					Abductors	Dorsal interossei				
					Abductor digiti quinti					
					Opponens digiti quinti					
				THUMB	M. P. flexor	Flex. poll. br.				
					I. P. flexor	Flex. poll. l.				
					M. P. extensor	Ext. poll. br.				
					I. P. extensor	Ext. poll. l.				
					Abductors	{ Abd. poll. br. { Abd. poll. l.				
					Adductor pollicis					
					Opponens pollicis					
				FACE:						

Additional data:

Fig. 318 (b).

KEY

5 N	Normal	Complete range of motion against gravity with full resistance.	S or SS	Spasm or severe spasm.
4 G	Good*	Complete range of motion against gravity with some resistance.	C or CC	Contracture or severe contracture.
3 F	Fair*	Complete range of motion against gravity.		* Muscle spasm or contracture may limit range of motion. A question mark should be placed after the grading of a movement that is incomplete from this cause.
2 P	Poor*	Complete range of motion with gravity eliminated.		
1 T	Trace	Evidence of slight contractility. No joint motion.		
0 0	Zero	No evidence of contractility.		

XXII

Neurologic Examination

Final

The nervous system assists in the adaptation of the human organism to changes, both in the outside world and in the inside world of the body. Perception of the outside world and interaction with it are accomplished primarily by means of the central nervous system, while changes within the body are mediated by the autonomic nervous system. This section will consider the examination of the voluntary motor system and the sensory system.

THE VOLUNTARY MOTOR SYSTEM

This complex but coordinated system governs not only voluntary control of muscles, but also control of tone and of coordination, and integration of the special senses, gnostic sensation and other sensory impulses. The role of each of these must be understood before the results of the clinical examination can be interpreted correctly.

Voluntary Motor Control. The basic unit of the voluntary motor system consists of two neurons. Each upper motor neuron has its cell body in the motor strip of the pre-rolandic[1] frontal cortex; the axon arises there. The axons traverse the subcortical white matter, the internal capsule and the brain stem (midbrain, pons, medulla) and cross in the lower part of the medulla to form the corticospinal (pyramidal; lateral) tract on the opposite side. Prior to reaching the medulla, some fibers cross the midline (corticobulbar tract) and end in the motor nuclei of the brain stem (third, fourth, sixth, seventh, tenth, eleventh, twelfth and the motor divisions of the fifth and ninth cranial nerves). The axons in the corticospinal portion end on anterior horn cells in the spinal cord at various levels.

[1] Luigi Rolando, Italian anatomist, 1773–1831.

414

Each lower motor neuron arises in one of the large diamond-shaped cells in the anterior horn of the spinal cord. It traverses the white substance of the cord on the same side; groups of axons then pass through the meninges to the intervertebral foramina as the roots. After emerging from the foramina the motor roots join with sensory components to form the peripheral nerves. The motor impulse is propagated along the nerve to the myoneural junction and ultimately to the muscle.

The lower motor neuron supplies nutritive tonic impulses to the muscles and maintains a degree of tonus, which is modified or inhibited by the upper motor neuron. It also constitutes the motor half of the reflex arc. In the final analysis, the lower motor neuron is responsible for the impulse necessary for the performance of a motor act; if it is destroyed, no impulse from the cortex can reach the muscle. Therefore, lesions of the lower motor neuron are characterized by loss of tone, motor weakness, atrophy, diminished or totally absent reflexes (*areflexia*) and changes in the response to electrical stimulation. If the lesion is in the region of the anterior horn cell, fibrillations will also be present.

The upper motor neuron acts as the inhibitor of the lower motor neuron in that it modifies tone and reflexes. The volitional component of the motor act is mediated through it. Lesions of the upper motor neurons inhibit the function of the corticobulbar and corticospinal pathways, but leave the lower motor neurons intact; they are characterized by hyperreflexia, pathologic reflexes, hypertonia and muscular weakness or paralysis, but not by marked atrophy or fibrillations. Irritative lesions of the upper motor neurons can give rise to contralateral convulsions.

Tone.   Certain phylogenetically older structures of the extrapyramidal system modify the function of the upper motor neuron. The better known parts of the so-called extrapyramidal system are the lenticular nucleus (globus pallidus putamen), the caudate nucleus, the substantia nigra, the red nucleus and the subthalamic nucleus luysi.[2] Like the corticospinal system, it is a crossed pathway. Discrete lesions of these structures may occur, as in Parkinson's[3] syndrome, and give rise to the phenomena of rigidity and tremor, either of which may be present alone.

Tone is essentially a clinical concept. It may be defined as a state of tension in a given muscle or group of muscles. Tone may be disturbed in lesions involving either the upper motor neurons (the spasticity of hemiplegia) or the lower motor neurons (the flaccidity of poliomyelitis). It is altered in sensory disturbances as in the hypotonia of tabes dorsalis or multiple neuritis, and frequently is disturbed in diseases of the cerebellum and its pathways. However, it is most characteristically altered with lesions of the extrapyramidal system.

[2] Jules Bernard Luys, French physician, 1828–98.
[3] James Parkinson, London physician and geologist, 1755–1824.

Coordination.   Synergic control is concerned with the proper forcefulness and timing of various antagonistic muscle groups in the interest of smooth performance of the motor act. Disturbances of synergic control can occur in the absence of any motor weakness or alteration of sensation or tone. Anatomically and physiologically, lack of control depends upon the disturbed function of the cerebellum and its major connections, especially the three cerebellar peduncles. The most striking examples of synergic disturbances are seen in tumors of the vermis of the cerebellum or of the cerebellar hemispheres; the patient has considerable difficulty in gait and in the use of his homolateral limbs, even though there is no motor weakness.

Special Senses.   The special senses, especially vision, are important in the smooth and purposeful performance of the motor act. Sight, hearing, and the less important functions of smell and taste are considered later.

Gnostic Functions.   These are concerned with the performance of highly skilled acts or the recognition of complicated sensory complexes for which there are centers in the cerebrum closely related to the known motor and sensory centers. There is the area for expressive speech (Broca's[4] area or convolution) near the motor cortex. There is a center in the upper temporal convolution for the reception of spoken speech, in the angular gyrus for reading, and in the supramarginal gyrus for recognition of objects placed in one's hand (stereognosis).

The loss of ability to speak or to comprehend spoken or written language (various *aphasias*), loss of a previously acquired ability to perform skilled acts (*apraxia*) and loss of power to recognize the significance of sensory stimuli (*agnosia*) depend upon a disturbance of the particular center, not on voluntary movement or sensory perception. Thus the patient with motor aphasia has no paralysis of the vocal cords or of the muscles of the larynx, tongue or lips, but still cannot express himself. Patients with lesions in the upper temporal convolutions can hear, but not understand; those with lesions of the supramarginal gyrus can feel all modalities of sensation, but cannot recognize objects placed in the hand.

The concept of cerebral dominance is significant, since most of the centers are unilateral and occur in that half of the brain that is opposite to the "handedness" of the person. Thus the center for expressive speech in a right-handed person is in the left frontal cortex (Broca's area).

Psychologic Component.   Both the reception of external stimuli and the subsequent motor response are markedly influenced by the level of intelligence and by the emotional stability of the person. One must ascertain his educational level and be able to understand what complexity of vocabulary and syntax would be normal for him. Even in a

---

[4] Paul Broca, French surgeon, neurosurgeon and anthropologist, 1824–80.

well educated patient, the degree of tension produced by the examination and the fact that he is having difficulties with one of his previously routine activities may substantially interfere with his performance. To evaluate accurately the degree of aphasia or other gnostic functions, several interviews may be necessary after a satisfactory relationship with the patient has been established.

Methods of Examination *read*

To perform a neurologic examination one needs to become proficient in a relatively small number of tests, and he should form the habit of making his observations in an orderly fashion. The gross divisions of the examination include: (1) observation of posture, gait and station; (2) notation of the presence or absence of various involuntary movements; (3) examination of the head, including the skull, the facial expression and the structures innervated by the twelve cranial nerves; (4) examination of the neck, including determination of the presence or absence of meningeal irritation; (5) examination of the trunk; (6) examination of the upper limbs; (7) examination of the lower limbs; (8) evaluation of the mental status, especially to determine organic thinking disorders (this has been discussed in Chapter II).

POSTURE, GAIT AND STATION

Posture.   Note the posture of the patient as he stands, sits or lies down. The position of the head in respect to the trunk, of the limbs to the trunk and to each other, and of the lower part of the limb to the upper part all give clues to motor function. The patient with Parkinson's disease stoops. The hemiplegic supports himself in standing and often has the affected upper extremity partially flexed at the elbow, with the hand turned out.

Gait.   This might be termed dynamic posture. Observe the ease with which the patient carries his head in relation to his trunk, the way in which he carries and swings his arms, the erectness of the trunk, and the relation of the hip, knee and ankle joints to each other in the movements of walking. Note the position of the patient's eyes; when an ataxic person tries to walk, he keeps his gaze fixed on the ground. There is considerable variation in the normal gait and often there is a family similarity. Local disease, especially of the feet, knees or hip joints markedly influences gait.

When a normal person walks, he swings his left arm forward as he advances his right foot, and vice versa. With pyramidal and extra-

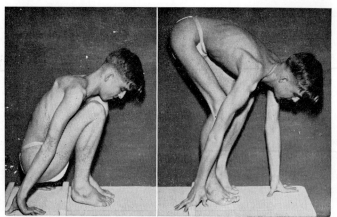

Fig. 319. Progressive muscular dystrophy. Typical maneuvers ("climbing up self") on arising. (Aird, R. B.: *In* Baker, A. B. (ed.): Clinical Neurology. New York, Paul B. Hoeber, Inc., 1955, Vol. 3.)

pyramidal disease these *associated movements* of the arms are decreased or lost. The hemiplegic may not lift his leg; he swings it forward with a circular motion (circumduction) or lets the paretic foot drag on the ground. In Parkinson's disease the gait is characterized by short steps, stooped posture, flexed neck, loss of associated movements of one or both arms and difficulty in stopping (*propulsion*); the patient often totters forward, often at an ever-increasing speed, to maintain his balance.

With cerebellar disease the patient walks with the feet far apart laterally (a wide base). The muscle movements are jerky and uncoordinated as in an intoxicated person, and there is danger of falling. In tabes, and less commonly in other diseases involving the posterior columns, there is hyperextension of the knee joint (*genu recurvatum*) as well as ataxia.

Infants and children with cerebral diplegia have bilateral spasticity that gives rise to the so-called "scissors gait." The right foot is swung forward and placed to the left of the left foot; then the left foot is swung around and planted to the right and in front of the right foot. This is maintained into adult life and is also known as the *marche à petits pas*. Patients with multiple neuritis or other diseases may be unable to dorsiflex the foot and toes (*foot drop*); they compensate by overflexion of the thigh and knee like a prancing horse (*steppage gait*).

In the muscular dystrophies, characterized primarily by degeneration of muscle fibers and replacement by connective tissue and fat, there is excessive forward curvature of the lumbar spine (lordosis); in walking the abdomen protrudes. If the glutei are affected, the gait is waddling.

With hysteria a variety of gait disturbances may occur. These may

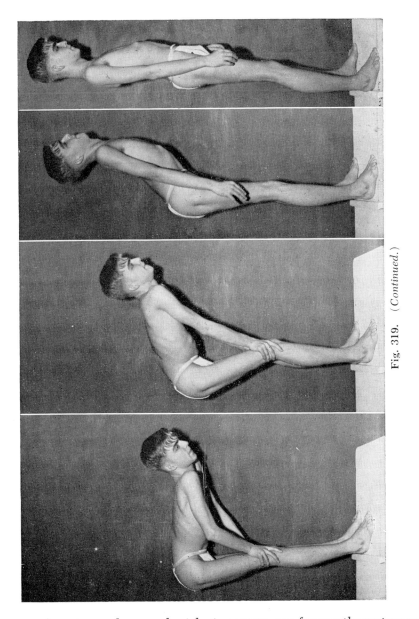

Fig. 319. (*Continued.*)

not conform to any known physiologic pattern, are frequently grotesque, and may be out of keeping with the other physical findings.

Station. Further information can be gained by having the patient stand in front of you, first with his eyes open, then with them closed. Note whether he can stand unsupported. If not, determine whether he always tends to fall to the same side (cerebellar hemisphere or cerebellopontile angle disease). Next, ask the patient to put his feet together and close his eyes, but be prepared to catch him. If he sways excessively or starts to fall, the Romberg[5] test is positive. This occurs with tabes or other posterior column diseases, with vestibular disturbances (eighth cranial nerve), with neuritis and occasionally with cerebellar disease.

Additional information can be obtained by asking the patient to squat and then stand again. By this maneuver early difficulties with co-ordination can often be detected, as can minor degrees of muscular weakness.

Watch the patient as he gets on or off the examining table. With muscular dystrophy, if you place your hands on the knees of the supine patient he will be unable to elevate his trunk. Unaided, such a person gets up by "climbing up his own body," grasping the ankles, knees and thighs.

INVOLUNTARY MOVEMENTS

Fibrillations (Fasciculations). These are slow, wormlike movements of individual muscle fibers or groups. These movements, especially when restricted to one area of the body, generally result from involvement of the anterior horn cells, and less frequently, of the roots or the peripheral nerves. Fibrillations occur predominantly in the shoulders and upper part of the arms, but may be seen in any part of the body. The most widespread fibrillations occur with amyotrophic lateral sclerosis, a degenerative disease that involves the anterior horn cells and the pyramidal tract. Fibrillations may also occur with states of tension or malnutrition, or from overindulgence in tobacco or other toxins. In these situations fibrillations are usually transient, whereas in organic disease they are fairly constant.

Tremors. These are fairly rhythmic oscillating movements of muscle groups. They may be coarse or fine, and may or may not be influenced by voluntary movement. Tremors occur as a normal reaction to cold, or may be due to fatigue or fear. Familial tremors of the head and extremities are not uncommon. Coarse tremors of the hands occur from intoxicants such as alcohol, cocaine or tobacco, and from large amounts of epinephrine or insulin. Fine tremors of the hands may occur with paresis, together with dysarthria and tremors of the lips and tongue, or in hyperthyroidism. Coarse tremors of the trunk and extremities occur with bromide intoxication. Bizarre tremors may be seen with hysteria.

In Parkinson's disease the upper extremities are involved more often than the lower. Coarse tremors of the extremities are present, together with a characteristic position and tremor of the hands. The forearm is

[5] Moritz Heinrich Romberg, Berlin physician, 1795–1873.

partially flexed and held in semipronation; the fingers are flexed almost at right angles to the palm; the thumb apposes the fingers and there is a rapid to-and-fro movement of the digits giving a "pill-rolling" appearance.

The intention tremor is mostly commonly seen with multiple sclerosis and is characterized by inability to perform purposeful acts with the upper extremities without marked oscillations as the hand nears the target. For example, if the patient attempts to reach for a glass of water the arm will be fairly steady until the hand nears the glass; then the amplitude of excursions of the hand increases. This is particularly evident in the so-called finger-to-nose test (p. 436).

Choreiform Movements. These are jerky, irregular, constantly changing movements of the face, trunk or extremities, and are usually associated with muscular hypotonia. Rheumatic (Sydenham's[6]) chorea occurs predominantly in young persons; hereditary (Huntington's[7]) chorea is a disease of middle life. Not infrequently choreiform movements beginning early in life may last for many months or years; it may be difficult to determine whether they reflect organic disease or a psychomotor situation, or both.

Athetoid Movements. These are slow, purposeless movements involving predominantly the fingers and toes, but occurring elsewhere. Movement is maximal at the metacarpophalangeal and metatarsophalangeal joints. They are usually congenital and are associated with cerebral spastic diplegia (Little's[8] disease). Choreiform and athetoid movements often occur together in the same individual and are described as choreoathetoid movements.

Dystonic Movements. These are larger than those discussed so far and spread around the long axis of the trunk or limb. *Hemiballism* consists of violent "throwing" movements of one half of the body; it is usually due to a lesion in the subthalamic area.

Spasms. These are repetitive movements involving various parts of the body, most often the muscles of the face and neck. They usually involve simultaneously several groups of muscles innervated by specific nerves or roots. They are rapid and stereotyped, and can often be checked voluntarily. If they are present, note whether the movements are tonic or clonic.

Tetanus ("lockjaw") can produce widespread spasm of muscle groups, in addition to spasm of the jaw muscles. Calcium deficiency may give rise to tetany, with spasmodic involuntary contractions of the hands

---

[6] Thomas Sydenham, English physician, 1624–89.
[7] George Sumner Huntington, American physician, 1851–1916.
[8] William John Little, English physician, 1810–94.

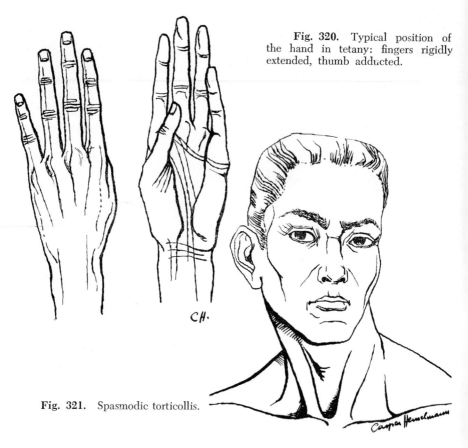

Fig. 320. Typical position of the hand in tetany: fingers rigidly extended, thumb adducted.

CH.

Fig. 321. Spasmodic torticollis.

and feet (*carpopedal spasm; main en griffe*); Chvostek's[9] sign may also be positive. To elicit this, tap the cheek along the course of the facial nerve; homolateral contraction of the facial muscles will occur. Pain, peripheral nerve lesions and nerve irritation can also produce muscular spasm. In spasmodic torticollis ("wryneck") there is forced turning of the head to one side because of tonic spasm of the opposite sternocleido-mastoid muscle or other neck muscles. Spasms of the muscles of one side of the face can result from irritation of the seventh cranial nerve. Recurrent diaphragmatic spasms (hiccup; singultus) are not uncommon and may be serious.

Tics (Habit Spasms).   These are repetitious, stereotyped movements involving generally one muscle mass; many different tics may occur in the same patient. A tic tends to mimic a physiologic action such as sticking out the tongue, blinking the eyelids or moving an extremity. These movements are generally considered to be psychologic in origin and are difficult to treat.

[9] Franz Chvostek, Austrian surgeon, 1835–84.

Table 1.   Differential Diagnosis of Convulsive Disorders*

LESION	CAUSE	TYPE OF SEIZURE
I. Convulsions occurring *with* demonstrable cerebral lesions:		
1. Expanding, space-occupying lesions	Neoplasm, chronic abscess, cyst, etc.	Focal (jacksonian) or generalized (grand mal)
2. Cerebral cicatrix	Trauma; infection	Focal; may become generalized
3. Local cerebral atrophy	Congenital ischemias, infections, compressions	Focal; may become generalized
4. Local microgyria	Infantile ischemia or compression	Focal; may become generalized
5. Diffuse cerebral disease	Degenerative disorders; infections, acute or chronic	Usually generalized
6. Diffuse cerebral vascular disease	Arteriosclerosis, syphilis or others	Usually generalized
7. Miscellaneous	Congenital lesions, etc.	Focal or generalized
II. Convulsions occurring *without* demonstrable cerebral lesions:		
1. Idiopathic	Abnormal cerebral physiology	Grand mal; petit mal Psychomotor attacks Epileptic equivalents (?)
2. Toxic and febrile	Extracerebral	Grand mal
3. Hypoglycemic	Extracerebral (pancreatic adenoma, etc.)	Grand mal or abortive grand mal
4. Miscellaneous	Extracerebral: syncope; carotid sinus abnormalities; circulatory impairment, etc.	Grand mal or abortive grand mal

* Modified from Penfield, W., and Erickson, T. C.: Epilepsy and Cerebral Localization. Springfield, Ill., Charles C Thomas, 1941, p. 20.

Convulsive Seizures.   These are of great clinical significance; the following classification may be helpful: (1) Seizures with gross muscular movements, which may be generalized or focal. In the generalized convulsion (*epilepsy; grand mal*) there are widespread clonic contractions of the extremities, face, jaws and trunk, followed by a period of tonic contractions, with eventual complete relaxation. Incontinence of feces and urine may occur. Focal (jacksonian[10]) seizures are associated with a localized disturbance in the electrical activity of the cortex. Initially there is clonic contraction of an extremity, half of the face or one side of the body. The seizure may then become generalized or may stop. The area of onset and the mode of spread should be recorded. (2) *Petit mal* attacks. In these there is momentary loss of consciousness but no abnormal movements except for occasional chewing motions or smacking of the lips. (3) Psychomotor attacks. Here one finds irrational behavior performed in a normal manner. For example, for no apparent reason the patient may carry a glass of water from one table to another, yet have no memory of this action. (4) Hysterical convulsions. Bizarre muscular movements occur; generally there is no loss of consciousness.

[10] John Hughlings Jackson, English physician, 1834–1911.

THE HEAD: CRANIAL NERVES

The general examination of the head and the more important anatomic abnormalities have already been considered (Chapter V). The integrity of the cranial nerves should now be determined.

First Nerve.   The *olfactory* nerves are tested by asking the patient to sniff one or more of the easily obtained volatile oils (lavender,
clove, wintergreen) or some substance such as coffee or tobacco, first
with one nostril closed, then the other. Sharp pungent odors such as
ammonia or acetic acid (vinegar) should be avoided; they may be perceived through common sensation (fifth nerve).

Loss of smell (*anosmia*) may be the result of a congenital lesion,
local nasal or sinus disease, basilar meningitis or a deep-seated intracranial tumor. The sense of smell is characteristically perverted with
lesions of the rhinencephalon and of the olfactory groove. Olfactory
hallucinations are common in toxic states, in schizophrenia and in hysteria; the patient insists that he smells pleasant or unpleasant odors
which others cannot perceive.

Second Nerve.   The appearance of the optic disks and the procedures for testing the function of the optic nerves were discussed under
The Eyes in Chapter V. From a neurologic standpoint it cannot be overemphasized that the examination of the eyes must be comprehensive.

Third, Fourth and Sixth Nerves.   These nerves are usually considered together because of their common function as the motor nerves
to the various extraocular muscles.

Each third cranial nerve (*oculomotor*) arises in the midbrain from
a complex intercommunicating group of nuclei. The fibers pass predominantly ipsilaterally through the midbrain and emerge at the upper
border of the pons. The nerve then passes forward and eventually bifurcates. The smaller superior division supplies the superior rectus muscle
and the levator palpebrae; the larger inferior portion supplies the medial
rectus muscle, inferior rectus muscle, inferior oblique muscle and the
constrictor of the pupil.

Complete paralysis of one oculomotor nerve results in ptosis, inability to deviate the affected eye upward, inward or downward, and fixed
dilatation of the pupil. Outward deviation alone is unaffected; the external rectus muscle is not involved (Fig. 322).

Unilateral complete paralysis is generally indicative of a peripherally located lesion. Because of the close proximity of the nerve to the
internal carotid artery, pressure from an aneurysm of the circle of Willis[11]
frequently produces this. Bleeding from such an aneurysm (subarachnoid hemorrhage) can also cause paralysis; it also occurs with syphilitic

---

[11] Thomas Willis, English anatomist and physician, 1621–75.

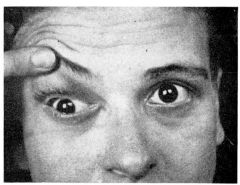

Fig. 322. Palsy of third nerve due to aneurysm of anterior part of circle of Willis. (Courtesy of Dr. A. M. Ornsteen.)

basilar meningitis, after head injury and occasionally in myasthenia gravis.

Incomplete oculomotor palsy is more commonly due to a lesion in the nucleus. This is usually vascular in origin; occasionally it is due to an invasive neoplasm of the midbrain.

The fourth pair of cranial nerves (*trochlear*) arise in the midbrain and each has a course similar to that of the oculomotor nerve. Each trochlear nerve innervates only the ipsilateral superior oblique muscle. Paralysis as an isolated finding is uncommon; it may be overlooked unless the examination is thorough. In the acquired form the lesion is usually in the nucleus. It may also be congenital and should be suspected if the child carries his head tilted toward the opposite shoulder.

The sixth pair of cranial nerves (*abducens*) arise from nuclei in the lower pons near the floor of the fourth ventricle. The fibers run freely in the subarachnoid space of the posterior fossa, pierce the dura and run under it along the petrous portion of the temporal bone.

Each abducens nerve innervates only the lateral rectus muscle on its own side. If it is damaged or destroyed the eye cannot be deviated laterally; such unilateral paralysis is the most common single extraocular palsy. Abducens paralysis may be congenital, probably due to birth injury. More commonly it is due to one of a multitude of diseases such as a vascular lesion of the nucleus, infection of the midbrain, meningitis, fracture of the wall of the orbit, periostitis of the orbit, fracture of the petrous portion of the temporal bone, injury to the posterior fossa, aneurysm of the internal carotid artery, a lesion in the posterior part of the pons, mastoiditis involving the tip of the petrous bone (Gradenigo's[12] syndrome), tabes dorsalis, myasthenia gravis or increased intracranial pressure irrespective of the cause.

Because of the long intracranial course of this nerve and the numerous conditions that may injure or destroy it, isolated sixth nerve palsy is of limited value in localizing neurologic diseases.

[12] Giuseppe Gradenigo, Italian physician, 1859–1926.

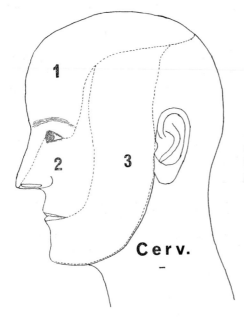

Fig. 323. Fifth cranial nerve (trigeminal): sensory distribution. 1, Ophthalmic division; 2, maxillary; 3, mandibular. Cerv., area supplied by cervical dermatomes.

Fifth Nerve. The *trigeminal* nerve has a major sensory and a minor motor component; the latter innervates the muscles of mastication. To test motor supply to the masseter and temporal muscles, place the fingers on the temples and mandibles and have the patient open and close his mouth forcefully; the two muscle groups should contract equally. To test the pterygoid muscles, ask the patient to open his mouth and then move the chin toward one side and then the other as you oppose this with your fingers. Unilateral pterygoid weakness is accompanied by deviation of the jaw toward the paralyzed side. Irritative lesions of the motor portion may occur in encephalitis or in tabes but reach their height in tetanus; the spasm of these muscles produces the "lockjaw."

The sensory portion of the fifth nerve subserves sensation to the entire face including the corneas, and common sensation to the tongue. The distribution of each of the three sensory divisions of this nerve is well established (Fig. 323). The integrity of each division on both sides of the face should be determined by testing the sense of touch and pain, and temperature also if indicated. Occasionally it may be necessary to attempt to differentiate anatomic from nonanatomic areas of altered sensation; hysterical anesthesia often stops exactly at the midline or extends below the jaw line into the area supplied by the cervical dermatomes.

In trigeminal neuralgia (*tic douloureux*) the lesion is usually in the gasserian ganglion; there is increased sensitivity over one or more of the three divisions of the nerve. Stimulation by pressure or even by a blast of air may initiate an attack of excruciating pain. Herpes zoster of the fifth nerve is not uncommon; corneal scarring may follow involvement of the first (ophthalmic) division of the nerve.

The corneal reflex is useful as a test of fifth nerve function. To elicit this, have the patient tilt his head backward and look up. Touch the cornea lightly with a small wisp of clean cotton; this must be brought up from below and out of the patient's visual field; otherwise he might wink when he sees it.

The efferent impulse is mediated through the ophthalmic division of the fifth nerve, the efferent through the seventh (facial) nerve. The reflex center is probably in the brain stem. The direct reflex is the blinking of the eyelids on the side tested; the consensual reflex is a similar movement of the opposite eyelids. With a unilateral disturbance of the sensory pathway of the fifth nerve, neither eye will react when the cornea on the affected side is touched; both eyes will react when the uninvolved eye is stimulated. With unilateral seventh nerve palsy both the direct reflex and the consensual reflex will be absent on the affected side; both will be normal in the other eye. Total absence of this reflex is strongly suggestive of a lesion in the course of the fifth nerve, and may be the earliest sign of a lesion in the cerebellopontile angle. In deep coma the reflex also disappears; this is frequently used to determine the stage of surgical anesthesia.

Seventh Nerve. Although the functions of the *facial nerve* are primarily motor, it also supplies sensation to the ear and part of the

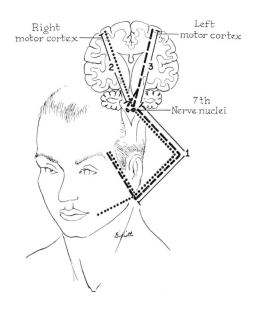

Fig. 324. Peripheral and central facial palsy: anatomical factors in differential diagnosis.

1. Lesion of peripheral nerve results in total paralysis of face on affected side, with inability to wrinkle forehead, close eye, puff out cheek, elevate corner of mouth or whistle.

2. Lesion of right motor cortex, or right subcortical fibers, results in paralysis of the lower two-thirds of the left side of the face, due to the interruption of the contralateral upper motor neuron. The upper third of the face receives fibers from both the right and the left motor cortex (2 and 3).

3. Lesion in the left motor cortex results in paralysis of the lower two-thirds of the right side of the face (not illustrated), but does not affect the upper third of the left side of the face because of bilateral innervation.

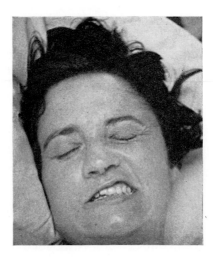

Fig. 325.   Right facial palsy due to tumor of the left frontal lobe. On the attempt to smile, the right side of the face remains immobile. The eyelids close normally. (Courtesy of Dr. A. M. Ornsteen.)

pharynx, taste to the anterior two-thirds of the tongue and secretory fibers to the salivary glands. It is frequently involved in neurologic diseases.

Motor function is studied by noting first the facial expression. Look for asymmetry, atrophy or flattening of the nasolabial folds and for fibrillations or other abnormal movements. Voluntary movement is then tested by having the patient wrinkle his forehead, close his eyes, show his teeth or whistle. The face should also be examined during emotional innervation; for this purpose have the patient smile or laugh.

Facial palsy is the most significant manifestation of seventh nerve damage; this may be central or peripheral, unilateral or occasionally bilateral. Central paralysis is due to a lesion in the contralateral cerebral cortex or subcortical white matter; it is most commonly seen following a cerebral vascular accident (a stroke). The lower two-thirds of the face is paralyzed, but the upper third shows little weakness because it receives fibers from both cortices through the corticobulbar tract. There is drooping of the angle of the mouth, flattening of the nasolabial fold and slight widening of the palpebral fissure on the affected side. There may be inability to elevate the angle of the mouth voluntarily, and often it cannot be elevated by emotional stimuli. However, the patient can usually frown or wrinkle the forehead, and can close his eyes (Fig. 325).

Complete peripheral facial nerve palsy may be produced by a lesion at any point along its pathway from the nucleus in the pons to the point at which it traverses the parotid gland and spreads over the face; flaccid weakness or paralysis of one entire side of the face results. The cheek is smooth, the eye is open, the corner of the mouth droops; both voluntary and emotional movements are practically lost. Tears may flow over the cheek; saliva may drool from the corner of the mouth; food tends to lodge between the cheek and the teeth, making eating difficult. Because the eye cannot be closed, there is danger of corneal injury or ulceration. Initially the face is drawn to the unaffected side; eventually there will be contractures, so that the face appears to be drawn to the affected side and the true site of the palsy may be apparent only when the patient attempts to smile, whistle or show his teeth.

Incomplete peripheral facial palsy is sometimes difficult to differentiate from the central type. One has to depend upon the relative weakness of the orbicularis oculi and frontalis muscles, on the flabbiness of the muscles of the affected side compared with those of the opposite side and on the response to electrical stimulation. The presence of fibrillary tremors is strong evidence that the lesion is either in the pons or distal to that point; with a cortical or subcortical lesion, atrophy and fibrillations do not appear.

TASTE SENSATION. This should be tested whenever peripheral facial palsy is present. This sensation (to the anterior two-thirds of the tongue) is supplied by the *chorda tympani*, a branch of the facial nerve that leaves the main trunk just distal to the facial canal. Thus a lesion in the canal or proximal to it is characterized by loss of taste sensation; if it is distal to that point, taste will be preserved.

There are four components of taste; only sweet, sour, salty or bitter substances can be distinguished. Sugar, vinegar, salt and quinine are commonly used as stimuli. Have the patient wet his tongue thoroughly, then protrude it and hold it out with a piece of gauze or tissue. A small amount of the test substance is placed on the anterior half of the tongue lateral to the midline or along the margin; this must not touch either the opposite half or the posterior third on the same side. The patient signals with his hand if he tastes anything.

The commonest form of peripheral facial palsy is called Bell's[13] palsy (Fig. 326). In these cases the nerve is involved either in the facial canal or, more commonly, distal to the stylomastoid foramen. Bell's palsy is presumably of viral origin but is frequently attributed to a sudden change in temperature—"I slept in a draft."

An uncommon but more specific type of peripheral facial palsy is seen in herpes zoster involving the geniculate ganglion (Ramsay Hunt[14] syndrome). In these cases there are herpetic lesions of the auditory canal and sometimes of the lateral surface of the pharynx, with tinnitus, impairment of hearing and vertigo.

Occasionally one encounters bilateral facial palsy (facial diplegia)

[13] Sir Charles Bell, Scottish physiologist working in London, 1774–1842.
[14] James Ramsay Hunt, American neurologist, 1874–1937.

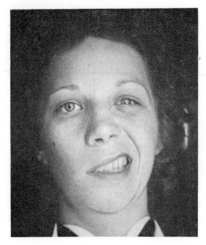

Fig. 326. Slight Bell's palsy. Weakness of all muscles on the right side of the face becomes evident when the patient tries to smile. (Courtesy of Dr. A. M. Ornsteen.)

with infectious polyneuritis (Guillain-Barré[15] syndrome). Motor weakness is present but the diagnostic feature is a cerebrospinal fluid that has a high protein content but a normal cell count (*albuminocytologic dissociation*). Facial diplegia also occurs with syphilis, especially in the secondary stage, with a tumor of the pons and from various lesions at the base of the skull involving the nerve. A pseudoplegia may be seen with myasthenia gravis, but the favorable response to appropriate drugs helps to differentiate this from true paralysis.

Eighth Nerve. The *auditory* nerve actually consists of two parts: auditory and vestibular. Both pass from the labyrinth to the pons and medulla. The auditory division is concerned with hearing. The chief functions of the vestibular division, in conjunction with the semicircular canals, the utricle and the saccule, are the maintenance of equilibrium and the orientation of the body in space while at rest and also during movement.

Tests of auditory acuity and integrity have been described (p. 96). From the neurologic standpoint, the Weber and Rinne tests are important. Symptoms referable to disease of the auditory or cochlear division include impaired hearing or deafness and "ringing in the ears" or other abnormal sounds (*tinnitus*).

Disturbances of the vestibular division may lead to nystagmus and vertigo. Seasickness and Meniere's[16] syndrome are examples of this; the latter is often accompanied by tinnitus and partial deafness. The cause of Meniere's syndrome is often in doubt; this form of labyrinthitis has been attributed to edema, inflammation or certain toxins such as DDT

[15] George Guillain, French neurologist, born 1876; J. A. Barré, French neurologist, born 1880. The name of A. Strohl also appeared on their paper; he seems to be the forgotten man—the one who probably did the work.

[16] Prosper Meniere, French physician, 1799–1862.

and formaldehyde. The condition of the temporal bone should always be evaluated in the presence of vestibular disturbances.

Clinically, the vestibular apparatus is difficult to examine, but a rough estimate of vestibular function can be obtained from the Romberg test (p. 420). The person with vestibular disease will sway excessively or may actually fall; be alert to prevent this. Nystagmus (p. 77) may also be indicative of vestibular disease. The test for *past pointing* should also be performed. Have the patient sit with one arm above his head, index finger extended. Hold your index finger in front of him. Tell him to bring him arm down and touch your index finger with his. Then have him close his eyes and repeat the maneuver; test both arms several times if necessary. When there is vestibular dysfunction his finger will deviate to the right or left and miss your finger completely.

The most accurate information is supplied by the Bárány[17] test. Bárány reported that when one external auditory canal is irrigated with cold water (20° C.) a normal person develops nystagmus with the quick component toward the opposite side; warm water reverses the direction of the nystagmus. With severe disease of the labyrinth or of the vestibular division of the eighth nerve, nystagmus does not develop when the involved side is irrigated. This procedure, with various additions and refinements, may be helpful in differentiating between such conditions as a cerebellopontile angle tumor and Meniere's disease, but it should be performed only by a trained person.

Ninth Nerve.   The *glossopharyngeal* nerve contains both motor and sensory fibers. It innervates the levator of the pharynx and the opening of the eustachian tubes, supplies taste to the posterior third of the tongue and common sensation to the hard and soft palate and tonsils. Motor function is tested by attempting to elicit the gag reflex; touch the posterior pharyngeal wall with a tongue blade if necessary. This reflex is extremely variable; it may be very active or it may be entirely absent without neurologic disease. In doubtful cases it may be necessary to test taste sensation of the posterior third of the tongue, using the substances previously mentioned but applying them to the posterior third.

Difficulty in swallowing (*dysphagia*) is the most common complaint with lesions of the glossopharyngeal nerve.

Tenth Nerve.   The *vagus* nerves have wide distribution. One or more of their many branches may be irritated, injured or destroyed, or one or both of the nuclei may be diseased. In the pharynx, unilateral damage results in deviation of the uvula toward the healthy side; bilateral disease can produce dysphagia or regurgitation of fluid into the nose. The recurrent laryngeal branches supply the vocal cords; the left branch loops under the aortic arch and the right passes beneath the subclavian artery. Either may be irritated or damaged by vascular lesions or by dis-

[17] Robert Bárány, Viennese otologist, 1876–1936.

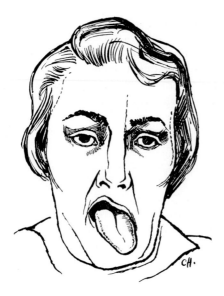

Fig. 327. Paralysis of the left hypoglossal nerve; deviation of the tongue *toward* the affected side.

ease of adjacent structures in the neck or mediastinum. Paralysis of one nerve allows the vocal cord to relax; it lies near the midline and does not move or vibrate with phonation. Hoarseness is commonly present; laryngoscopy is indicated. Bilateral paralysis will cause serious respiratory difficulties.

Stimulation of the fibers going to the heart will produce bradycardia; with impaired function or complete paralysis tachycardia develops. Many drugs affect the vagus nerves; often the pulse rate is a clue to their efficacy or toxicity. Disorders of gastric secretion and of gastrointestinal peristalsis and motility may also be due to vagal disturbances; here again the effects of drugs may be striking.

Bilateral involvement of certain branches may occur in postdiphtheritic neuritis, bulbar palsy (amyotrophic lateral sclerosis), Guillain-Barré syndrome and polioencephalitis. Complete destruction of both vagi is incompatible with life.

Eleventh Nerve. The *spinal accessory* nerves innervate the sternocleidomastoid muscles and the upper portion of the trapezii. To test the integrity of each nerve, have the patient rotate his head while you oppose this with your fingers. With the other hand, palpate the sternocleidomastoid muscle on the opposite side. The head cannot be turned if the muscle is weak or paralyzed. To test the trapezius, have the patient shrug his shoulders against resistance, but remember that this muscle (other than the upper portion) is also innervated by various cervical cord segments.

The spinal accessory nerve may be damaged or destroyed by infections such as polioencephalitis, by degenerative diseases such as amyotrophic lateral sclerosis, by a spinal cord tumor, by a herniated disk or as a result of trauma. An irritative lesion of the eleventh nerve results in muscular spasm. It can be responsible for congenital wry neck; more frequently it is seen as spasmodic torticollis (pp. 119; 422).

Twelfth Nerve.   The *hypoglossal* nerves innervate the muscles of the tongue; abnormalities of motor function have been discussed (The Tongue, p. 102).

The Peripheral Motor System

The examination of the neck, trunk and extremities must be complete, but the routine to be followed is optional. Each area may be examined completely as a unit, or the procedures can be subdivided into three broad classifications: testing the voluntary motor system, the sensory system and the reflex arcs. The latter method of examination will be discussed here.

The general procedure for examining the various muscles and muscle groups of the neck, trunk and extremities was outlined in Chapter XXI. Whenever muscular weakness, paralysis, atrophy or hypertrophy is present it should be charted, and certain tests that have important neurologic implications should be performed.

THE NECK

In the neurologic examination one is interested in the movements of the neck, in abnormal masses and pulsations, and in localized areas of tenderness. The neck should be passively flexed and extended; any limitation should be noted. The cervical vertebrae should be palpated as carefully as possible, seeking areas of tenderness. The supraclavicular areas should then be palpated, especially in the region of the scalenus muscles. Look for undue sensitivity of the subclavian vessels and adjoining components of the brachial plexus (neurovascular bundle). When there is a history of pain in the arm, some procedure such as Adson's[18] maneuver should be performed. The patient is asked to take a deep breath and hold it; the examiner forcibly turns the patient's chin as far as possible toward the affected side while palpating the radial pulse. When there is compression of the neurovascular bundle by a tight scalenus muscle or by a cervical rib, the volume of the radial pulse is diminished or it is completely obliterated. This maneuver should be performed bilaterally, even though the pain is unilateral, and the radial pulses compared.

In the presence of cerebral symptoms palpate the carotid arteries

[18] Alfred W. Adson, Rochester, Minn., neurosurgeon, 1887–1951.

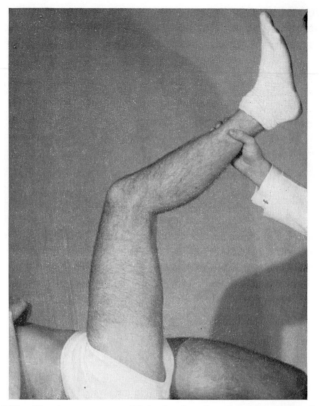

Fig. 328. Kernig maneuver. With the leg flexed at the knee, the thigh is raised to a vertical position; the leg is then gradually elevated. Normally it can be extended considerably farther than shown.

gently and one at a time; simultaneous bilateral compression may lead to cerebral anoxia or to cardiac disturbances from stimulation of the carotid sinus. If there is marked inequality of the pulsations, or if the pulse is absent on one side, cerebral arteriography may be desirable; surgical intervention can often relieve obstruction.

Whenever there is headache, fever, vomiting or neck pain, the results of tests for meningeal irritation are especially important (p. 119). Nuchal rigidity caused by meningeal irritation must not be confused with that due to arthritis of the cervical spine. In the former, rotation of the head is not restricted and does not cause pain. With arthritis there is usually pain and limitation of motion when an attempt is made to move the head in any direction.

For the Kernig[19] maneuver, have the patient lie on his back with both legs extended. Raise one thigh until it is vertical, allowing the leg to flex at the knee; then extend the leg gradually (Fig. 328). Kernig's

[19] Vladimir Kernig, Russian physician. 1840–1917

sign is considered positive when the leg cannot be extended on the thigh more than 135 degrees. A positive Kernig sign is due to stretching of the posterior roots, which are involved in the presence of meningeal irritation.

Lasegue[20] described a closely related sign. The initial procedure is the same; the thigh is raised to a vertical position to rule out hip joint disease, and then lowered. Grasp the foot or ankle and elevate the leg *without* flexion at the knee until pain in the lumbar area or in the sciatic nerve inhibits further elevation or causes flexion at the knee. If positive, this sign is usually indicative of cord tumor, herniated disk or other lesion impinging on the nerve roots.

Patrick's[21] test is also helpful. With the patient supine, flex the hip and knee and place the ankle as high as possible on the opposite leg, preferably above the patella. Then press the knee laterally and downward toward the bed. This combines lateral rotation and abduction of the hip joint, forcing the head of the femur into the acetabulum. With sciatic nerve involvement the knee can be made to approximate or touch the bed. With arthritis of the hip joint, or with sacroiliac disease, lateral deviation of the knee will be limited by pain.

THE TRUNK

The deep muscles of the back cannot be tested individually, but the general development and tonicity of the two sides should be compared with the patient lying face downward (prone). Then have him turn over. The muscles of the shoulder girdle, thorax and abdomen are examined with particular reference to fibrillations, atrophy, weakness or paralysis. Alterations may be unilateral or bilateral; the probable site of the lesion (central or peripheral) should be determined. Ask the patient to cough; a weakened or paralyzed area of the abdominal wall will bulge when he does this. Have the patient raise his head from the pillow and then sit up; look for inequality of muscular contractions.

THE UPPER EXTREMITIES

Examination usually starts with the upper extremities. Each is examined as a unit, and the various tests for motor power, tone and coordination are performed.

The arms should be in a relaxed position, either hanging by the sides or resting on the lap. Look for atrophy, hypertrophy or fibrillation of muscle groups and for any involuntary movements. Then have the patient extend the hands and arms with the fingers outstretched. This will

---

[20] Ernest Charles Lasegue, French physician, 1816–83.
[21] Hugh Talbot Patrick, Chicago neurologist, 1860–1939.

give some information concerning muscle power; a paretic upper extremity cannot be extended, and any marked weakness is immediately apparent. Look for tremors of the outstretched fingers; these may be the fine tremors of hyperthyroidism or the coarse pill-rolling tremors of Parkinson's disease. When the latter is suspected, have the patient approximate the thumb and forefinger rapidly for 45 to 60 seconds. The affected fingers will move more slowly than normal and the excursion will be smaller. If bilateral involvement is present, use your ability to perform this maneuver as a control.

Coordination Tests.   Ask the patient to pronate and supinate the upper extremities rapidly, with the elbows extended. Normally this will be done rapidly and smoothly. With cerebellar disease, posterior column disease or generalized weakness due to chronic disease of any type, the patient is unable to perform this movement smoothly, especially on the affected side. For the finger-to-nose test, have him extend one arm laterally, and then touch the tip of his index finger to the tip of his nose, first with the eyes open and then with them closed. Then test the other arm. Inability to do this reasonably accurately, or the appearance of a marked tremor when he tries, is commonly found in a person with multiple sclerosis; it is also seen with cerebellar disease, posterior column disease and generalized weakness. If previously omitted, the test for past pointing (p. 431) should be done at this time.

Muscle Tone.   To test muscle tone, have the patient place his hands loosely in his lap; grasp the wrists and then flex and extend each forearm. In hypotonic states there is little resistance; in spastic conditions such as hemiplegia the resistance is markedly increased. In a person with Parkinson's disease, if a joint (particularly the elbow) is passively flexed and extended, you may feel a series of abrupt jerks which alternately seem to stop and then release the moving portion (*cogwheel phenomenon*). When performing this test for tone, be sure that the apparent resistance is not due to disease of the elbow joint.

Muscle Strength.   Determine muscle strength by the procedures described in Chapter XXI, noting the general development and power of the various muscles and comparing the right side with the left. Occasionally a person's occupation will lead to much greater development of the muscles of one extremity. When testing the muscles of the hand, the patient is asked to "shake hands" and then squeeze; if great strength is suspected, have him squeeze one or two fingers of your hand instead. Atrophy of the intrinsic muscles of the hand or of the thenar or hypothenar eminence develops in amyotrophic lateral sclerosis, progressive muscular atrophy, syringomyelia, and with herniated disk or a cord tumor; it may also occur as a sequel of poliomyelitis or with a destructive lesion of the brachial plexus, the ulnar or the median nerve.

Then ask him to flex and extend the wrists and forearms against resistance; estimate the strength of the various muscles involved. Have him raise his arms sidewards, first to 90 degrees and then to 180 degrees. Abduction to 15 degrees is accomplished by the supraspinatus, from 15 to 90 degrees by the deltoid, and from 90 to 180 degrees by the combined action of parts of the trapezius plus the serratus magnus. Ordinarily, if the person can perform these procedures satisfactorily, and if there is no difficulty in holding the outstretched arms steady, there is no need to do more detailed muscle studies. However, if specific nerve injuries are suspected, or if there is any history or finding suggestive of spinal cord disease or involvement of the brachial plexus, each individual muscle or group should be tested.

Motor Nerve Lesions. The ulnar nerve innervates many of the intrinsic muscles of the hand, the adductor pollicis, the flexor carpi ulnaris, the flexor profundus of the fourth and fifth fingers and the skin of the ulnar portion of the hand. A lesion of this nerve produces a characteristic attitude of the hand. The fourth and fifth fingers are hyperextended at the metacarpophalangeal joints and flexed at the interphalangeal joints. There may be atrophy of the interossei and of the thenar and hypothenar areas. Hypesthesia or anesthesia will also be present in the cutaneous distribution of this nerve.

A simple test may disclose an ulnar nerve lesion. Have the patient grasp a piece of paper or cardboard between the thumb and index finger of each hand and attempt to pull the hands apart. Normally the terminal phalanx is extended and the thumb is flat. With paralysis of the adductor pollicis (ulnar nerve), the thumb is flexed at the interphalangeal joint during this test by involuntary contraction of the flexor pollicis longus and the opponens pollicis, which are supplied by the median nerve.

The median nerve innervates the abductor brevis, opponens and flexor brevis of the thumb and the long flexors of the first two fingers. In lesions of this nerve the thumb cannot be apposed to the other fingers and there is loss of many of the flexor movements.

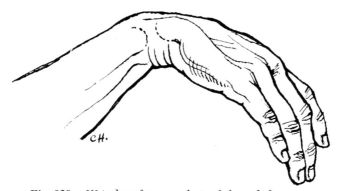

Fig. 329. Wristdrop from paralysis of the radial nerve.

The radial (musculospiral) nerve supplies the extensors of the arm, forearm, hand and fingers. When this is damaged the hand hangs down and cannot be dorsally extended (*wrist drop*) and there may be weakness of the triceps muscle (Fig. 329).

THE LOWER EXTREMITIES

Examination of the lower extremities is conducted in a similar manner. The motor power of the ambulatory patient is exhibited as he walks, stands or squats. With a bedfast patient, some estimate of strength can be gained by asking him to raise both lower extremities. Normally, a person can hold the extended lower extremities at an angle of 40 to 50 degrees for 15 to 30 seconds. The hemiplegic will be unable to raise the involved leg from the bed.

When there is any question of neurologic disease, it is necessary to test the strength of the flexors, extensors, adductors and abductors of the thigh, the flexors and extensors of the knee, the flexors, extensors and evertors of the ankle and the flexors and extensors of the toes. Change in tone is detected by passively flexing and extending the leg on the thigh and the thigh on the trunk.

Coordination in the lower extremities, or the lack thereof, can be observed as the patient walks. Another method is to have the recumbent patient close his eyes and place one heel on the opposite knee, and then run the heel rapidly down the shin. Inability to perform the heel-to-knee test accurately may be due to muscular weakness or joint disease; it also occurs in multiple sclerosis, with a cerebellar tumor or other lesion involving the cerebellar pathways, or with pyramidal tract disease associated with spasticity.

THE SENSORY NERVOUS SYSTEM

The four special senses (sight, smell, taste and hearing) have already been discussed; touch and other sensations concerned with the cutaneous surface will be considered here. From the clinical standpoint the chief divisions are touch, pain, temperature discrimination, position or joint sense and the perception of vibration. These various stimuli converge from receptors in the periphery by way of the sensory nerve fibers, which unite to form the sensory roots. After entering the spinal cord, fibers carrying pain, temperature and light touch sensations diverge to reach the thalamus through the spinothalamic tracts of the contralateral half of the cord, while the so-called deep sensations (position, vibration, joint sense and deep touch or pressure) proceed to the thalamus through the posterior columns of the homolateral half of the cord. The various pathways thus diverge upon entering the spinal cord, but again converge after leaving the thalamus on their way to the parietal lobe.

Certain adjuncts are used for testing common sensation. For touch, a wisp of cotton or a small camel's hair brush is convenient. For superficial pain a needle is preferable but a sharp pin or short hatpin is often adequate; this will provide both a "sharp" and a "dull" test object. For thermal discrimination two test tubes are employed; one is filled with hot water, the other with ice or ice water. To test vibratory sense a tuning fork of relatively low pitch (128 cycles per second) is needed. The patient should keep his eyes closed while these tests are being performed.

Touch. Using the wisp of cotton, touch the skin lightly. Over hairy areas it is not necessary to touch the skin; merely move one or more of the hairs slightly. Ask the patient to say "now" or "yes" each time he feels the touch. Compare similar areas on each side of the midline, and proceed in an orderly manner from head to foot. When the results are conflicting or in doubt, it may be necessary to retest the area several times.

Alterations include decreased sensitivity (*hypesthesia*), total loss (*anesthesia*) and abnormally increased sensitivity (*hyperesthesia*). With the latter the patient may also have perversion of sensation (*paresthesia*); a light touch may cause a painful or burning sensation.

Pain. The pin is then used; touch the skin lightly with the point or the head. Ask the patient to state whether it is "sharp" or "dull." With decreased sensation (*hypalgesia*) the point will be "dull"; with total loss of pain sensation (*analgesia*) the patient will feel nothing, or merely a sense of pressure if you press too hard. With increased sensitivity (*hyperalgesia*) even the head of the pin will feel sharp. When an area of abnormal sensation is encountered, the pin should be touched to that area and then drawn outward with a light stroking motion. Have the patient indicate the exact point at which sensation changes.

Temperature. When either of these procedures shows an area of altered sensitivity or seems inconclusive, the area should be tested for temperature sensation by momentarily touching various spots with the hot or cold tube in a random manner and asking the patient to indicate what he feels.

Position. A normal person can tell the position of his extremities even when his eyes are closed; a slight change in position is perceived at once. For a rapid check of position sense, grasp the sides of a toe or finger and quickly flex or extend it *slightly*. The patient should know immediately whether it is "up" or "down."

Vibratory Sensation (Pallesthesia). If the handle of the vibrating tuning fork is placed over a bony prominence where there is little overlying tissue such as the malleolus, tibia, olecranon or clavicle, a

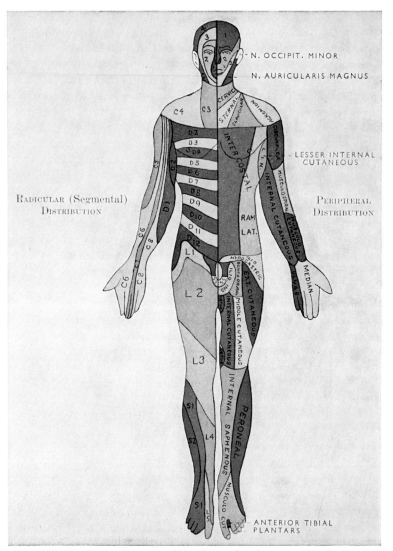

Fig. 330. Radicular (segmental) and peripheral sensory distribution, anterior view. (After Dejerine, Head, Villiger and Stewart. Nelson Loose-Leaf Medicine, Vol. VI. New York, Thomas Nelson & Sons.)

"buzzing" or "tingling" sensation should be felt. Loss of vibratory sense is one of the first neurologic changes in addisonian (pernicious) anemia; it is also altered in certain neuropathies.

Many neurologists recommend that pain sensation should be determined first, using the pin. If abnormalities are found, touch, temperature and other special tests are then used. Regardless of the order of testing, each dermatome and the sensory distribution of the main peripheral nerves must be tested. This must not be done haphazardly; a definite plan must be followed.

All areas of altered sensation should be carefully outlined and charted. Altered sensation may be radicular (segmental) in distribution if the root is involved, or it may occur in the distribution of a peripheral nerve. The charts (Figs. 330 and 331) indicate the areas supplied by the spinal roots (dermatomes) and also by the main peripheral nerve trunks.

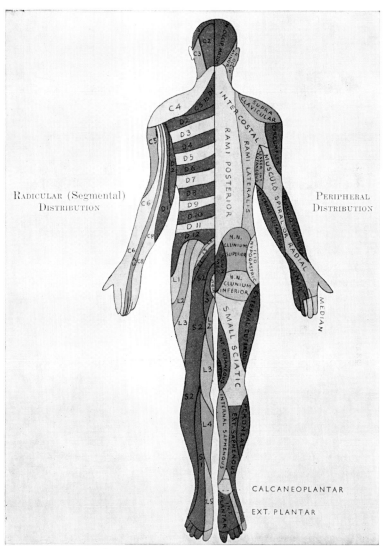

Fig. 331. Radicular (segmental) and peripheral distribution, posterior view. (After Dejerine, Head, Villiger and Stewart. Nelson Loose-Leaf Medicine, Vol. VI. New York, Thomas Nelson & Sons.)

These will be helpful in determining the probable site of damage when alterations in sensation are found.

The Sensory Examination; Procedure

Start at the side of the neck. Touch the point of the pin to several areas on the shoulder, the lateral aspect of the arm and forearm, thumb, middle finger and little finger; then bring it up the ulnar side of the hand, forearm and arm to the axilla, thus circling the arm in its long axis. Select an area near the middle of the arm and draw the pin around the arm at right angles to its long axis; repeat this maneuver in the mid-forearm. In this way you can be sure that you have tested all the dermatomes from C 4 to T 2, which supply sensation to the upper extremity. If an area of altered sensation is found, test for touch and thermal discrimination. When abnormalities are present or suspected the examination may have to be repeated several times, preferably in a quiet room; you and the patient may both become fatigued during the examination. To determine the integrity of the posterior columns, place the handle of the vibrating tuning fork over bony prominences such as the wrist or elbow, or test for position sense.

When a lesion of the contralateral cerebrum is suspected, the ability of the patient to identify objects by touch sensation (stereognosis) should be tested. The patient's eyes must be closed or covered; then hand him a series of small objects such as a key, paper clip, book of matches, coin or short pencil. Allow him to move each one around with the fingers of that hand, and then ask him to name the object. A patient with impaired common sensation will be unable to feel the object at all; the test is useless in such a case. However, if common sensation and posterior column function are normal, failure to recognize such objects is suggestive of a lesion in the opposite parietotemporal lobe.

Common sensation of the thorax, abdomen, perineum and lower extremities is then tested in a similar methodical manner; be sure that the test points selected include all of the spinal cord segments and major peripheral nerves.

In the lower extremities it is important to test for nerve trunk tenderness. Make pressure over the sciatic nerve in the posterior portion of the thigh, and squeeze the calf muscles and the midportion of the foot. Nerve trunk tenderness occurs in peripheral neuritis of all types except that due to lead poisoning; it is a particularly useful sign in alcoholic neuritis.

Proprioceptive sensation is tested with the tuning fork and by determining the integrity of position sensation. Place the vibrating tuning fork over the shin or the lateral malleolus; ask the patient to tell when the vibrations stop. This may be compared with the other leg or with the upper extremities. Vibration perception is generally lost over the tibia after the age of sixty; in younger persons this loss is usually a sign of posterior column disease. To test position sense, move the great toe slightly and ask the person to identify its position.

REFLEXES

A reflex is the response, usually motor, that follows a stimulus arising from some other source. It depends upon the integrity of the sensory receptors and afferent pathways, the synapses in the brain or the spinal cord, the efferent motor nerve and the muscle itself. It will be absent if there is a break anywhere in this arc, and will be modified by other changes in the arc itself or in the upper motor neuron system. Since the pathways of many reflexes are well established, alterations are helpful in determining the site of organic neurologic disease.

Two important reflexes have already been described (pupillary reflex; gag reflex); other normal reflexes that should always be tested will now be considered. These can be classified as superficial or deep. The former are elicited by stimulation of the skin or mucosa. A deep reflex, tendon reflex or muscle stretch reflex follows a stimulus which produces a rapid stretch of the muscle with subsequent reflex contraction.

In testing reflexes two points are important: the quality or activity of the reflex and the equality of similar reflexes on the right and left sides. There will be unilateral decrease (*hyporeflexia*) or absence of a reflex (*areflexia*) if there is a cord lesion at the level of the reflex arc, dysfunction or disruption of the motor or sensory nerve or nerve root, or an abnormality in the muscle itself. Unilateral exaggeration (*hyperreflexia*) is indicative of an upper motor neuron lesion somewhere above the level at which the reflex is mediated. Bilateral changes in activity are much less significant than unilateral alterations. Structural disease of the central nervous system may be present, but more commonly this is the physiologic response of a nervous individual.

In recording reflexes during a routine physical examination, use parallel columns ("Right"; "Left") and indicate the activity of each reflex tested by using "0" for an absent reflex, "+" if diminished, "++" if normal, "+++" if moderately increased and "++++" if extremely active.

Deep ("Tendon") Reflexes

Biceps Reflex.   Whether the patient is erect or recumbent, the arm and forearm must be in a relaxed position with the forearm mod-

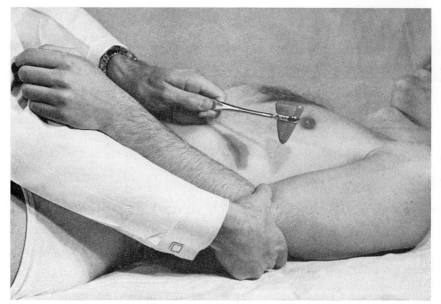

Fig. 332. Eliciting biceps reflex in a recumbent patient.

erately flexed at the elbow. Place your thumb against the biceps tendon; support the elbow with the fingers if necessary. Tap your thumb with a reflex hammer; you should feel tensing of the tendon. There may be visible contraction of the belly of the muscle and further flexion of the forearm if the reflex is hyperactive or the blow is sharp. This reflex is mediated by segments C 5 and C 6 of the spinal cord and by the musculocutaneous nerve.

Triceps Reflex.   Flex the patient's arm to an angle of about 90 degrees; be sure that it is properly supported and relaxed. Tap the triceps tendon directly; you should feel or see contraction of the belly of the muscle and slight extension of the arm. This reflex depends upon the integrity of C 7 and the radial nerve. It is more difficult to elicit than the biceps reflex and is more liable to be misjudged. Normally, the biceps and triceps reflexes are more difficult to elicit than the knee and ankle reflexes.

Quadriceps Reflex (Knee Jerk; Patellar Reflex).   If the patient is ambulatory, have him sit in a chair with the thighs well supported and extend his legs moderately but keep his toes on the floor. A bed patient should sit with his legs hanging freely over the side of the bed. If he is unable to sit, place your forearm under the lower third of his thighs and raise them slightly from the bed (Fig. 334). Be sure that the muscles are relaxed; it may help if you have him close his eyes. Tap the quadriceps tendon between the patella and the tibial tubercle.

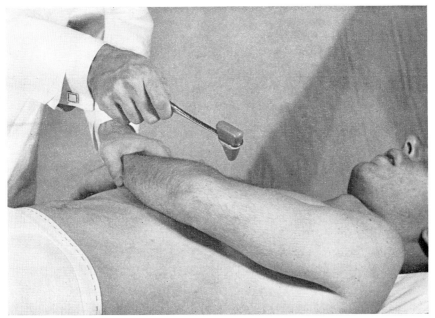

Fig. 333. Eliciting triceps reflex in a recumbent patient. As the forearm is drawn across the chest (to the right, in this case) the biceps tends to contract, thus relaxing the triceps.

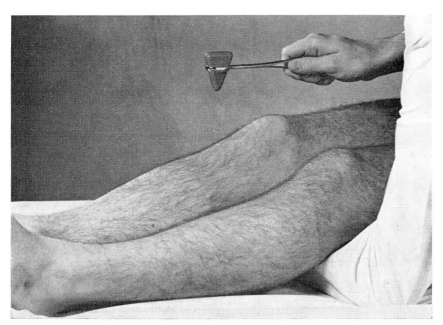

Fig. 334. Eliciting quadriceps reflex in a recumbent patient. Slip one forearm under the lower part of the thighs to raise them slightly from the bed, then wait until you feel the tendons relax.

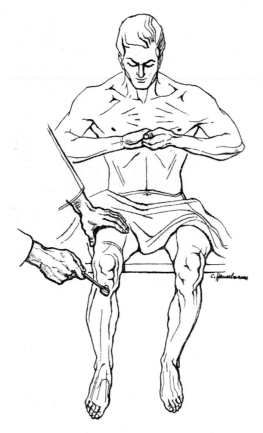

Fig. 335. Reinforcement. As the patient attempts to separate his clasped hands, tap the tendon.

Normally, the quadriceps will contract and slight extension of the leg will occur; a hyperactive reflex will result in marked extension, but there is a considerable range of normal activity of the quadriceps reflex. If the reflex is depressed or seems absent, place one hand on the quadriceps muscle; a slight contraction is more easily felt than seen. If this fails, reinforcement should be tried. Ask the patient to hook his fingers together and then attempt to pull his hands apart; tap the tendon as he is doing this (Fig. 335).

This reflex is mediated through segments L 2, L 3 and L 4 of the spinal cord and the femoral nerve.

Triceps Surae Reflex (Ankle Jerk; Achilles Reflex).   This is often difficult to elicit. If possible, have the patient kneel on a padded chair or on the bed with his feet hanging freely over the edge. The feet must be relaxed; the Achilles tendon is then tapped. Plantar extension of the foot should occur.

In a bedfast patient the reflex may be sought by having him lie on his abdomen and flex his legs to a vertical position; then tap the tendon. An alternate method is to have him supine; flex the leg about 30 degrees

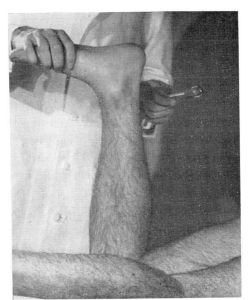

Fig. 336. Eliciting Achilles reflex. With the patient prone, the leg is flexed and the foot slightly dorsiflexed.

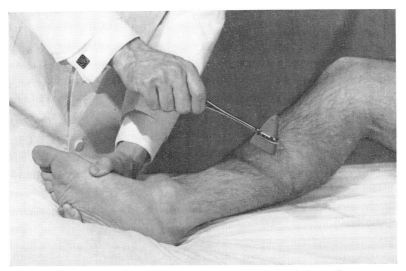

Fig. 337. Alternate procedure for eliciting Achilles reflex.

and rotate the entire extremity externally. Dorsiflex the foot slightly and tap the tendon.

This reflex is mediated through segments S 1 and S 2 and the sciatic nerve. It is diminished or lost in a variety of lower motor neuron diseases, including neuritis and pressure on the motor roots by herniation of a nucleus pulposus, and with various motor disorders. The sensory side of the arc may be broken in tabes dorsalis. In hypothyroidism both the contraction and the relaxation phase may be markedly slowed.

Superficial Reflexes

Abdominal Reflexes.   To elicit the abdominal reflexes, the skin over the upper portion of each rectus muscle is stroked with a pointed object in a direction parallel to the costal margin and toward the midline. Normally, the underlying muscle will contract and the umbilicus will be drawn toward the stimulated area. Repeat the maneuver over the lower part of each muscle, stroking parallel to Poupart's ligament; a similar response should be obtained.

The upper abdominal reflex is mediated largely through dermatome T 7, and the lower through T 11 and T 12. The abdominal reflexes disappear early in multiple sclerosis and are absent in other pyramidal tract diseases.

Cremasteric Reflex.   In males, this reflex should be tested routinely. Stroke the upper inner aspect of the thigh longitudinally; the cremasteric muscle on that side should contract and draw the testis upward. This reflex is mediated through dermatome L 1 of the spinal cord.

Anal Reflex.   Fecal or urinary incontinence should have been noted in the history or during the general physical examination, but the rectal examination is also an essential part of the neurologic survey. Normally there will be momentary contraction of the anal muscles when the finger touches the skin. If in doubt, the skin around the anus should be stimulated by stroking or pricking with a pin. This reflex is mediated through S 2–5; loss of tone of the rectal sphincter may indicate spinal cord disease in this area.

Abnormal Reflexes

Digital Reflex.   To elicit the Hoffmann[22] (Trömner[23]) reflex, support the patient's palm loosely with one hand, with his fingers relaxed. Extend his middle finger and sharply flex the terminal phalanx by flicking the nail of that finger. If the thumb is adducted the reflex is positive. With a strongly positive response, the fingers will also flex.

The Hoffmann reflex is suggestive but not diagnostic of pyramidal or extrapyramidal tract disease. It may also be present and of no significance in a tense person with generalized hyperreflexia. A unilateral positive reflex accompanied by other evidence of pyramidal tract disease is significant.

[22] Johann Hoffmann, Heidelberg neurologist, 1857–1919.
[23] Ernest L. O. Trömner, German neurologist, born 1868.

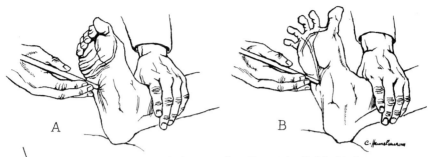

Fig. 338. *A*, Normal plantar reflex; *B*, positive Babinski sign.

Plantar Reflex (Babinski[24] Sign). Grasp the foot firmly and stroke or scratch the lateral border of the sole from the heel toward the toes and across the ball of the foot mesially; use increasing pressure if necessary, but avoid painful stimuli. Normally, the toes and sometimes the entire foot will undergo plantar flexion (Fig. 338 *A*). An abrupt withdrawal reflex may occasionally occur; the leg and thigh will be sharply flexed in an attempt to remove the foot from the source of irritation.

Dorsiflexion of the great toe and fanning of the other toes constitute a positive Babinski reflex. Except in infants this is considered pathognomonic of pyramidal tract disease. With minimal involvement one may see only dorsiflexion of the great toe or nothing but fanning of the other toes; this is an equivocal response and should be so recorded. If there is paralysis of the ventral flexors of the great toe, a false positive response may occur.

Various modifications of this test have been described. Oppenheim[25] reported that if the examiner ran his fingers forcefully down the tibia, the great toe would dorsiflex. Chaddock[26] recommended stroking around the external malleolus and along the dorsum of the foot laterally. Throckmorton[27] preferred to scratch the inner side of the great toe.

Clonus

Clonus is an exaggerated stretch reflex due to loss of pyramidal tract inhibition of the reflex arc. It might be considered as a "5+" tendon reflex. It consists of repeated rhythmic contractions of a muscle subjected to stretch. Its duration is roughly proportional to the degree of release of inhibition. It may be "abortive" and consist of only a few contractions

---

[24] Joseph François Felix Babinski, Paris neurologist, 1857–1932.
[25] Hermann Oppenheim, Berlin neurologist, 1858–1919.
[26] Charles Gilbert Chaddock, St. Louis neurologist, 1861–1936.
[27] Thomas Bentley Throckmorton, American neurologist, 1885–1961.

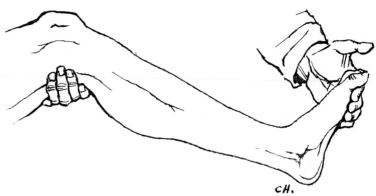

Fig. 339.   Method of eliciting ankle clonus.

of decreasing strength, or it may be continuous and persist as long as pressure is exerted to maintain the stretch.

Quadriceps Clonus (Patellar Clonus).   The patient should be recumbent with the leg extended and relaxed. Grasp the upper portion of the patella between your thumb and index finger; push it quickly downward toward the foot to stretch the muscle, and maintain the pressure. Alternate contraction and relaxation of the muscle will result in rhythmic movement of the patella.

Triceps Surae Clonus (Ankle Clonus).   After testing the Achilles reflex, grasp the ball of the foot and quickly dorsiflex it; with clonus, alternate plantar flexion and dorsiflexion will follow.

After you have completed the neurologic examination, record the abnormalities and then make an attempt to determine the anatomic site of the lesion. Needless to say, the interpretation requires adequate knowledge of the anatomy and physiology of the nervous system. With a good history and definite neurologic signs, and with the help of special diagnostic procedures, one eventually should be able to make at least an anatomic and often an etiologic diagnosis. For a detailed discussion of cerebral localization and for descriptions of the more common neurologic syndromes a textbook of neurology should be consulted.

XXIII

Pediatric Examination

Examination of infants and children might logically be considered to be not one but three different procedures. Examination of the newborn is performed primarily to detect gross anatomic abnormalities. The examination of a sick child is a second problem; the general procedure outlined in previous chapters will be applicable here, with certain modifications that will be mentioned later. The majority of examinations are performed on healthy infants* and children to determine and record their rate of development and to discover any variations from normal or average physical and mental growth. In this chapter no attempt will be made to cover the entire field, but a few of the differences between the child and the adult will be mentioned, as well as problems that are of importance primarily in this age group.

THE HISTORY

Although the general outline in Chapter I should be followed, certain modifications are necessary. For a newborn the important points are the health of the parents and especially of the mother during the pregnancy, the length of gestation and the details of labor and delivery. The condition at birth, the need for resuscitation and the presence of cyanosis or of obvious bleeding should be recorded, as well as the initial weight and length of the infant.

As the months pass additional facts should be added. Some of these are: postnatal weight loss and time required to regain this; jaundice or easy bruising; breast feeding and time of weaning; acceptance of the bottle and various formulas, with exact details of the proportions, amount taken and interval of feedings; reaction to solid foods; bowel habits; weight gain at various periods. Food allergy may occur at an early age;

* An infant is a child less than 2 years old.

451

the infant refuses his feedings or develops vomiting, diarrhea or eczema when certain items are offered. Cow's milk, egg and orange juice are the most common offenders at an early age; wheat and chocolate enter the picture later.

Physical development and activity of various types should also be noted. When did the infant hold his head erect, turn over, sit upright without support, stand, creep, walk and talk? If this is the first baby, don't be surprised if the parents report that these actions were noted at a somewhat earlier age than average.

When the child returns for periodic checkups more attention should be devoted to the general physical, mental, emotional and sociologic development, but items such as diet, rest and sleep must not be forgotten. Here the problem of obtaining an accurate history from the mother may become more complicated. In an attempt to prove that she is a good mother and training her child properly, she may forget that the child has his radio under his pillow at bedtime, or that cake and candy seem to disappear rapidly. It is often helpful to have the child seated on the mother's lap or somewhere beside or behind her so that as she talks you can see the child's face, but she can't. His expression may be revealing; young children are inherently honest.

If an infant or young child is sick you may have to rely largely upon the mother's story. Again you will have to estimate the accuracy of the information. Important facts may be minimized or even denied; unimportant details may be grossly exaggerated. If you have known the family, the problem is much simpler than if this is the first visit.

THE EXAMINATION

Fear is often the predominating emotion in a child who is taken to the doctor's office. After squirming in the unfamiliar surroundings of the waiting room he is taken into another room where a strange man seems to tower over him and threatens him. Later, an array of peculiar instruments catches his eye as he is unceremoniously stripped of his clothing. If this is not the first visit he probably remembers vaguely or vividly that previous meetings may have been friendly at first, but always seemed to end abruptly with the sharp jab of a hypodermic needle.

To be successful you must win the confidence of the child and hope to win his friendship also, even though you may be forced to hurt him at times. Knowledge of child psychology is helpful but cannot substitute for patience, tact, kindness and gentleness. As soon as the child is old enough to understand, the various instruments and procedures should be explained in such a manner that he can comprehend them. "Let's see

how wide you can open your mouth." "I wonder what my telephone will
tell me about your heart." "How high will your leg jump when I tap
your knee?" A few minutes thus "wasted" during the first examination
may save hours at subsequent visits.

The exact order in which the various procedures are performed will
vary with the circumstances. With the very young it is advisable to
examine the heart, lungs, abdomen and extremities first; then do the
things that are more liable to be annoying, upsetting or painful such as
checking the blood pressure, inspecting the ears, nose and throat or
doing a digital rectal examination.

The use of force is not justifiable if the child is undergoing a
checkup examination; if he is ill it may be necessary. If a child has a
high fever and a sore throat but persistently refuses to open his mouth,
you may finally be forced to use something more than persuasion to
obtain material for bacteriologic study.

VITAL SIGNS

Temperature.   This should be determined by the axillary or rectal
method with infants and young children; it may be safe to use the oral
method with a cooperative child of six or older.

In a newborn infant the normal axillary temperature may range
from 92° to 97° F.; after the first week it tends to stabilize at about
97° F. but is subject to considerable fluctuation. It may be slightly increased after a meal or because of excitement or exercise. Until the age of
six or even eight a rise to 104° may occur with a relatively minor illness;
this should be considered equivalent to 100° or 101° in an adult. When
the axillary temperature is higher than 104° a convulsion may occur
without other evidence of convulsive disorders or central nervous system
disease. A rapid rise of temperature in a child who looks healthy otherwise may occur in the prodromal stage of one of the exanthems, especially
roseola infantum (exanthema subitum), a disease of relatively brief
duration. In infants, as in the aged, a normal or subnormal temperature
may be found with an overwhelming infection.

Blood Pressure.   A narrow cuff must be used; its width should
be less than two-thirds the length of the upper arm. Too wide a cuff will
result in a low reading; with too narrow a cuff the reading will be too
high. If auscultation is unsatisfactory, palpation of the radial pulse may
have to be substituted; the reading will be about 10 mm. lower. Occasionally it may be necessary to estimate the systolic pressure by another
procedure. The hand, wrist and forearm are wrapped with an elastic
bandage. The cuff is then inflated to a pressure well above the expected
level and the bandage is removed. As the cuff is deflated, the hand will

suddenly become flushed; this point is approximately equal to the reading obtained by palpation.

In a newborn infant the systolic pressure ranges from 60 to 80 mm. and the diastolic from 20 to 40 mm. The pressure rises 2 to 5 mm. each year; adult levels are reached at or after puberty. Elevation of both the systolic and the diastolic pressure occurs with various types of renal disease, increased intracranial pressure, vitamin A or D poisoning or hyperfunction of the adrenal cortex. An increase in the systolic pressure may be due to exercise, excitement or fever; it is also found with patent ductus arteriosus and other abnormal arteriovenous communications and occasionally with aortic insufficiency. Elevation of the diastolic pressure, with normal or low systolic pressure, suggests some type of aortic stenosis, either congenital or acquired. Both the systolic and the diastolic pressure will be low with circulatory collapse, shock, heat exhaustion, blood loss, adrenocortical deficiency and various chronic or wasting diseases.

Height and Weight.   The exact height and weight are of less importance than the rate at which these figures change as the months pass. A variety of charts, tables and graphs are available that give normal or average values for such measurements; the child's progress can be judged by these.

THE SKIN

The skin of a newborn is covered with cebum and desquamated epithelial cells (*vermix caseosa*). A flame-colored capillary nevus on the back of the neck is physiologic; it usually disappears in infancy but occasionally it persists. Similar lesions may be present elsewhere, as well as raised vascular nevi.

Cyanosis is often present at birth; if it persists it suggests poor expansion of the lungs (fetal atelectasis) or other pulmonary disease, or some congenital cardiovascular anomaly. In older children cyanosis occurs with breath-holding, temper tantrums or convulsions because of apnea during these states. The color in the upper and lower extremities should be compared; with coarctation of the aorta or with patent ductus arteriosus and pulmonary hypertension the lower limbs may be more cyanotic than the upper ones.

Jaundice at birth is rare; it may be due to Rh or A-B-O blood group incompatibilities or to developmental defects in the liver or biliary system. Most newborn have an excessive number of erythrocytes; within a week or two hemolysis may lead to a mild degree of icterus because the liver is as yet unable to handle this excessive load of pigment. In older children jaundice may accompany a hemolytic crisis of congenital ictero-anemia (hereditary spherocytosis) or sickle cell disease; occasionally these attacks lead to the formation of gallstones at an early age. Hepatitis must also be considered when jaundice develops.

Seborrheic dermatitis starts in the scalp and produces yellow, greasy scales; this is often called "cradle cap" or "milk crust." It may spread to the face or body. Infantile eczema usually begins on the cheeks, then spreads to the scalp, the ears and down the neck. Contact dermatitis, often complicated by infection, produces erythema and scaling in the diaper area ("diaper rash").

Eruptions of many types are not uncommon. Retained sebum in the sebaceous glands produces tiny white nodules (*milia*). Excess warmth and moisture can lead to a papular eruption involving the sweat glands (*miliaria*); the itching or burning sensation which this produces justifies the common name "prickly heat." Measles, German measles, scarlet fever, roseola infantum, chickenpox and other infections produce characteristic skin lesions.

Petechiae may be present with meningococcemia or other severe forms of bacteremia, with subacute bacterial endocarditis or with scurvy, purpura or leukemia. More commonly they are seen as a result of severe paroxysms of cough in pertussis; similar hemorrhages can also occur in the brain. Hemophilia or other blood dyscrasias may lead to ecchymoses.

Hair often covers the shoulders of a newborn; this disappears within a few weeks. Thereafter hair is present only on the scalp and as eyebrows and eyelashes until puberty. Excessive hairiness, especially of the arms and legs, is usually a familial characteristic but may occur with hyperthyroidism, vitamin A poisoning, Cushing's syndrome or drug sensitivity (diphenylhydantoin). A patch of alopecia may develop if the infant lies in one position for long periods of time; this is not permanent. A nervous child may pull out one or several hairs when upset; occasionally this becomes excessive (trichotillomania).

Pubic hair may appear at eight to twelve years of age; axillary hair develops about six months later, and facial hair in boys soon starts to grow. Delayed development or decreased amounts of pubic and axillary hair may be due to endocrine disturbances—hypothyroidism, hypopituitarism, Addison's disease or gonadal dysfunction. Premature or excessive development suggests testicular, ovarian or pituitary tumor, adrenal hyperplasia or the ingestion of corticosteroids, androgens or estrogens.

In texture, the skin may be coarse and rough in a child with vitamin A deficiency, hypothyroidism or eczema; the latter most commonly begins in the flexor folds, especially the antecubital and popliteal areas but may spread to involve large areas.

An infant rarely sweats until he is at least one month old. Thereafter, profuse perspiration may be due to external heat, fever, hypoglycemia, hyperthyroidism or hypocalcemia, and sometimes to congenital heart disease. Abnormal dryness occurs with dehydration, hypothyroidism or eczema; drugs like atropine will also inhibit sweating. Occasionally the sweat glands fail to develop (*hereditary ectodermal dysplasia*).

To determine tissue turgor, grasp the skin and subcutaneous tissues of the anterior abdominal wall between the thumb and index finger, squeeze it gently and then release it. With dehydration the skin will remain elevated and wrinkled. With malnutrition there will be little palpable subcutaneous tissue. With chronic wasting disease or diffuse peritonitis the tissues may feel doughy. Edematous skin will retain the depressions produced by the pressure of the thumb and finger.

THE HEAD

Skull. The skull of an infant is relatively much larger than that of an adult; it constitutes one-fourth the body length, instead of the adult one-eighth. In circumference it is as large as the abdomen or chest, or larger, during the first 18 to 24 months; thereafter the thorax and abdomen enlarge more rapidly.

Asymmetry in the newborn may be due to molding of the skull during birth, edema of the scalp over the site of the presenting part (*caput succedaneum*) or subperiosteal bleeding (*cephalhematoma*). The anterior fontanel should be easily palpable as a defect in the bone measuring up to 4 or 5 cm. in diameter; the posterior fontanel will be much smaller or closed. With dehydration the fontanel will be visible as a depression. Bulging may occur during expiration if the child is straining or crying, but persistent bulging indicates increased intracranial pressure from hydrocephalus or some other disease. The anterior fontanel is usually completely closed before the age of 24 months; premature closure may be associated with brain atrophy.

Eyes. A newborn apparently has light perception but nothing more. By two months the infant will follow moving objects, and after six months he should be able to focus for short periods. In an older infant a rough estimate of vision can be obtained by observing his interest in brightly colored objects, both stationary and moving. Determination of visual acuity with test charts is rarely satisfactory or accurate before the age of 4 or 5, but may be desirable before the child enters school.

The external examination of the eyes is performed much as in an adult (Chapter V). Sinus thrombosis, a cerebral vascular lesion or a retro-orbital tumor may cause bulging of one or both eyeballs; exophthalmos due to hyperthyroidism is rare. Enophthalmos in an infant is usually the result of cervical sympathetic nerve damage; chronic malnutrition or severe dehydration will simulate this. An obstructed lacrimal duct may be undiagnosed for the first month or two, by which time tears are usually formed.

Strabismus is frequently present during the first few months; if it persists appropriate treatment is indicated. Paralytic strabismus may develop with meningitis or increased intracranial pressure. Nystagmus may be congenital or due to blindness; it also accompanies various neurologic disorders.

The pupils of a newborn are constricted for two weeks or more; then the light reflex becomes demonstrable. Opacity of the lens may indicate glaucoma; it can also occur if the mother had rubella during the first trimester of the pregnancy.

The red reflex will be absent if there are cataracts or retrolental fibroplasia; the latter is a form of retinopathy developing in a premature baby placed in an atmosphere containing too much oxygen. At times it is possible to visualize the fundus fairly adequately, with or without the cooperation of the patient. Retinal hemorrhage in a newborn can be due to trauma, to prolonged anoxia during birth or to subdural bleeding.

Ears. The size, shape, symmetry and position of the auricles will be obvious at a glance; congenital variations are not uncommon. A small sinus just in front of the ear, often accompanied by slight swelling just inside the canal, represents the remnant of the first branchial cleft. In children the auricle may be displaced by mumps or by disease of the mastoid; the latter has become rare since antimicrobial agents became available.

At birth the external auditory canal is directed upward; the tympanic membrane appears almost horizontal and the light reflex is diffuse. As the child grows these structures assume the normal adult position and the light reflex becomes cone-shaped and sharply outlined.

Infection in one or both ears is a common cause of fever in infants and children. The drum may be only slightly reddened or it may be intensely congested, with either retraction or bulging. Always test for sensitivity over the mastoid area when the drum appears inflamed.

A rough estimate of hearing can be obtained even in infants; a sharp noise such as snapping the fingers near the ear will cause the eyelids to blink. Older children can be tested as adults are. Congenital deafness is frequently found in children whose mothers had rubeola during the first trimester of the pregnancy. Pseudodeafness may be found with mental deficiency or psychoses. A mother will frequently believe that her child is becoming deaf when actually he is merely engrossed with his own thoughts and activities, or has become so bored with adults and their unpredictable behavior that he chooses to ignore any words that do not threaten punishment or promise pleasure. Audiometry can be useful when the child is old enough and intelligent enough to cooperate.

Nose.   The patency of the nasal passages and of the posterior choanae in a newborn infant is determined by passing a small soft catheter through each side. Obstruction may be due to displacement of the cartilage of the vomer during delivery or to a congenital anomaly. A common cause of nasal obstruction in a young child is hypertrophy of the pharyngeal tonsil (adenoids). This is characterized by breathing through the partially opened mouth, a narrow pinched nose, high palate, nasal voice and general appearance suggestive of slight mental retardation.

Cleft palate associated with regurgitation can produce chronic nasal irritation or infection. Children love to put small objects in the nose; a retained foreign body may be responsible for nasal discharge, infection or epistaxis.

Mouth.   It may be advisable to defer inspection of the mouth until late in the examination, especially if a tongue blade is to be used or palpation of the adenoids is indicated. Cleft lip, more commonly occurring on the left, is obvious; cleft palate may also be present. Delayed dentition or poor formation of the teeth that are erupted should be recorded; cretinism, rickets, mongolism, hypocalcemia or congenital syphilis are some of the diseases responsible for such changes. Severe jaundice at birth or prolonged ingestion of iron may produce abnormal pigmentation or staining of the teeth.

Small white patches that adhere to the buccal mucosa are thrush; milk curds may look the same but are easily wiped or scraped off. Thrush may lead to shallow ulcers or may spread to other parts of the gastrointestinal tract. Koplik's spots (p. 106) also develop here and are considered diagnostic of measles.

There is little production of saliva during the first three months; total absence of secretion is seen with congenital ectodermal dysplasia. Drooling is normal during the first two years; the amount of saliva increases with teething or other conditions causing oral irritation in older children.

Macroglossia suggests cretinism or severe hypothyroidism; it can also be congenital or due to lymphangioma or hemangioma. A thyroglossal cyst located at the base of the tongue will force a normal tongue forward and make it appear large. If the frenum is so short that the tip of the tongue cannot be raised (tonguetie) it may have to be cut.

A longitudinal cleft may be present in the palate; the mouth is in direct communication with the nasal cavity. This should be differentiated from palatal perforation, which is rare but may occur in older children. Vesicles or ulcers of various types may be present; Coxsackie virus, herpes simplex, fungi or low-grade bacterial infection can produce these. An ulcer on the hard palate may result from trauma in nursing (Bednar's[1] aphthae) or from thumb-sucking.

[1] Alvis Bednar, Viennese physician, 1816–88.

The uvula may be cleft (bifid) or very short; if very long it can irritate the pharynx and cause coughing or gagging. In children with repeated head colds it may be the site of chronic inflammation and may give rise to the complaint of "sore throat."

Tonsils cannot be recognized in the newborn but may become very large during the next two years. The maximum is usually reached by the age of 5 or 6; thereafter they tend to decrease in size. In some young children they become so large that they interfere with swallowing, oral breathing and speech. The adenoid mass may obstruct nasal breathing or partially occlude the eustachian tube; this can lead to repeated attacks of serous otitis media or partial deafness. The size of the adenoids in a young child cannot be determined accurately by inspection of the oropharynx, and posterior rhinoscopy is difficult; digital palpation is necessary. To do this, some form of mouth gag must be used to prevent an uncooperative or unappreciative child from biting the examining finger. One relatively atraumatic procedure is to have the child stand in front of you or sit on your lap with his back to you. Hold his head against your body with your left forearm and wrist. With a finger, make pressure on his left cheek until he opens his mouth; the right index finger quickly explores the nasopharynx. He may gag but he will not bite his own cheek or your finger.

Larynx. In a newborn or infant the character of the cry can be significant. Hoarseness may be due to abnormality or injury of the larynx or laryngeal nerves, to an anomalous vascular ring surrounding the trachea, or to infection, hypothyroidism or hypocalcemia. In older children infection is the most common cause, but hoarseness may be merely the result of prolonged shouting as a child cheered his team with unrestrained exuberance. Unless the hoarseness is temporary or the cause is found elsewhere, laryngoscopy is necessary.

Stridor is a harsh, high-pitched, crowing sound heard during inspiration and occasionally during expiration. It is associated with partial obstruction of the larynx, trachea or a large bronchus. It is not uncommon in young infants and is usually due to delayed development of cartilage in the larynx, trachea or epiglottis. In older children acute laryngitis or laryngeal edema is generally the cause.

An infant should start to say a few words by the time he is ten months or a year old; by the age of two he speaks phrases or short sentences. Delayed or limited speech occurs when there is deafness or mental retardation, and with neurologic or anatomic abnormalities; it may also be physiologic if his every wish is anticipated. A speech defect may be noticed at an early age; this tends to become more obvious during the third or fourth year. There may be stammering, stuttering, lisping or other changes that should be investigated. A low-pitched voice suggests sexual precocity or the adrenogenital syndrome. A nasal quality is heard when the child has large adenoids, sinusitis or some other process that interferes with proper resonance in the nasal cavities.

NECK

The neck normally appears short during infancy and begins to lengthen during the second or third year. A persistently short neck is seen with various dystrophies and congenital anomalies. Flexion, extension and rotation should be tested; meningeal irritation may limit flexion. Impaired rotation or torticollis can be due to spasm of the muscles, especially the sternomastoid, from acute infection or trauma. In an infant, a hematoma of the sternomastoid occasionally develops during or shortly after birth; unless this is recognized and treated promptly it can result in fibrosis and permanent shortening of the muscle.

To elicit the tonic neck reflex, place the baby on his back and then turn his head sharply to one side. The ipsilateral arm will extend and the contralateral one will flex; usually the legs also show similar movements. This reflex is physiologic during the first few months; if present in an older infant it indicates brain damage or faulty development of the nervous system.

Other abnormalities such as a large thyroid, venous congestion, enlarged lymph nodes or swollen salivary glands should be recorded and the cause determined if possible.

CHEST

In a premature the ribs are very thin and soft; respiration is largely diaphragmatic and the chest may seem to be retracted with every inspiration. In an infant the chest is relatively short, almost circular and approximately of the same circumference as the head and the abdomen. After the second year it enlarges more rapidly, especially in the transverse diameter, and slowly assumes the adult configuration.

Various deformities of the thorax may be present. Midsternal depression gives rise to funnel chest; when the lower portion is involved it is often called cobbler's chest. A prominent protruding sternum produces keeled chest or pigeon breast deformity. The xiphoid process may be visible and palpable as a fairly mobile cartilaginous projection in the epigastrium. A rachitic rosary or Harrison's groove may be present. A precordial bulge in an older child suggests heart disease with cardiomegaly; an area of retraction may be the result of pulmonary fibrosis.

Respiration in a newborn child, and especially in a premature one, will tend to be of Cheyne-Stokes type; this becomes normal within a few weeks. The rate is more rapid than in adults; at birth it may be 40 to 60 per minute but this does not persist. With infection and fever, and especially with respiratory tract disease, the rate increases markedly. A very slow rate suggests increased intracranial pressure or central nervous system depression due to sedatives or other drugs.

When you first examine the lungs of infants and young children you will think that palpation, percussion and auscultation are of little value. You must remember that the chest contour is different, the wall is very thin and the lungs themselves are small. Everything has been "miniaturized" and your examination must be adapted to this. As the child matures the procedures can approach those used in an adult.

In percussing the chest the force normally used in an adult will set up vibrations in an entire hemithorax. Very light percussion must be used to outline organs or to detect changes in the lung parenchyma. Even with this precaution the note will seem hyperresonant, and over areas with lesions such as pneumonic consolidation, atelectasis or pleural effusion the resonance will be decreased but rarely dull or flat.

Tactile and vocal fremitus are difficult to elicit in a happy baby; if he cries, or if you unintentionally or deliberately make him cry, you may be able to detect slight changes. As the child learns to speak the problem is less troublesome and the findings are more reliable. You can palpate or auscultate the chest as he chats with you.

For auscultation of an infant's chest it is essential that you use a small bell, preferably one rimmed with soft rubber. The diaphragm will be too large and too rigid to make complete contact with the chest wall.

The normal breath sounds in an infant or young child have characteristics that would seem to warrant classifying them as bronchovesicular; a hypothetical explanation for this has been suggested (p. 194). With atelectasis, pleural effusion, empyema or pneumothorax the breath sounds may be decreased, rather than absent. With consolidation they tend more toward the bronchial type, but rarely have the characteristics of pure bronchial breath sounds as heard in an adult.

Adventitious sounds such as rales, rhonchi, wheezes or friction rubs have much the same significance as they do in adults. Because the lumina in the tracheobronchial tree are small, a very slight amount of swelling or a minimal amount of fluid can give rise to palpable or audible vibrations.

As in adults, cough can be helpful in diagnosis. Paroxysmal cough followed by inspiratory stridor is characteristic of pertussis (whooping cough); vomiting may occur in the very young and may lead to nutritional difficulties. A sharp, brassy, nonproductive cough should suggest tracheal compression, a foreign body in the tracheobronchial tree or diphtheria, tuberculosis or croup. Intermittent paroxysms of cough often accompany the initial stage of an attack of asthma.

It is very difficult to obtain sputum from infants and young children. Because the ribs are so soft the expulsive force is not great, and small amounts of secretion are promptly swallowed if they reach the pharynx. Bacteriologic studies can sometimes be obtained by holding a culture plate near the mouth and collecting the droplets that spray out as the infant coughs.

BREASTS

Enlarged breasts are not uncommon at birth, and secretion from the nipple may occur ("witch's milk"); this is due to stimulation by hormones derived from the mother's blood and lasts only a few weeks at most. In girls, normal development begins somewhere between the tenth and fourteenth years. Inequality in size is common at this stage but is rarely permanent. Precocious development may be physiologic; it can also be due to an ovarian tumor. Lack of development or marked hypoplasia may be normal or due to endocrine disturbances. In boys there is usually a slight increase in the size of the breasts at puberty; marked enlargement (gynecomastia) is rare. In an obese child of either sex, pads of fat may mimic enlargement of the breasts.

HEART

Tachycardia is physiologic in young children. The rate may be 140 or more per minute at birth; this gradually falls as the child grows older and reaches adult rates during adolescence. Sinus arrhythmia is common; premature contractions occasionally occur but other disturbances of rhythm are unusual in the absence of some congenital defect.

During infancy the heart is situated more horizontally than in older children; this should not be mistaken for cardiac enlargement. A murmur is frequently heard; the tachycardia may make it difficult to determine timing and other characteristics. The criteria previously discussed (Chapter XIV) should be applied. Many of these murmurs are of no significance (functional murmurs) but others may be due to congenital heart disease. An accurate diagnosis is important so that surgical correction of the latter may be undertaken at the proper time. In older children a murmur may be due to rheumatic heart disease or to some other infection such as diphtheria, pneumonia or scarlet fever.

ABDOMEN

In an infant the abdomen is relatively long compared to the thorax, but its circumference is slightly less. When the child is supine the abdomen should be flat, but since the abdominal musculature is not well developed it will protrude when he stands. This bulging decreases in older children and normally disappears during puberty. A scaphoid abdomen may be due to malnutrition, marked dehydration or high intestinal obstruction; in a newborn it may signify the presence of a large diaphragmatic hernia or eventration of the diaphragm.

An umbilical hernia is not uncommon at birth, but during the first two years of life it usually disappears; in Negro children it may persist for several years. Infection of the umbilicus may be present; sometimes this is associated with a patent urachus and intermittent discharge of urine. A cherry-red cellulitis of the umbilicus and the surrounding skin is said to be pathognomonic of inflammation of Meckel's[2] diverticulum; this sign appears only if a remnant of the vitelline duct is still present.

Visible peristalsis is a sign of obstruction until that possibility has been excluded. Pyloric stenosis is the most common cause in the first few months of life; intussusception occurs in older infants and children.

To demonstrate a hernia it may be necessary to have an infant cry; if possible, this should be postponed until other parts of the examination have been completed.

Because the chest is relatively short the liver edge may be palpable 1 or 2 cm. below the costal margin during childhood, and the tip of the spleen may be felt during early infancy. The abdominal aorta is usually easily felt; other masses should be fully described. Tenderness or rigidity have the same significance as in adults.

GENITALIA

In girls, patency of the urethral and vaginal orifices should be determined; sometimes there are fibrous adhesions between the labia minora during infancy. The clitoris may appear large because the labia are relatively small. A newborn girl may have a slight amount of serosanguineous vaginal discharge for a week or two; a persistent discharge is abnormal. In an older child profuse vaginal discharge may be due to a foreign body in the vagina, to infection (including gonorrhea) or to an ovarian tumor, which usually produces precocious puberty as well. A variable amount of mucoid discharge appears at puberty.

---

[2] Johann Friedrich Meckel, Jr., anatomist in Halle, 1781–1833.

In the male, one should look for epispadias, hypospadias, phimosis or firm adhesions between the glans and the prepuce; circumcision or other corrective measures may be necessary. The scrotum should be palpated and the testes identified. With an active cremasteric reflex they may be drawn up to the inguinal canal; this must be differentiated from cryptorchidism. A congenital hernia or hydrocele may be found in the scrotum. Acute swelling may be due to trauma or infection, or to torsion of the spermatic cord or testis.

ANUS AND RECTUM

The anal region must be inspected but digital examination is not done routinely. An imperforate anus is a congenital defect that requires prompt correction. An anal fissure may be responsible for constipation or rectal bleeding. Pinworms (*Enterobius vermicularis;* seat worms) may cause pruritus and may lead to excoriation from scratching. A pilonidal cyst or sinus may be visible over the lower sacral region.

Ordinarily the fifth finger is used for rectal examination of infants or young children; preferably the child should lie on his back with the legs and thighs flexed.

SPINE

In the newborn the spine has one long dorsal curve from the head to the coccyx. The anterior curve in the cervical spine develops when the infant begins to hold his head up; the lumbar curve appears when he starts to walk. Structural or postural changes in the physiologic curves may be apparent in older children.

EXTREMITIES

The hands are small and fat in an infant, and the fingers appear short. The lower extremities are also short and fat and the musculature is poor. There may be congenital dislocation of one or both hips; fracture of a humerus or femur may occur during birth. Clubfoot may also be present; this must be differentiated from the intrauterine position that the feet tend to assume. The former can be straightened only by force;

the latter will assume a normal position if the feet are gently scratched or stroked.

A moderate degree of bowlegs or knock knees is not uncommon when the infant starts to walk; this may persist for a year or two. A fat pad under the arch of the foot is normally present for the first year or two; only after this disappears can the presence of abnormalities of the arches be determined by inspection and palpation.

REFLEXES

The Moro[3] reflex (startle reflex; embrace reflex) is very important in infants. If the patient is startled by a loud noise, bright light or other stimulus, his thighs and legs flex, his fingers fan and then clench, and his arms are first thrown outward and then flexed and brought together with jerky movements, as if to embrace something. Absence of this reflex in a newborn is indicative of severe central nervous system damage or deficiency; persistence of this after the fifth or sixth month has the same significance. Absence of the reflex in one arm occurs with fracture of the clavicle or arm, or with brachial plexus injury; absence in one leg accompanies low spinal injury or a dislocated hip. A hyperactive reflex is found with tetany or with central nervous system irritation.

The sucking reflex is usually present at birth or appears within a day or two; this enables the infant to obtain necessary nourishment. The grasp reflex is normally demonstrable in an infant from the age of one to three months; any small object that touches the palm or fingers will produce this. By the sixth month a normal infant will reach for objects; in another month or two he will transfer them from one hand to the other. Purposeful release appears later, usually about the tenth month. These responses are delayed in a child with mental deficiency or with a lesion of the pyramidal tract.

The deep tendon reflexes are variable in infants and their presence or absence is of little significance. During the ensuing years they gradually assume adult characteristics and can be helpful in the diagnosis of neurologic disorders. For about the first ten months, extension or dorsiflexion of the toes is the normal response in testing the plantar reflex (Babinski); thereafter flexion occurs.

[3] E. Moro, Heidelberg pediatrician, 1874–1951.

INDEX

Folio numbers in *italics* refer to illustrations;
n. following a folio number refers to a footnote.